Critical Realism, Feminism, and Gender: A Reader

In assessing the current state of feminism and gender studies, whether on a theoretical or a practical level, it has become increasingly challenging to avoid the conclusion that these fields are in a state of disarray. Indeed, feminist and gender studies discussions are beset with persistent splits and disagreements. This reader suggests that returning to, and placing centre-stage, the role of philosophy, especially critical realist philosophy of science, is invaluable for efforts that seek to overcome or mitigate the uncertainty and acrimony that have resulted from this situation. In particular, it claims that the dialectical logic that runs through critical realist philosophy is ideally suited to advancing feminist and gender studies discussions about *broad ontological and epistemological questions and considerations*, *intersectionality*, and *methodology, methods, and empirical research*. By bringing together four new and eight existing writings this reader provides both a focal point for renewed discussions about the potential and actual contributions of critical realist philosophy to feminism and gender studies and a timely contribution to these discussions.

Michiel van Ingen is an Associate Lecturer at Anglia Ruskin University and a Visiting Lecturer at the University of Hertfordshire, United Kingdom.

Steph Grohmann is a Leverhulme Early Career Fellow at the Centre for Homeless and Inclusion Health at the University of Edinburgh, United Kingdom.

Lena Gunnarsson is a Researcher and Teacher in Gender Studies at Örebro University and Lund University, Sweden.

Routledge Studies in Critical Realism

Critical Realism is a broad movement within philosophy and social science. It is a movement that began in British philosophy and sociology following the founding work of Roy Bhaskar, Margaret Archer and others. Critical Realism emerged from the desire to realise an adequate realist philosophy of science, social science, and of critique. Against empiricism, positivism and various idealisms (interpretivism, radical social constructionism), Critical Realism argues for the necessity of ontology. The pursuit of ontology is the attempt to understand and say something about 'the things themselves' and not simply about our beliefs, experiences, or our current knowledge and understanding of those things. Critical Realism also argues against the implicit ontology of the empiricists and idealists of events and regularities, reducing reality to thought, language, belief, custom, or experience. Instead Critical Realism advocates a structural realist and causal powers approach to natural and social ontology, with a focus upon social relations and process of social transformation.

Important movements within Critical Realism include the morphogenetic approach developed by Margaret Archer; Critical Realist economics developed by Tony Lawson; as well as dialectical Critical Realism (embracing being, becoming and absence) and the philosophy of metaReality (emphasising priority of the non-dual) developed by Roy Bhaskar.

For over thirty years, Routledge has been closely associated with Critical Realism and, in particular, the work of Roy Bhaskar, publishing well over fifty works in, or informed by, Critical Realism (in series including Critical Realism: Interventions; Ontological Explorations; New Studies in Critical Realism and Education). These have all now been brought together under one series dedicated to Critical Realism.

The Centre for Critical Realism is the advisory editorial board for the series. If you would like to know more about the Centre for Critical Realism, or to submit a book proposal, please visit www.centreforcriticalrealism.com.

Social and Ethnic Inequalities in the Cypriot Education System
A Critical Realist View on Empowerment
Areti Stylianou and David Scott

The Space that Separates: A Realist Theory of Art
Nick Wilson

Critical Realism, Feminism, and Gender: A Reader
Edited by Michiel van Ingen, Steph Grohmann and Lena Gunnarsson

For more information about this series, please visit:
www.routledge.com/Routledge-Studies-in-Critical-Realism-Routledge-Critical-Realism/book-series/SE0518

Critical Realism, Feminism, and Gender: A Reader

Edited by Michiel van Ingen, Steph Grohmann, and Lena Gunnarsson

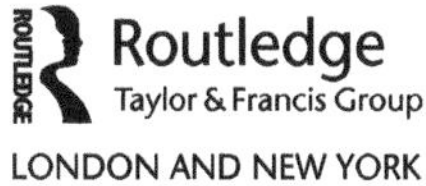

LONDON AND NEW YORK

First published 2020
by Routledge
2 Park Square, Milton Park, Abingdon, Oxon OX14 4RN

and by Routledge
605 Third Avenue, New York, NY 10017

First issued in paperback 2021

Routledge is an imprint of the Taylor & Francis Group, an informa business

British Library Cataloguing-in-Publication Data
A catalogue record for this book is available from the British Library

Library of Congress Cataloging-in-Publication Data
Names: Ingen, Michiel van, editor. | Grohmann, Steph, editor. |
Gunnarsson, Lena, editor.
Title: Critical realism, feminism, and gender : a reader / edited by Michiel van Ingen, Steph Grohmann, and Lena Gunnarsson.
Description: Abingdon, Oxon ; New York, NY : Routledge, 2020. |
Series: Routledge studies in critical realism | Includes bibliographical references and index.
Identifiers: LCCN 2019058584 (print) | LCCN 2019058585 (ebook) |
ISBN 9781138083707 (hardback) | ISBN 9781315112138 (ebook)
Subjects: LCSH: Feminist theory. | Critical realism.
Classification: LCC HQ1190 .C754 2020 (print) |
LCC HQ1190 (ebook) | DDC 305.42–dc23
LC record available at https://lccn.loc.gov/2019058584
LC ebook record available at https://lccn.loc.gov/2019058585

ISBN 13: 978-1-03-223595-0 (pbk)
ISBN 13: 978-1-138-08370-7 (hbk)

DOI: 10.4324/9781315112138

Typeset in Times New Roman
by Swales & Willis, Exeter, Devon, UK

Contents

Acknowledgements

This volume came perilously close to never being published. It is only because of the generosity and emotional support of others that this fate was ultimately avoided. In particular, we are extremely grateful for the financial backing that was provided by both the *Centre for Critical Realism* (Dave Elder-Vass, Angela Martinez Dy, Alan Norrie, Sean Vertigan, and Nick Wilson) and the *Bhaskar Commemoration Fund* (Mervyn Hartwig and Hilary Wainwright). Also deserving of special mention are Marijke Borstel, Kim van Ingen, Martin van Ingen, Marcel Steenhuis, Ella Steenhuis, and Sam Steenhuis.

Chapter 1 was originally published as: Tony Lawson. 1999. "Feminism, Realism, and Universalism." *Feminist Economics* 5(2): 25–59. © IAFFE 1999, www.feministeconomics.org.
Chapter 2 was originally published as: Carrie Hull. 2006. "Poststructuralist and Constructivist Feminism," in Hull, C. *The Ontology of Sex*. Routledge, pp. 54–82.
Chapter 3 was originally published as Caroline New. 2005. "Sex and Gender: A Critical Realist Approach." *New Formations* 56: 54. © Lawrence and Wishart.
Chapter 4 was originally published as Lena Gunnarsson. 2011. "A Defence of the Category 'Women.'" *Feminist Theory* 12(1): 23–27. © Sage. DOI: 10.1177/1464700110390604. © Sage.
Chapter 6 was originally published as Angela Martinez Dy, Lee Martin and Susan Marlow. 2014. "Developing a Critical Realist Positional Approach to Intersectionality." *Journal of Critical Realism* 13(5): 447–466, DOI: 10.1179/1476743014Z.00000000043. © Taylor & Francis Ltd, www.tandfonline.com.
Chapter 7 was originally published as: Sue Clegg. 2016. "Agency and Ontology within Intersectional Analysis: A Critical Realist Contribution." *Journal of Critical Realism* 15(5): 494–510, DOI: 10.1080/14767430.2016.1210470. © Taylor & Francis Ltd, www.tandfonline.com.
Chapter 8 was originally published as Lena Gunnarsson. 2017. "Why We Keep Separating the 'Inseparable': Dialecticizing Intersectionality," *European*

Journal of Women's Studies 24(2): 114–127. © Sage. DOI: 10.1177/1350506815577114.

Chapter 11 was originally published as: Sadie Parr. 2015. "Integrating Critical Realist and Feminist Methodologies: Ethical and Analytical Dilemmas." *International Journal of Social Research Methodology* 18(2): 193–207, DOI: 10.1080/13645579.2013.868572. © Taylor & Francis Ltd, www.tandfonline.com.

The authors thank the publishers for their permission to include this material in *Critical Realism, Feminism, and Gender: A Reader.*

Contributors

Sue Clegg is Emeritus Professor of Higher Education Research at Leeds Beckett University, United Kingdom. Her research draws on critical realist philosophy and feminist theory and explores the social and pedagogical significance of the gendering of information technology. She developed a critique of the debate about the nature of evidence-based practice, was Editor of *Teaching in Higher Education* between 2006 and 2014, and sits on the Editorial Boards of *Studies in Higher Education* and *Higher Education Quarterly.*

Amber J. Fletcher is Associate Professor in Sociology and Social Studies at University of Regina, Canada. Her research combines sociology, gender studies, and public policy studies to examine the everyday effects of macro-level changes in policy and climate. She currently leads a research project on the social dimensions of climate hazards and is involved in a project on policy engagement strategies for gender issues in Canada. Her publications include *Women in Agriculture Worldwide: Key Issues and Practical Approaches* (with Wendee Kubik, 2016).

Steph Grohmann is a Leverhulme Early Career Fellow at the Centre for Homeless and Inclusion Health at the University of Edinburgh, and Research Affiliate at the School of Anthropology and Museum Ethnography, University of Oxford, United Kingdom. She is an anthropologist with research interests in ethics, spatial existence, and cognition. Her work uses critical realist philosophy to explore how conscious experience is shaped at the intersection of evolved behaviour and cultural symbolism. She is the author of an ethnographic monograph entitled *The Ethics of Space: Homelessness and Squatting in Urban England* (2019).

Lena Gunnarsson is a researcher and teacher in Gender Studies at Örebro University and Lund University, Sweden. Her key research interests are feminist theory, philosophy (of science), love and intimacy, and sexual violence and consent. She currently leads a research project on sugar dating. Along with articles in feminist and critical realist journals, she has written two books: *The Contradictions of Love* (2014), for which she was awarded the Cheryl Frank Memorial Prize, and *Samtyckesdynamiker* (*Dynamics of Sexual Consent*, 2020).

Carrie Hull taught at Wilfrid Laurier University, the University of Waterloo, and the University of Toronto, Canada. Aside from her book, *The Ontology of Sex* (2006), her articles have appeared in *Philosophy and Social Criticism*, *Radical Philosophy*, *New Political Science*, and *Environmental Values*.

Tony Lawson is Emeritus Professor of Economics and Philosophy at Cambridge University, United Kingdom. His key areas of research include philosophy of science, political economy, the history of economic thought, alternative approaches to economics, social ontology, and methodology. Among his numerous publications are *The Nature of Social Reality: Issues in Social Ontology* (2019), *The Nature and State of Modern Economics* (2015), *Reorienting Economics* (2003), and *Economics and Reality (1997).*

Susan Marlow is Professor of Entrepreneurship at the University of Nottingham, United Kingdom. Her research is concerned with entrepreneurship and adopts a particular focus on gender issues. Her work has been published in leading U.K. and U.S. journals. She is holder of the *Queens Award for Enterprise*, consulting editor for the *International Small Business Journal*, and Distinguished Visiting Professor at Manchester Metropolitan University.

Lee Martin is Associate Professor of Creativity and Culture at the University of Warwick, United Kingdom. His work critically explores the links between creative production, sustainable cultures, and cultural policy. He was Chair of the Creative and Cultural Industries track and the Organisational Psychology track for the *British Academy of Management* and acted as co-editor of the *Journal of Critical Realism*. He has advised on the development of creative potential and sustainable practices within public, private and charitable organisations.

Angela Martinez Dy is a lecturer and researcher at the Institute for Innovation and Entrepreneurship at Loughborough University London, United Kingdom. She is a trained anti-racist and intersectional feminist organiser with substantial experience of building community-based organisations. Her research interests include digital entrepreneurship, intersectional feminism, and critical realism. She adopts this perspective to analyse social dynamics and the ways in which technology impacts society, especially the world of work/entrepreneurship.

Caroline New taught sociology at the Faculty of Education and Human Sciences, Bath Spa University College, United Kingdom. Her research focused on gender and social theory and her publications include both a monograph entitled *Agency, Health and Social Survival: The Eco-Politics of Rival Psychologies* (1996) and articles in the *Journal for the Theory of Social Behaviour*, *Sociology*, *Alethia*, and *The Sociological Review*.

Sadie Parr is Research Fellow at the Centre for Regional Economic and Social Research, Sheffield Hallam University, United Kingdom. Her research (and publications) are concerned with the experiences of multiply-disadvantaged adults, children and families. Through this research, she developed a sustained interest in engaging with social theory to critically understand governing practices, policy implementation processes, political agency, and the role of state institutions in the lives of people and families deemed 'troublesome'.

Wendy Sims-Schouten is Associate Head (Research and Innovation) and Reader in Childhood Studies at the University of Portsmouth, United Kingdom. Her research and publications are in the areas of bullying, childhood obesity, female employment, and early years care and education. She is co-editor of the interdisciplinary journal *Children and Society*, set up the *Mental Health in Childhood and Education Hub*, and works with local partners and academics on research concerned with mental health in childhood and education.

Michiel van Ingen is an Associate Lecturer at Anglia Ruskin University and a Visiting Lecturer at the University of Hertfordshire, United Kingdom. His research sits at the intersection of a range of disciplines, ranging from International Relations to conflict studies, development studies, (global) political economy, anthropology, and philosophy. The main thematic areas with which his research has engaged are violence, the philosophy/methodology of (social) science, and feminism/gender-studies. He has taught at the University of Cambridge, King's College London, the London School of Economics, and the University of Westminster.

Making waves, and beyond

Michiel van Ingen, Steph Grohmann, and Lena Gunnarsson

In evaluating the current state of feminism and gender studies it has become increasingly challenging to avoid the conclusion that these fields are in a state of disarray; or, less calamitously, that they are at least in a state of considerable flux. Despite the fact that important victories have been won around the world, after all, many feminist and gender studies theorists and practitioners have continued to express significant dissatisfaction with the contemporary status quo. This discontent has obvious roots in the fact that patriarchal gender norms and relations, while weakened in some contexts, have by no means been entirely done away with (e.g. Enloe 2017). Indeed, it may well be the case that – rather than just experiencing a 'stalled revolution' (Hochschild 2012 [1989], p. 11) – feminist and gender studies theory and practice are at present undergoing a range of reversals and defeats. Whether these fields are currently on the back foot or not, however, political events in recent years should serve as a sobering reminder that whatever gains or progress have been made can be swiftly and matter-of-factly overturned whenever the political winds change direction.

While this initial conclusion is sufficiently troubling on its own, the problem runs deeper than this; it is not just that social structures have often proven to be resilient against feminist critiques but also that the feminist movement is itself far from being a unified force for liberation. If feminism is still struggling with the fact that patriarchy has not been eradicated 'out there', it also faces a new and more troubling set of problems that derive from the fact that it is currently beset with persistent 'internal' differences, tensions, and splits.

While this situation is not wholly negative – after all, the presence of a diverse range of theoretical/political positions may simply reflect the vitality of the feminist movement – it does raise any number of fundamental questions. For example, what role (if any) should the second wave distinction between (biological) sex and (social/cultural) gender play in twenty-first-century feminism and gender studies? What consequences does any negation or affirmation of this opposition have for the place of trans-politics within feminism? If – as some proponents of third wave feminism have argued – biological sex (along with the related notions of sex roles/classes and sex/gender systems) are to be gotten rid of as a potential basis for solidarity and political struggle, what should replace it? If biological sex is to be purged in this manner, who/what exactly are feminism and gender studies for? Should these fields simply be absorbed into a more encompassing field of critical theory/practice? What role (if any) should the 'intersectional imperative' (Wiegman 1999, p. 376) play in feminism and gender studies? Does – and should – this imperative, along with any potential deconstruction of the male/female opposition, displace the traditional feminist concern with sex-based exploitation/oppression with a focus on hierarchies that are rooted in class, 'race', age, sexual orientation, etc.? Are these different social axes, vectors, or locations analytically separable or inseparable?

Such questions – and many more like them – suggest that feminism and gender studies are not just experiencing challenges that have emerged from the conduct of hostile, 'external' agents, and neither are they simply lacking clear 'directions' or a good 'map'; rather, *their 'destination' has become obscured as well.* While it is of importance to proceed with caution – specifically, we must remain vigilant against the threat of blaming only the (feminist) victim for our political fate – it is therefore appropriate to ask how we might move past this impasse?

The present volume – from this general introduction to the section introductions and the twelve individual chapters that it contains – suggests that returning to, and placing centre-stage, the role of philosophy, especially the philosophy of science, is invaluable for any such effort. Certainly, in some feminist and gender studies circles this claim is likely to be received with suspicion or even outright hostility. Such responses would not, in any case, be without historical precedent, as the relationship between philosophy (of science), feminism, and gender studies has long been characterised by mutual suspicion.

First, many authors working in the fields of feminism and gender studies have stressed that science, like philosophy, continues to be numerically-dominated by men. Second, rather than endeavouring to change this *contingent* state of affairs, some of these authors have claimed that science is *necessarily*, *inherently*, *unavoidably*, and/or *wholly* androcentric. Sandra Harding, for instance, leans towards (but does not fully commit to) this kind of stance when she argues that 'the epistemologies, metaphysics, ethics, and politics of the *dominant* forms of science are androcentric and mutually supportive; [...] [and] science today [therefore] serves primarily regressive social tendencies' (1986, p. 9, emphasis added). In contrast, Virginia Woolf is unequivocal when – in *Three Guineas* – she claims that 'science [...] is not sexless' but 'a man, a father, and infected too' (2000 [1938], p. 267). From this perspective, then, the objectivity, universality, neutrality, rationality, etc. that are conventionally associated with science are to be understood as manifestations of a masculinist, androcentric, or patriarchal logic. Third, while numerous feminist/gender studies theorists have self-evidently drawn on philosophy, their writings have also prioritised a concern that is arguably less ubiquitous within it; in particular, like the work produced by most forms of specifically *critical* theory, they have commonly echoed Marx's claim that philosophers have only sought to understand or interpret the world, whereas the real point is to change it. This is not to say, of course, that feminism and gender studies have had nothing (of merit) to say about philosophical questions; rather, it is to suggest that their primary motivation for engaging with philosophy has been to inform emancipatory practices. Indeed, in accordance with this contrasting motive, theorists and practitioners in these areas have commonly sought to question, deconstruct, and/or overturn the prioritisation of *facts* over *values* which, they claim, is inherent to science, and which has resulted in feminism being side-lined as 'merely' a normative or political project.

In turn, philosophers (of science) have also played their part in ensuring that the relationship of philosophy with feminism and gender studies has remained fractious. While individual proponents of (neo-)positivist philosophy of science have demonstrably been motivated by a desire to bring about positive social change (see e.g. Creath 2017), for instance, there can be little doubt that the approach which their work advances shows a far greater concern with verifying and/or falsifying facts than it does with providing a basis for values (and broader normative/political struggles). Further to this – and adding to the aforementioned charge that it is often too focused on interpreting/understanding the world and insufficiently attentive to the task of bringing about emancipatory change – it is plain to see why some forms of philosophy are considered irrelevant or nothing more than narcissistic self-absorption. It is little wonder, for instance, that – in the face of e.g. persistent sex- and gender-based violence, or the dirty, dangerous, and demeaning working conditions which many female 'sweatshop' labourers face – feminist and gender studies theorists/practitioners have generally not endorsed the solipsistic claim that we cannot be certain that other minds exist. Finally, philosophy has commonly reinforced the cleavage between these fields by unthinkingly assigning labels like 'feminist scholar' to any philosopher whose work incorporates the concerns that are typically associated with feminism and gender studies; as such, this field has habitually *excluded* work of this kind from the realm of 'philosophy proper' and *downgraded* it to specialist status.

In circumstances such as these it may well appear that – by proclaiming the need for feminism and gender studies to both return to and place centre-stage the role philosophy (of science) – we are reheating old debates that have long since been resolved. Indeed, we may well be thought of as inviting scorn by suggesting that these fields would benefit from engaging with, or being rooted in, specifically *critical realist* philosophy of science. After all, it remains true, as Caroline New noted more than twenty years ago, that (critical) realism is undergoing an extended period of 'resounding unpopularity among feminist theorists' (1998, p. 366).

Such observations should, to be sure, serve as a caution that we are fighting what is unequivocally an uphill battle; they should not, however, be allowed to divert our attention from the fact that – in numerous important ways – the histories of feminism and gender studies just *are* the history of philosophy (of science). This is readily apparent when we take note of the fact that even the seemingly most practical debates within feminism and gender studies can usually be traced back to underlying philosophico-methodological splits. These include, most prominently, the splits between (1) *positivism* and *post-positivism*, (2) *foundationalism* and *anti-foundationalism*, (3) *naturalism* and *anti-naturalism*, (4) (scientific, causal) *explanation* and (humanistic, interpretive) *understanding*, (5) *essentialism* and *anti-essentialism*, (6) *materialism* and *idealism*, (7) *objectivism* and *subjectivism*, and (8) *facts* and *values*. Divides such as these are not just at the heart of key *theoretical* debates – say, those between post-structuralist, standpoint, socialist, and new materialist (neo-vitalist) approaches to feminism and gender studies – they are also central to key *practical* discussions, for instance the far-reaching dispute over whether activists should (primarily) engage in 'consciousness raising' or prioritise the subversion/disruption of gender norms. As a result, it seems ill-advised to imagine that it would be possible to develop a satisfactory understanding of the three 'waves' that are conventionally held to make up the history of feminism without taking into consideration the role that philosophical and methodological fissures have played in bringing about and solidifying them. In fact, any account of the relationship between these fields may be said to fail insofar as it portrays them as developing in perfect isolation; while non-identical, their histories self-evidently intertwine, entangle, and – at times – even run in parallel.

If this is the case, however, it follows both that philosophy (of science) has likely contributed to the impasse that was alluded to above, and – at the same time – that it is central to any future programme which seeks to move past or alleviate it. It is exactly in terms of providing the basis for such a programme that we envisage an important role for critical realist philosophy. Specifically, we contend that the philosophical resources which this approach provides hold significant promise for any effort that seeks to overcome or mitigate the uncertainty and acrimony which – at present – characterises much of feminism and gender studies.

It deserves emphasis, however, that – in making this claim – we are emphatically not suggesting the need to make a 'clean break' with current or past theoretical and practical traditions, and neither are we attempting to pave the way for a new, fourth 'wave'. Rather, our intentions are much more closely aligned with the broader aims of critical realist philosophy. As will become clear, this approach – while developing trenchant critiques of philosophical traditions like positivism and interpretivism/hermeneutics – is inherently *preservative* in nature; that is to say, it both *negates* the positions of other philosophical traditions and proposes a dialectical *synthesis* of their various strengths and insights. Likewise, this volume foregrounds the need to adopt a dialectical understanding of the various rifts and splits that plague feminism and gender studies. This means, first, that – at an historical level – it seeks to move past or go beyond accounts of these fields which are centred on discrete, discontinuous, and incompatible 'waves'. Second, it means that – at a philosophical level – it aims to show that critical realism, though certainly not without its own set of problems, challenges, complications, and dilemmas, provides valuable resources for theorists and practitioners who wish to circumvent or bypass the antinomies inherent to the 'problem-field' (Bhaskar 1998 [1979], p. 21) that curbs progress in these fields. As such, this reader is ultimately rooted in the idea that returning to, and placing centre-stage, the role of philosophy (of science), specifically the tenets of critical realism, can facilitate the generation of 'light' rather than just 'heat'. Indeed, the dialectical logic which runs through it – sometimes explicitly, at other times implicitly – suggests that moving past the 'historical see-saw' and 'oscillation to-and-fro' (ibid., p. 20) of feminist and gender studies debates is feasible; while it is clearly necessary to remain attentive to the risk of falling victim to epistemological foundationalism or absolutism it *is* possible to provide a basis for these fields that is both inclusive and philosophically- and methodologically-robust.

If it is true – as we claim it is – that re-examining, and directing attention towards, the role of philosophy (of science) need not generate further animosity, however, neither is it our intention to suggest that critical realism – or any other philosophical approach – can simply put an end to disagreements among feminist and gender studies theorists/practitioners. Not only do the proponents of this approach – including those brought together in this volume – wholeheartedly disagree on a range of key issues, after all, there are also good reasons to believe that philosophical reflections, no matter how sophisticated, can never substitute for analyses of concrete spatiotemporal settings. In fact, from a critical realist perspective, philosophy simply operates at a different level of abstraction than do such contextual analyses.[1] An approach to feminism and gender studies that is rooted in, or informed by, critical realist philosophy therefore provides significant space for theoretical and practical pluralism, and – by extension – for the substantive debates and disagreements that result from them. This is not to say, of course, that critical realist philosophy cannot contribute to developing more nuanced, coherent, and reflexive work in these fields. Rather, this reader should be understood as making a concerted effort to show that – while our philosophical positions may not *determine* our theoretical reflections and practical activities – they clearly do *speak to them*.

In making the case for this position, the three individual sections that follow this general introduction will discuss the relevance of critical realist philosophy of science for feminist and gender studies debates about (1) broad ontological and epistemological questions and considerations, (2) intersectionality, and (3) methodology, methods, and empirical research.

In exploring these sections, we encourage readers to remain cognisant of the fact that – out of a total of twelve chapters – only four were written specifically for this reader; in particular, these are Chapter 4 (by Angela Martinez Dy), Chapter 9 (by Amber J. Fletcher), Chapter 10 (by Michiel van Ingen), and Chapter 12 (by Wendy Sims-Schouten). The remaining eight chapters, then, pre-exist this volume and they are here set side-by-side for the first time. While this serves an important purpose – specifically, the bringing together of existing resources on critical realism, feminism, and gender that are currently scattered around (sometimes inaccessible) physical and virtual spaces – it also has a number of clear drawbacks. In particular, the fact that two-thirds of the chapters which follow were not written for the purpose of being included in this reader means that its contents are less integrated than they otherwise would have been. This applies especially to the second chapter, by Carrie Hull, as – in contrast with the other chapters, all of which were intended to be read as stand-alone pieces – this section reproduces one part of a larger book, namely Hull's *The Ontology of Sex: A Critical Inquiry into the Deconstruction and Reconstruction of Categories* (Hull 2006).

To counteract the adverse effects of this situation, each of the abovementioned sections begins with an extended introduction to the topic at hand. It is our hope that these contribute both to fusing-together/contextualising their claims and providing broader forms of sign-posting. More generally, we hope that this reader will (1) prove to be a useful resource for readers who wish to explore the various intersections of critical realist philosophy, feminism, and gender, and (2) provide something of a focal point and impetus for the development of both a much more sizable and a much richer literature on these topics. At the time of writing it is incontestable that conversations between critical realists and the fields of feminism and gender studies have remained stunted. This is deeply regrettable, as the potential for theoretico-practical 'cross-pollination' – and more generally, for a renewal of critical realist philosophy, feminism, and gender studies – is arguably very significant. Indeed, critical realists and feminist and gender studies theorists/practitioners *already* share much in common. For one, both unmistakably have a strong interest in, and commitment to, furthering critical and emancipatory theory and praxis. As dark political clouds continue to gather all around us, it would surely be both negligent and foolhardy to disregard such resonances.

Note

1 While, from a critical realist perspective, philosophy investigates the same reality as such contextual (feminist and gender studies) analyses, its focus differs; specifically, philosophy operates at a higher level of abstraction or generality. For example, critical realist philosophy asserts that social structures are real, emergent features within being as a whole. A feminist analysis might build on this *philosophical* ontology by developing a *social scientific/theoretical* ontology. Such an analysis might claim, for instance, that the specific social structures in concrete spatiotemporal context 'A' should be considered patriarchal for reasons 'B', 'C', and 'D'.

References

Bhaskar, R. 1998 (1979). *The Possibility of Naturalism*. London: Routledge.

Creath, R. 2017. "Logical Empiricism," in E. N. Zalta (Ed.) *The Stanford Encyclopedia of Philosophy*, available at: https://plato.stanford.edu/archives/fall2017/entries/logical-empiricism/.

Enloe, C. 2017. *The Big Push: Exposing and Challenging the Persistence of Patriarchy*. Oakland, CA: University of California Press.

Harding, S. 1986. *The Science Question in Feminism*. Ithaca, NY: Cornell University Press.

Hochschild, A. 2012 [1989]. *The Second Shift: Working Families and the Revolution at Home*. London: Penguin Books.
Hull, C. 2006. *The Ontology of Sex: A Critical Inquiry into the Deconstruction and Reconstruction of Categories*. London: Routledge.
New, C. 1998. "Realism, Deconstruction and the Feminist Standpoint." *Journal for the Theory of Social Behaviour* 28(4): 349–372.
Wiegman, R. 1999. "What Ails Feminist Criticism: A Second Opinion." *Critical Inquiry* 25(2): 362–379.
Woolf, V. 2000 [1938]. *A Room of One's Own/Three Guineas*. London: Penguin Books.

Part I

Philosophical preliminaries

Critical realism, feminism, and gender

The first section of this reader – consisting of five chapters – examines those features of critical realist philosophy that are of most general relevance to feminism and gender studies. In accordance with this aim it begins with Tony Lawson's early insistence on the urgent need for greater ontological reflection in these fields. As Lawson shows, 'explicit ontological analysis is conspicuously [...] down-played in much of feminist theorizing' (p. 15). This is unfortunate, as 'ontology matters for any would-be projects of illumination and emancipation' (p. 37). Such claims – claims *for* ontology – are the nuts-and-bolts of critical realist philosophy. Rather than stopping there, however, both Lawson's chapter and the four chapters that follow it (by Carrie Hull, Caroline New, Lena Gunnarsson, and Angela Martinez Dy) also argue for a *new* ontology; an ontology, that is, which places centre-stage notions like depth, structure, emergence/stratification, differentiation, complexity, systemic openness/closure, and process.

As the abovementioned authors make clear, their focus on the importance of (developing/adopting a new) ontology unequivocally does *not* amount to a wholesale rejection of the epistemological stance that significant parts of the feminist and gender studies literature have adopted in recent decades. Lawson stresses, for instance, that 'there is nothing essential to scientific or ontological realism that supposes or requires' that knowledge 'is other than fallible, partial and itself transient, or that scientists or researchers are other than positioned, biased, interested, and practically, culturally and socially conditioned' (p. 17, emphasis removed). Rather, the proponents of critical realist philosophy have commonly regarded 'the necessity of knowing *from a particular place* as enabling knowledge rather than hindering it' (New, p. 82). In Lawson's chapter this epistemological stance takes the specific form of a theory of contrastive explanation which 'does not merely support the thesis [...] that interested standpoints are inevitable' but 'goes further in suggesting that interested standpoints [...] are [...] actually indispensable *aids* to the explanatory process' (p. 29). More generally, critical realist feminism and gender studies clearly does *not* negate the views of standpoint feminists in favour of epistemological foundationalism or absolutism and it *rejects* the idea that a god's-eye view is achievable; its various advocates subscribe, though admittedly in a qualified sense (see e.g. New 1998), to the epistemological perspective that standpoint feminists favour and – in some cases (e.g. Lawson's) – they have sought to build on it.

Instead, perhaps the primary motivation behind the critical realist emphasis on (developing/adopting a new) ontology is to both oppose and overcome the pernicious influence of the *epistemic fallacy*, or the view that 'statements about being can be reduced to or analysed in terms of statements about knowledge' (Bhaskar 2008 [1975], p. 26). In Hull's chapter this opposition results in a compelling critique of the nominalism and relativism which – despite time-honoured but well-worn protestations to the contrary – is an inherent feature of much post-structuralist feminist and gender studies work.[1] In particular, Hull takes issue with the work of third wave feminist authors like Judith Butler and Anne Fausto-Sterling who – inspired, in part, by the idea that the category of 'race' is very largely a scientific fiction, a social construct that lacks any morally significant biological referents – reject dimorphic understandings of sex differentiation in favour of the idea that sex should be understood as a continuum, a rainbow, or akin to the colour spectrum. While Hull – like New, Gunnarsson, and Martinez Dy – accepts that intersexuality is real and significant, she disputes both the *scientific evidence* of which post-structuralist authors have made use to accentuate the prevalence of this phenomenon and *the nominalist and relativist philosophical orientation* that has caused them to be 'too deeply vested in uncovering relatively high rates of sexual nondimorphism' (p. 61).

In contrast, critical realist feminist and gender studies authors have generally maintained (1) that 'human beings are (almost all) sexually dimorphic, female and male', and (2) that '[t]his dimorphic structuring is *active*, causally powerful, enabling (in certain contexts) different reproductive roles and certain (hetero and homo) sexual possibilities and pleasures, while rendering others less likely (elbow as erogenous zone) and ruling others out (male parturition)' (New, p. 83). In the prevailing intellectual climate – which, despite an ever-expanding range of alternatives to it, continues to be dominated by approaches to feminism and gender studies that are rooted in the cultural turn – such assertions are likely to be received with scepticism or even hostility. As Hull remarks, 'any expression of doubt about the figures or the leap in logic' can either 'land the sceptic in the camp of reactionaries' (p. 59) or at least expose them to risk of being ridiculed as the sort of person who is 'somehow against freedom itself' (p. 49). And yet, as she adds, 'larger philosophical and scientific points' *are* 'being promulgated in these feminist arguments' (p. 49). As such, Hull's chapter does not just provide its readers with a powerful critique of the nominalism and relativism that inheres in many examples of post-structuralist work, but it also takes them on a whistle-stop tour of intellectual terrain that is occupied both by natural scientists and by prominent philosophers/social theorists like Quine, Goodman, Foucault, Kant, and Hegel.

If an opposition to the epistemic fallacy results in a rejection of third wave claims about sexual non-dimorphism, however, this emphatically should not be mistaken for warm feelings regarding the determinism of reductionist approaches to evolutionary biology. Such approaches are wholeheartedly rejected by critical realists. Rather, the aforementioned opposition to post-structuralist feminist claims – which, importantly, is a feature of Martinez Dy's chapter on gender theory non-conforming, trans-politics, and affordance theory as well – reflects a commitment to the emergentist version of ontological realism that critical realist philosophy favours; specifically, it reflects a commitment to (1) the *realist* claim that reality exists, for the most part, independently of the individual researcher/scientist who seeks to understand/explain it, and (2) the *emergentist* claim that biological powers/mechanisms, while real, only ever *co*-determine outcomes alongside physical, chemical, psychological, sociocultural, etc. powers/mechanisms. In line with this perspective, all five authors take seriously the thoroughgoing complexity that characterises concrete (sexed and gendered) reality, especially by giving psychology (and hence agency/intentionality, consciousness, reflexivity, etc.) and the social/cultural sciences (and hence rules, relations, positions, discourses, ideologies, etc.) pride of place in their work. While they suggest that the dimorphic structuring of biological sex is 'active', these authors therefore repeatedly insist on extending the same privilege to a wide range of other causal factors as well.

Further to this, and in contrast with the post-structuralist feminist tendency to reduce discourse to a phenomenon which is formative or constitutive of reality, the ontological realism that informs the work of these authors points to the possibility of reference. In so doing they echo, albeit implicitly, Bhaskar's claims about *referential detachment*, or 'the detachment of the act by which we refer to something from that to which it refers' (2010 [1994], p. 12). As Bhaskar notes, referential detachment 'is a presupposition of *discourse* which must be *about* something other than itself, of *praxis* which must be *with* something other than itself or of *desire* which must be *for* something alterior to itself' (ibid., p. 198). To be sure, such references are never simple, direct, or socially/culturally unmediated; this is why, in addition to making the case for *ontological realism*, critical realist feminists also subscribe to the idea of *epistemic relativism*, or the notion 'that all beliefs are socially produced, so that all knowledge is transient and neither truth-values nor criteria of rationality exist outside historical time' (Bhaskar 1998 [1979], pp. 62–63). Not only does critical realist philosophy insist that the sociocultural context in which knowledge-production takes place has significant effects on this process, therefore, it also stresses that '[t]here are no self-evident criteria, [and] no uncontested standards' because 'what constitutes good evidence for an account is, of course, itself part of the argument' (New 1998, p. 366).

Despite this – or, rather, *because of* both their opposition to the epistemic fallacy and their partnering of ontological realism with epistemic relativism – critical realist feminists also endorse the principle of *judgmental rationalism*; that is to say, they subscribe to the idea that there are rational grounds for preferring one explanatory account over another. This claim is rooted in the realist position that 'the real world puts limits on knowledge so that not all interpretations are equally plausible' (McCall 2005, p. 1793) and hence makes for a significant contrast with the *judgmental relativism* of much post-structuralist work. Rather than conceiving of judgmental rationalism as a reckless attempt to reinstate the 'philosopher/scientist king' that is now commonly associated with hubristic forms of modernism, however, this principle should be understood as an alternative both to such perspectives and to the post-structuralist merger/collapse/inversion of 'active knowing subject' and 'passive object known'. Specifically, critical realists tend to conceive of the subject-object relationship in dialectical terms. As such, they both *separate them* – by stressing the non-identity of knowledge/knowledge claims (the 'transitive dimension') and the largely independent reality to which they refer ('intransitive dimension') – and *connect them* by stressing that knowledge (claims) are always part of this same reality; knowing, from the anti-anthropocentric perspective which critical realist philosophy favours, is a particular way or state of being. This means both that causal interactions between subject and object are likely to occur and that the lines which divide them are often blurry or fuzzy; the transitive dimension has an intransitive aspect, and vice versa. In contrast, this does *not* mean that submitting to the either/or (dualism/identity) logic that characterises much of the modernism/post-structuralism debate is required; rather, the both/and logic of epistemological dialectics provides the proponents of critical realist philosophy with a robust alternative to such dichotomous framings.

Gunnarsson's chapter shows the value of this alternative; it begins by highlighting that, when it comes to the use of categories like woman/female (and man/male), feminist theorising has increasingly resorted to a framing which relies on a dualistic contrast between a universalising 'before' and a particularising/singularising and intersectional 'after'. This is, from Gunnarsson's perspective, a fruitless stand-off. At an *historical* level she counters that 'much of the rhetorical force of intersectional arguments has come to depend upon caricature-like representations of "earlier", "Western" or "hegemonic" feminist theories' (p. 101). At a *philosophical* level she develops an alternative approach to theorising the abovementioned terms that, first, conceives of them as abstractions and, second, is rooted in the work of Bertell Ollmann and Andrew Sayer. As a result, Gunnarsson claims – in a statement that is developed in much greater detail in her second contribution to this reader – that '[w]e must question the very dualism between sameness and difference that rejections of commonality are so often premised upon' (p. 103). More generally, and reflecting the both/and logic that characterises critical realist philosophy, she stresses that theorising is unavoidably messy, often paradoxical, and necessarily takes place 'in the dialectic between the concrete and the abstract, the subjective and the objective, the specific and the general, and [...] the fundamentally processual character of concrete reality and the irredeemably static quality of the words and signs which we employ to understand and explain it' (p. 110).

Overall, the picture of critical realist feminism and gender studies that emerges from these five chapters is both preservative and heterodox. This is the case, primarily, because it provides *both* natural scientific (especially biological/bio-chemical) *and* human/social scientific (especially psychological and sociological/anthropological/etc.) approaches to understanding reality with a 'seat at the table'. For instance, critical realist philosophy allows us to talk – as both Lawson (ch. 1) and New (ch. 3) do – of human nature *without* succumbing to biological determinism, and it allows us to talk of socialisation/enculturation – as all five authors do – *without* deconstructing the subject into a haphazard collection of fragmented identities. As such, an approach to feminism and gender studies that is rooted in critical realism is able to incorporate the strengths of earlier approaches (or waves) into an ontologically grounded synthesis that (1) avoids their weaknesses, and (2) provides valuable resources for those who wish to circumvent or bypass the antinomies inherent to the 'problem-field' (Bhaskar 1998 [1979], p. 21) which currently curbs progress in these fields. Of particular importance in this regard is what is now increasingly referred to – plainly tongue-in-cheek – as the 'holy trinity' of critical realism: *ontological realism*, *epistemic relativism*, and *judgmental rationalism*. As the second and third parts of this reader will show, this trinity – along with the depth ontology that results from critical realist critiques of the epistemic fallacy – form a robust support structure that allows us to develop a sophisticated understanding of, and approach to, both intersectionality and methodology/methods/empirical research.

Note

1 While the larger book (2006) from which it is taken does explicitly reference the epistemic fallacy, this concept does not feature in the chapter that is reproduced here.

References

Bhaskar, R. 2008 [1975]. *A Realist Theory of Science*. London and New York: Verso.

——. 2010 [1994] *Plato Etc. The Problems of Philosophy and their Resolution*. Abingdon, Oxon: Routledge.

——. 1998 [1979]. *The Possibility of Naturalism: A Philosophical Critique of the Contemporary Human Sciences*, third edition. London: Routledge.

Hull, C. 2006. *The Ontology of Sex: A Critical Inquiry into the Deconstruction and Reconstruction of Categories*. Abingdon, Oxon: Routledge.

McCall, L. 2005. "The Complexity of Intersectionality." *Signs: Journal of Women in Culture and Society* 30(3): 1771–1800.

New, C. 1998. "Realism, Deconstruction and the Feminist Standpoint." *Journal for the Theory of Social Behaviour* 28(4): 349–372.

1 Feminism, realism, and universalism[1]

Tony Lawson

Introduction: the practice of *a priori* universalising

Feminist contributions can claim a good deal of the credit for modern social theory displaying increasing sensitivity to the dangers of overgeneralising. Fundamental here is the recognition that values, experiences, objectives, and common-sense interpretations of dominant groups may be merely that; there is nothing especially natural or necessarily universal about them. All claims, whether made from within the academy or without, whether cautiously or boldly formulated, etc., are made from particular positions by interested parties. No person or group can reasonably profess a neutral, detached, unbiased perspective; all understandings achieved are partial (as well as fallible and likely to be transient). The practice of universalising *a priori*, of merely asserting/assuming the widespread validity/relevance of some position is now widely recognised as, at best, a methodological mistake, and one that can carry significant political consequence.[2]

As is well known, however, it has proven all too easy to slide from a position of opposing the practice of *a priori* universalising to one of more or less opposing the endeavour of generalising altogether. In particular, once the basis for treating a dominant stance or approach as universally legitimate has been successfully called into question it has often proven difficult to avoid concluding that all approaches or stances are as legitimate as each other.

With regards to some issues this sort of reaction is unproblematic, even facilitating. But this is not the case with all matters, and especially, I think, with respect to broader projects of illumination and human emancipation. In particular, theorists have found it difficult to defend a notion of objectivity or progress in knowledge, or to sustain any basis for an emancipatory politics, where these objectives are of central concern to many feminists. The conclusion too often drawn is that, even in regard to matters such as these, all we can safely say is that there are differences.

My limited objective here is to argue that, in addressing these latter sorts of difficulties, there are possible advantages to feminist explanatory and emancipatory projects from engaging (or engaging more fully) in the sort of explicit ontological analysis associated with modern versions (at least) of scientific realism.

In encouraging this sort of stance I do not wish to suggest that scientific realism or ontological considerations are entirely absent from feminist thought. Indeed, I think it is impossible that they could be. But I think it possible that ontological commitments are too rarely rendered explicit. And when the question of realism is raised (in whatever form) at all, the latter, it seems to me, is mostly treated in an overly guarded way in much feminist thought, as if accepting any explicitly realist perspective is necessarily problematic.

I am not alone in this perception. Caroline New (1998, p. 2), for example, recently records that in modern feminist thought 'realism' seems 'tainted', and writes of 'realism's current resounding unpopularity among feminist theorists' (ibid., p. 12). She also suggests that providing a reasonably 'robust' defence of feminist standpoint theory's realism is more 'than its current proponents seem willing to risk' (ibid., p. 6).

Others caution distance. Martha Nussbaum (whose argument for grounding ethical theory in the nature of human capacities is undoubtedly realist) finds the standing of realism to be sufficiently low as to caution 'that it would appear strategically wise for an ethical and political view that seeks broad support not to rely on the truth of metaphysical realism' (Nussbaum 1995, p. 69).[3]

Some feel the need to include a forthright disclaimer. Donna Haraway provides a prominent example. Despite setting out a perspective that seems so clearly to embrace scientific or ontological realism,[4] Haraway seemingly feels that credibility rests upon expressly denying that this is so: 'The approach I am recommending is not a version of "realism", which has proved a rather poor way of engaging with the world's active agency' (Haraway 1988, p. 260).

My worry is that this negative or distancing orientation can result in legitimate realist considerations being played down to an extent that may actually be debilitating for the feminist project, not least in preventing it from dealing as effectively as it might with the sorts of tensions or difficulties already noted. My aim here, then, is to caution against any blanket rejection of realist-type analysis as ultimately unnecessarily constraining of feminist thinking and advance.

I start, though, by defining some of my terms. Following this I move, in the main part of the paper, to indicate the sorts of differences that I think explicit realist/ontological analysis can make.

Feminism and realism

There are, in fact, numerous interpretations or types of realism. In the broadest philosophical sense of the term relevant here, any position can be designated a *realism* that asserts the existence of some (possibly disputed) kind of entity (such as black holes, quarks, gender-relations, Loch Ness monsters, utilities, probabilities, men, women, truth, tables, chairs, etc.). I think it is clear there are very many conceivable realisms of this sort and all of us are realists of some kind or other.

In science, a realist position, i.e., *scientific realism*, asserts that the ultimate objects of enquiry exist for the most part independently of, or at least prior to, their investigation. (My primary concern here is indeed with scientific realism. But significant amongst other types of realism relevant here are *perceptual realism*, maintaining the existence of material objects in space and time independently of their perception, and *predicative realism*, maintaining the existence of universals either independently of particular material things, as in *Platonic realism*, or as their properties, as in *Aristotelian realism*. Clearly, scientific realism reduces to perceptual or predicative realism if the objects of scientific knowledge just are material objects or Platonic – or Aristotelian – forms.)

Realism so interpreted is inherently bound up with ontology, with the nature of existence or being. And indeed it is an explicit concern with ontology that I want to promote here. Not all questions traditionally of interest to scientific realists have turned on the explicit study of ontology. Indeed, until very recently discussions about realism have turned to a large extent on the epistemological question of the truth of our knowledge, rather than the ontological question of the reality of structures and things.[5] The debate, though, has moved on in recent years, and in ways that I think has relevance for feminist concerns.[6]

Of course, scientific realism, even when recognised as first and foremost a theory *not* of knowledge or truth, but of being, is nevertheless bound to possess epistemological implications. But it warrants emphasis that *there is nothing essential to scientific or ontological realism that supposes or requires that objects of knowledge are naturalistic or other than transient, that knowledge obtained is other than fallible, partial and itself transient, or that scientists or researchers are other than positioned, biased, interested, and practically, culturally and socially conditioned.*

I emphasise this aspect just because I suspect that it may be central to the distancing orientation to realism that I detect in much feminist thought. My concern is that there is a tendency in the feminist literature for a particular and naive form of realism to be made to stand in for all (and specifically scientific) realisms. This is a version which does treat all reality as fixed, science and knowledge as somehow value- and interest-free or neutral, as well as *necessarily* convergent on truth regarded as objective. To the extent that scientific realism is so conceived its rejection in feminist thought is explicable.[7]

My primary concern here though is not with explaining the phenomenon in question but with indicating some of its consequences. My starting point remains the perception that, for whatever reasons, scientific realism, as an explicit orientation, is to a significant extent excluded from, or downplayed in, the mainstream feminist discussion, including that now occurring in economics.[8] But my intention here, the main purpose of this paper, is to suggest that this situation, whatever its explanation, is unfortunate; a rehabilitation of explicit realist reasoning in feminist thinking not only does not necessitate a slide into absolutism but actually carries the potential to make a constructive difference, to serve to advance feminist epistemological and emancipatory projects.[9]

An indication that realism/ontology matters

In the remainder of the paper I want to give a set of schematic illustrations to help ground my claim that realist thought, and in particular explicit ontological analysis, can be beneficial to, and is probably indispensable for, any would-be revelatory and emancipatory projects. In particular, I want to indicate that such analysis is most likely essential to sustaining revelatory and emancipatory projects in the face of problems or difficulties of the sort I noted at the outset – turning on the need to oppose ungrounded *a priori* universalising without altogether abandoning the possibility of generalist or collective endeavour.

I start with a specific issue of method confronting contemporary economics, before moving, for my second illustration, to topics more widely discussed within feminist epistemology, and, for my third, to assessing the possibility of projects of human emancipation. In the first illustration, which lays the basis for the two illustrations that follow it, I join the 'deconstructive' strand of feminist thinking by bringing ontology to bear in questioning the general relevance of certain methods of economics that have in practice been universalised in an *a priori* fashion. In the second and third illustrations I indicate how ontological analysis can help ground projects of epistemology and emancipation of the sort pursued by feminists.

Illustration 1: the formalistic modelling of social processes

Consider first the case of method in modern economics. The dominant feature here is the widespread reliance upon the practice of formalistic modelling.[10] This approach has certainly been universalised within the economics discipline, and with little if any grounding or argument, and despite its record of failure. Feminists have also criticised it as masculinist. I think it is (albeit an approach that is also perhaps race and class, etc., specific). But what follows for the feminist critic? Is it that all other approaches, including any preferred by feminists, be given greater emphasis?[11] Or should more feminists do formalistic modelling?[12] Perhaps both responses follow; or are they largely incompatible? Is it, say, that the scarcity of feminist modellers entails that the set of questions currently addressed is unnecessarily limited, or is it, perhaps, that formalistic methods themselves are undesirably limited in their usefulness, and possibly even debilitating of revelatory and emancipatory progress? How do we begin to decide?

Answering such questions, questions that may or may not involve a false dichotomy, requires at the very least that the revelatory potential of formalistic methods be investigated. And this, I will argue, necessitates an attention to ontology. Specifically, I want to indicate that by briefly examining both the nature of social material and the ontological presuppositions of the procedures of formalistic modelling, it can be demonstrated that the latter procedures are not at all well equipped for illuminating the social realm. This conclusion is easily established, but rarely is so precisely because of the widespread reluctance to engage in ontology. It is just this reluctance that I wish to call into question.

The particularity of formalistic modelling

But is formalistic modelling really so restricted in its usefulness? As I say, I think it is *and that it can be shown to be so*. Let me briefly sketch my argument. First consider the sort of conditions under which formalistic modelling has relevance. Basically such modelling attempts to relate one (measurable) set of events or states of affairs to others. It presupposes correlations in surface phenomena, that is strict (possibly including probabilistic) regularities of the form 'whenever event (or state of affairs) *x* then event (or state of affairs) *y*'. Let me refer to situations in which such regularities occur as *closed systems*. Formalistic modelling, to have general relevance, presupposes the ubiquity of such closures.

Now an observation often recorded but rarely reflected upon is that outside astronomy such event regularities, or at least those found to be of interest and significance in science in general, are mostly confined to situations of well-controlled experiments. An additional observation is that the results of controlled experiments are regularly successfully applied outside the experimental laboratory where event regularities are not in evidence.

A recognition of this situation, then, already casts doubt on the rationality of ploughing ever more resources into producing yet additional formalistic economic models. Certainly the failure of the econometrics project over the last fifty years or so is indicative that the social world is open, that event regularities in the social realm are far from ubiquitous. The usual response, of course, is to pronounce that we must try harder: to formulate ever more complex models using larger data sets, or to dig deeper in the expectation of finding the sought-after invariances at a more micro, or anyway different, level. However, the recognition that even in the natural realm significant event regularities are systematically restricted, and largely found only in situations of experimental control, encourages a suspicion that significant successes in the social realm may not be possible even in principle. It is clearly essential at this stage that the observed patterning of event regularities be explained.

But how *can* we make sense of the observed *confinement* of most event regularities to the experimental set-up? Notice first that this observation generates immediate tensions for any program that insists that such event regularities are essential to science (as the indispensable objects of scientific laws including laws of nature, or some such). For it follows that science (if thought to necessitate the elaboration of event regularities) is after all not only far from universal but, outside astronomy, mostly confined to experimental set-ups; it is actually fenced off from most of the goings-on in the world. Moreover, one is bound to conclude from this that (many) laws of nature (if event regularities are essential to them) depend upon human actions (in setting up the experimental situation), which is at least counterintuitive. But it also follows that the further familiar observation that science is efficacious outside the experiment, where event regularities do not occur, is unintelligible.

How, then, are we to make sense of these considerations? How is it that scientists, in their experimental activities, can (frequently) codetermine a particular pattern of events that would not have come about but for their intervention? And how can we make sense of the successful application of science outside of the experimental laboratory, and specifically in conditions in which event regularities do not necessarily occur? What must the world be like for such experimental practices, results, and their successful nonexperimental application to be possible?

A structured ontology

In order to provide a satisfactory set of answers to such questions it is necessary to abandon not only the presumption, implicit in a good deal of economic modelling practice and debate, that event regularities of the sought-after sort are ubiquitous in nature, but also the equally widely held view that the scientifically significant generalisations of nature consist of event regularities. Instead, we must accept a conception of the objects of science as structured (irreducible to events) and intransitive (existing and acting independently of their being identified). That is, experimental activity and results, and the application of experimentally determined knowledge outside of experimental situations, can be made intelligible only through invoking something like an ontology of structures, powers, generative mechanisms, and their tendencies that lie behind and govern the flux of events in an essentially open world.

The fall of an autumn leaf, for example, does not conform to an empirical regularity, precisely because it is governed in complex ways by the actions of different juxtaposed and counteracting mechanisms. Not only is the path of the leaf governed by gravitational pull, but also by aerodynamic, thermal, inertial, and other mechanisms. According to this conception, then, experimental activity can be understood as an attempt to intervene in order to insulate a particular mechanism of interest by forestalling all other potentially counteracting forces. The aim is to engineer a system in which the actions of any mechanism being investigated are more readily identifiable. *Thus, experimental activity is rendered intelligible not as the production of a rare situation in which an empirical law is put into effect, but as an intervention designed to bring about those special circumstances under which a non-empirical law, a mechanism or tendency, can be empirically identified.* The law itself (now understood as a description of the workings of an underlying tendency) is always operative; if the triggering conditions hold, the mechanism is activated and in play whatever else is going on. On this understanding, for example, a leaf is subject to the gravitational tendency even as I hold it in the palm of my hand or as it 'flies' over roof tops and chimneys. Through this sort of reasoning we can make sense of the successful application of experimentally established scientific knowledge outside experimental situations. The context in which a mechanism is operative is irrelevant to the law's specification.

Conditions for closure

If, then, we are to make sense of the largely experimental confinement of event regularities, along with the wider application of experimentally determined results, it seems that we must recognise that reality is (1) *open* (event regularities are not ubiquitous – openness is required in order that closure, the occurrence of an event regularity, is a human achievement); and (2) *structured* (constituted by underlying powers, mechanisms, and so forth as well as the actual course of events and states of affairs); with (3) some features of it being **both** (i) *separable* (allowing the experimental manipulation and insulation of some mechanisms from the effects of others) and (ii) *intrinsically stable* or *'atomistic'* (allowing the production of definite repeatable and predictable consequences once/if the mechanism is triggered).

Under these conditions it is at least feasible that human intervention can bring about a situation in which a mechanism which can act both inside and outside the experimental laboratory, is insulated under controlled experimental conditions and triggered. In these circumstances a predictable correlation between triggering conditions, and the effects of the mechanism is feasible and a modelling strategy legitimate.

The social domain

To what extent do these ontological conditions, conditions whose regular satisfaction seems essential if we are to persevere in a generalised fashion with methods of formalistic modelling, carry over to the social realm? I pose this question, of course, merely to determine whether the methods of formalistic modelling have much relevance to the social realm at all. We shall see that this is unlikely.

First of all what is meant by the social realm? I follow standard practice here and interpret it as the domain of phenomena whose existence depends at least in part on (intentional) human agency.

So understood the social world is clearly structured. For example, a condition of our speech acts, but irreducible to them, are rules of grammar and other structures of language. It is easy to see that social life in general is governed or facilitated by social rules, rules that lay down rights, obligations, prerogatives, and other possibilities and limits.

Although the fact of the social realm being structured seems a necessary condition for social event regularities of the sort pursued by econometricians to be guaranteed, it is not, as we have seen, sufficient for such an outcome: social structures including mechanisms need also to be intrinsically stable and amenable to insulation. I now want to suggest that the regular satisfaction of the latter two conditions is unlikely, and that this in large part explains the widespread failure of the econometrics project to date.

Notice, first of all, that because social structure both depends upon human agency and in turn conditions it, a switch of emphasis in social analysis is necessitated, away from those (extreme) conceptions, familiar in economics, of creation and determination, to notions of *reproduction* and *transformation*. For human intentional activity does not *create* social structure if the latter is presupposed by such activity. Instead, individual agents draw upon social structure as a condition of acting, and through the action of individuals taken in total, social structure is *reproduced* or (in part, at least) *transformed*. Equally, though, social structure cannot be reified. For it is itself dependent upon always transformative human agency, and only at the moment of acting can aspects of social structure be interpreted as given to any individual. In short, through individuals drawing upon it in action, structure is continually reproduced or modified in form.[13]

Social positions and relations as integral to social reality

Social life, then, is not only structured but intrinsically dynamic. In emphasising its structured nature I have so far focused upon social rules. But this is not all there is to it. Specifically, social being is also constituted in a fundamental way by both *social relations* and *positions*. These features are essential to understanding the precise manner in which human agency and structure come together.

The significance and fact of social relations and positions are easily recognised once we take note (and inquire into the conditions) of a general feature of experience: that there is a systematic disparity across individuals regarding the practices that are, and apparently can be, followed. Although most rules can be utilised by a wide group of people it by no means follows that all rules are available, or apply equally, to everyone, even within a given culture. To the contrary, any (segment of) society is highly segmented in terms of the obligations and prerogatives that are on offer. Teachers, for example, are allowed and expected to follow different practices than students, government ministers to follow different ones than lay-people, employers than employees, men than women, landlords than tenants, and so on. Rules as resources are not equally available, or do not apply equally, to each member of the population at large.

What, then, explains the differentiated ascription of obligations, prerogatives, privileges, and responsibilities? This question directs attention to the wider one of how human beings and social structure, such as rules, come together in the first place. If social structure such as rules is a different sort of thing to human beings, human agency, and even action, what is the point of contact between human agency and structure? How do they interconnect? In particular how do they come together in such a manner that different agents achieve different responsibilities and obligations and thereby call on, or are conditioned in their actions by, different social rules and so structures of power?

If it is clearly the case that teachers have different responsibilities, obligations, and prerogatives than students, and government ministers face different ones than the rest of us, then it is equally apparent that these obligations and prerogatives exist independently of the particular individuals who happen, currently, to be teachers, students, or ministers. If I, as a university teacher, were to move on tomorrow, someone else would take over my teaching responsibilities and enjoy the same obligations and prerogatives as I currently do. Indeed, those who occupy the positions of students are different every year. In short, society is constituted in large part by a set of *positions*, each associated with numerous obligations, rights, and duties, and into which agents, as it were, slot.

Something more about this system of societal positions can be expressed if we take note of the additional observation that practices routinely followed by occupants of any type of position tend to be oriented towards some other group(s). The rights, tasks, and obligations of teachers, for example, are oriented towards their interactions with students (and vice versa), towards research-funding bodies or governing institutions, and so forth. Similarly the rights and obligations of landlords are oriented towards their interactions with tenants, and so on.

The importance of internal relations

Such considerations clearly indicate a causal role for certain forms of *relation*. Two types of relation must be distinguished: *external* and *internal*. Two objects or aspects are said to be externally related if neither is constituted by the relationship in which it stands to the other. Bread and butter, coffee and milk, barking dog and mail carrier, two passing strangers, provide examples. In contrast, two objects are said to be internally related if they are what they are by virtue of the relationship in which they stand to one another. Landlady/landlord and tenant, employer and employee, teacher and student, magnet and its field are examples that spring easily to mind. In each case it is not possible to have the one without the other; each, in part, is what it is, and does what it does, by virtue of the relation in which it stands to the other.

Now the intelligibility of rule-governed and the rule-differentiated social situation noted above requires that we recognise, first, the internal relationality of social life and, second, that the internal relationality in question is primarily not of individuals *per se* but of social positions. It is the positions that are defined in relation to others, say of teachers to students. The picture that emerges, in other words, is of a set, or network, of positions characterised by the rules and so practices associated with them, where the latter are determined in relation to other positions and their associated rules and practices. According to this conception, the basic building blocks of society are *positions*, involving, depending upon, or constituted according to, social rules and associated tasks, obligations, and prerogatives, along with the practices they govern, where such positions are both defined in relation to other positions and are immediately occupied by individuals.

Notice, finally, that notions of social *systems* or *collectivities* can be straightforwardly developed using the conceptions of social rules, practices, relationships, and positions now elaborated. Specifically, the conception of social systems and collectivities that is supported in this framework is precisely of an ensemble of networked, internally related, positions with their associated rules and practices. All the familiar social systems, collectivities, and organisations – the economy, the state, international and national companies, trade unions, households, schools, and hospitals – can be recognised as depending upon, presupposing, or consisting in, internally-related position-rule systems of this form.

Formalistic modelling as a generalised tool of social science

What follows for the practices of economic modelling? We know that econometrics and other projects concerned with detecting social-event regularities of interest have so far been rather unsuccessful. We now have an explanation: the social world is a highly internally related, intrinsically dynamic process, and one that is dependent upon, if irreducible to, transformative human agency. Certainly the experimental isolation of stable separable social structures and processes seems infeasible. Nor is it surprising that event regularities of sufficient stability to facilitate a successful practice of economic modelling have not been found to occur spontaneously, that is behind the backs of human intentional actions. It can be admitted that there are numerous regularities that are *made* to happen but that are thereby of limited scientific interest. For example, in certain parts of the world Christmas is celebrated on the same day each year (although even here, in specific families say, there can be exceptions due to illnesses, the need for members of the family to be away from home on 25 December, or whatever.) But regularities such as this hardly constitute the sort of result that formalistic modellers seek to uncover.

In short the social realm seems to be constituted of stuff that is largely not *separable* and *intrinsically stable*, so that the lack of successes of the formalistic modelling project in economics is quite explicable, and future successes are seemingly improbable.

It follows, I think, that feminists may have been too cautious in their criticisms of formalistic modelling. Certainly, there are grounds for supposing that those empirically oriented feminists in economics insistent upon applying standard econometric methods in all contexts are proceeding wholly in the wrong direction.

But it may even be the case that feminists have been largely in error in identifying the primary direction of causation of the errors involved. I have in mind here the tendency of feminist economists to interpret as fundamental the disposition of male economists to portray human agents as relatively isolated, self-contained individuals. The latter is seen as a peculiarly masculinist view, counterpoised with the feminist emphasis on social relations. I think it is. But it may be indirectly and subconsciously achieved.

For I am suggesting that the primary problem with mainstream economists, which differentiates them from other social researchers, is their largely uncritical passion for formalistic modelling. And once it is realised that, to guarantee results that take the event-regularity form, it is necessary to formulate conceptions of separable, stable (intrinsically constant) entities – basically of isolated crypto-atoms – the mainstream emphasis falls into place. For the individualistic agents of mainstream constructions are just that: individual optimising atoms set in situations where a unique optimum of sorts is feasible, guaranteeing stable predictable results. It may thus be the modelling strategy *per se* that is the chief masculinist error here, and the substantive formulations a secondary implication.[14]

In any case, ontological analysis is seen to be consequential. It follows from it that formalistic modelling is not only overly partial: it may actually be misplaced.[15] Economists can pursue the same sorts of goals as the *ex posteriori* successful natural sciences; that is, be concerned to identify causes of surface phenomena. But when mainstream economists insist that we should all work more or less exclusively with procedures of formalistic modelling, they succeed not only in marginalising without investigation all alternative approaches to doing economics (those that are not based on closed systems modelling), they also succeed in universalising a practice that even in natural science is found to be but a special case (confined mainly to the well-controlled experimental situation), and a special case that, in the social realm, conceivably has no legitimate counterpart at all.

Illustration 2: positioned interests as essential to epistemic practice

If event regularities of the sort that are sometimes produced in the experimental sciences are so elusive in the social sciences, how is the systematic investigation of social phenomena possible? If ontology has helped us understand the *ex posteriori* failures of the formalistic modelling approach in the social sciences, as well as the intrinsic limitations of the latter as a method for illuminating the open social system, can it take us further and also help guide us towards a more fruitful alternative way of proceeding? I want now to suggest that it can, and that in doing so it necessarily joins, and contributes to, the discussion, prominent in feminist theory, concerning the situatedness of knowing.

An epistemology for an open system

If social reality is open and complexly structured, being intrinsically dynamic and highly internally related, with a shifting mix of mechanisms lying beneath the surface phenomena of direct experience, how can we begin even to detect the separate effects of (relatively) distinct (aspects of) mechanisms or processes? This is the question I turn to address here. And it is only through ontological reflection that it is apparent that this *is* the question that needs addressing.

In motivating my answer let me quickly take note of the fact that controlled experiments do not *all* take the form of insulating single stable mechanisms in ‘repeated trials’ with the intention of generating event regularities. That is, although event regularities of the sort required by mainstream modelling approaches are mostly produced in well-controlled experimental situations, not all experimental situations are concerned with producing event regularities of this form. An alternative project, illustrated, for example, by plant-breeding experiments, involves the use of control groups to help identify the effects of specific mechanisms of interest. Where, for example, crops are grown in the open there can be no expectation that all the causal factors affecting the yields are stable, reproducible, or even identifiable. Yet progress in understanding *can* be achieved, through ensuring that two sets of crops receive broadly similar conditions except for one factor that is systematically applied to one set but not to the other. In this case systematic differences in average yields of the two sets of crops can with reason be attributed to the factor in question.

In other words, experimental control frequently takes the form of comparing two different groups or populations with common or similar (if complex, irreversible, and unpredictable) histories and shared (if nonconstant) conditions, excepting that one group is 'treated' in some definite way that the second, control, group is not.

In the plant-breeding scenario just described, of course, the aim is to experiment with some compound that is already suspected of possessing yield-increasing causal powers. Our primary concern, however, is with detecting the effects of hitherto unknown or unrecognised mechanisms. But it is easy enough to appreciate the relevance of this scenario for a situation wherein, say, the yield of a given crop was expected *a priori* to be roughly the same in all parts of the field but discovered *ex posteriori* to be systematically higher at one end. In this case an experimentalist has *not* actively treated the relevant end of the field. But it seems prima facie that there is an additional causal factor in operation here, even if we are as yet unaware of its identity.

The general situation I am suggesting as being relevant for social-scientific explanation in open systems, then, is one in which there are two or more comparable populations involved. Our background knowledge leads us to expect a specific relation between outcomes of these populations (frequently a relationship of similarity, but not always), but we are *ex posteriori* surprised by the relation we actually discover. Under such conditions it is prima facie plausible that there is at work a previously unknown yet identifiable causal mechanism, or aspects of a mechanism. Outside these conditions, however, it is difficult to see how, in an open system, projects of identifying hitherto unknown causal processes can even begin.

Contrastive explanation

The open and structured nature of social reality, then, means that we might resort to something like *contrastive explanation*, with explaining descriptive statements that take the form 'this rather than that'. Contrastive explanation is concerned not with questions such as 'why is the average crop yield *x*?' but with 'why is the average crop yield in that end of this field significantly higher than that achieved elsewhere?' Explaining the latter contrast is much less demanding than explaining the total yield. While accounting for the total yield requires an exhaustive list of all the causal factors bearing upon it, the contrastive question requires only that we identify the causes responsible for the difference. But the import of relatively systematic contrasts here lies not so much (or just) in the fact that the task delineated is less demanding, but in the fact that contrasts alert us to the situation that there is something of interest to be explained at all.[16]

Of course, it could have turned out that contrasts of the sort in question were nowhere to be observed. But *ex posteriori* this has not been the case; they are everywhere in evidence. Women usually get worse jobs than men, or are paid less for the same contribution; a car journey from Cambridge to London is usually quicker by night than by day; currently in the U.K. many women wear make-up whereas most men do not; currently in the U.K. schoolgirls perform better academically in single-sex schools than in mixed schools; and so on.

I am suggesting, then, that, in a highly internally related, dynamic (and so typically nonseparable, and nonrepeatable) reality, the effects of causal mechanisms can be identified through formulating interesting contrastives at the level of actual phenomena. This means identifying differences (or surprising relations) between outcomes of two groups whose causal histories suggest that the outcomes in question ought to stand in some definite anticipated or plausible relationship (often one of rough equality or similarity) that is systematically at odds with what we observe. We do not and could not explain the complete causal conditions of any social or other phenomenon. To do so would presumably mean accounting for everything back to the 'big bang' and beyond. Rather, we aim to identify single sets of causal mechanisms and structures. And these are indicated where the observed relationship between outcomes or features of different groups is other than was, or might have been, expected or at least imagined as a real possibility.

Notice, incidentally, that I am not (of course) presuming that any factor or set of factors most directly responsible for a surprising contrast inevitably (or even mainly) combines with all others in a mechanistic fashion. A causal factor present in one situation but not another may well combine with other factors in an organic or internally related fashion and so affect the manner of functioning of any or all causal conditions. This is merely something to be determined in the course of the investigation. Here I am mainly focusing on the usefulness of contrasts of interest for getting potentially successful projects of illumination initiated.

Now it may seem that I am recommending a reasonably general approach here. And indeed I am, although I am making no claims about how generalised is its relevance. Certainly, I do not wish to claim other than a partial perspective. But in truth there is no getting away from generalities. Claims that everywhere there are differences, or that differences matter, or that knowledge is situated, partial and so forth, are no less general. The relevant point is that (unlike, say, formalistic modellers in economics) I am identifying an approach for which the claim of being widely applicable seems *ex posteriori* to have some grounds: there is both reason (as seen in the first illustrative example above) to suppose that the social world is not only open but intrinsically structured, and evidence that contrasts of interest abound in the social domain.

We can note, parenthetically, that the dominant approach of mainstream economics, namely formalistic modelling, is in the end a special case of that which I am defending anyway. For under certain experimental conditions stable mechanisms can be, and often are, insulated and empirically identified. These moments are significant just because (or when) the event patterns produced within the experimental conditions *contrast* in a systematic way with those that emerge 'outside'. In other words, the experimental scientist is able to make an advance precisely by, and when, addressing the contrastive question: 'why is this event regularity achieved under these (specific experimental) conditions but not others?' The problem that remains for mainstream economic modellers, of course, is that whilst interesting contrasts abound in the social realm, few if any seem to involve the discovery of surprising event regularities of a degree of strictness that can be regarded as satisfactory for their intended ('explanatory'/predictive/policy) purposes.

We might also note that the broader argument for reality being open and structured, sustained in the discussion of formalistic modelling above, is itself a further example of contrastive explanation. The contrast in question in this case is the generalised fact of experience that, outside astronomy, event regularities of interest in science are mostly confined to experimental situations. Explaining this contrastive phenomenon leads to the structured ontology I have elaborated. Thus it can be seen that if particular contrasts of interest lead to hypotheses about specific mechanisms, generalised contrasts of interest lead to philosophical ontologies. Given the *ex posteriori* pervasiveness of interesting contrasts, the fact of open systems is seen to be debilitating neither for science nor for philosophy.

Situated knowing

Now all this has a bearing on the situatedness of knowledge emphasised in feminist theorising. For it follows from the emphasis upon contrastive explanation that the sorts of issues addressed in science, and the manner of their treatment, will necessarily reflect the perspectives, understandings, and personal-social histories, in short the 'situations', of the scientist/investigator. It is hardly a novel insight that in the process of choosing a primary phenomenon for explanatory analysis (scientific and other) interests necessarily come to bear. But it is now apparent, once we recognise the contrastive nature of social scientific explanation, that the interests of the researcher necessarily determine which causal mechanism is pursued as well. For when phenomena in an open system are determined by a multiplicity of causes, *the particular one singled out for attention depends upon the contrast identified as puzzling, surprising, unusual, undesirable, or of interest in some other way. And this in turn will reflect the interests and understandings of the individual or group of researchers or interested onlookers involved.* It may be that only the interested farmer can recognise that her or his animals are behaving strangely, only the parent can perceive that all is not well with the child, and only the marginalised group can appreciate the full nature or extent/effects of certain dominant structures or processes or of inequalities, and so forth.

In this way, if amongst others, the situatedness of the investigator comes to the fore in science and explanation, in bearing upon the sorts of contrasts found surprising and warranting of explanation. It influences the direction or location of investigatory practice and so, ultimately, such discoveries or contributions to understanding as are made. In fact, I now want to suggest that insights into the situatedness of knowing achieved by reflecting on the multiple causation of phenomena serves not only to reinforce the feminist insistence on the situated nature of knowing but also to throw further light on certain related issues raised in feminist epistemology. Let me briefly indicate a few of the ways in which contrastive explanation theory and feminist epistemology join together.

Contrastive explanation and feminist epistemology

I should emphasise, first of all, that the theory of contrastive explanation does not merely support the thesis, argued by many feminists, that interested standpoints are inevitable. Certainly the latter insight is sustained. And this insight is sufficient to undermine the conventional presumption whereby, as Sandra Harding critically summarises: 'socially situated beliefs only get to count as opinions. In order to achieve the status of knowledge, beliefs are supposed to break free of – to transcend – their original ties to local, historical interests, values and agendas' (Harding 1993, p. 236).

The position I am defending, however, goes further in suggesting that interested standpoints (including acquired values and prejudices) are not only unavoidable but actually indispensable *aids* to the explanatory process.[17] The task of detecting and identifying previously unknown causal mechanisms seems to require the recognition of surprising or interesting contrasts, and the latter in turn presupposes people in positions of being able to detect relevant contrasts and to perceive them as surprising or otherwise of interest and to want to act on their surprise or aroused interest. The initiation of new lines of investigation requires people predisposed, literally prejudiced, to looking in certain directions.

It follows that science, or the knowledge process more generally, can benefit if undertaken by individuals who are predisposed in different ways, who are situated differently. It is thus the case, as other feminists have already argued (for example, Seiz 1995; Harding 1995; Longino 1990), that the endeavour to attract diverse voices into the scientific community or any prominent (or other) discussion can be supported on grounds not just of democracy or fairness but also of good methodological practice.

Second, contrastive explanation theory appears capable of reinforcing the claim of *standpoint theorists* that marginalised positions can facilitate significant insights. Let us recall that standpoint theories or 'epistemologies' claim that *certain* positioned ways of knowing are in some sense or manner privileged. In early feminist standpoint formulations the emphasis was upon women's ways of knowing.[18] In more recent accounts, the viewpoint of any group that has been marginalised is regarded as privileged. My specific thesis here is that such claims of standpoint theory can be given a good deal of backing if we see the relative advantage of the marginalised arising (in part or whole) just in their being *better able to recognise contrasts of some significance.*

How might being marginalised, meaning being constrained from the centre of some form of social life, confer a relative epistemic advantage? More specifically, why do I suppose it can facilitate the detection of contrasts that are (in a manner yet to be explicated) highly significant? The answer, I believe, lies in that dual feature of being marginal: that it denotes both an insider and outsider position. To be marginalised you are outside of the centre. But equally in order to be marginalised you first have to belong. British women usually are, but the Hopi Indians are not, marginalised in many spheres of modern British society. Feminist economists, post-Keynesians, (old) institutionalists, Austrians, and Marxian economists are, but physicists and chemists are not, marginalised in modern university economics departments.

It is this duality of belonging and yet being constrained from the centre, I think, that is essential to the epistemically advantaged situation of the marginalised. It facilitates an awareness of contrasts of significance. For unlike the dominant group, the marginalised are forced both to be aware of the practices, belief systems, values, and traditions of the dominant group as well as to live their own. And with this being the case there is a greater opportunity, at least, for marginalised people to be aware of contrasts between the two, contrasts that can lead ultimately to the understanding of both sets of community structures, and the relevance of the two, and their interrelatedness (and so ultimately the functioning of the totality). It is in this way and sense in particular, that contrasts more readily available to the marginalised are likely to be especially significant in a given context.[19]

I cannot elaborate on this thesis here. But even from the above brief sketch we can see how this thesis, and the theory of contrastive explanation more generally, can support some of the insights of 'feminist epistemology' and specifically standpoint theory, whilst avoiding many of the tensions often associated with the latter position. Specifically, *contrastive explanation theory* accommodates the principle, widely accepted by feminists, that all voices be admitted to the conversation, *and* can do so in a manner that *neither* supposes that marginalised voices necessarily provide truer accounts, *nor* necessitates that the result will be (a) a plethora of contradictory voices, (b) possibly backed up by a judgmental relativism (i.e., a relativism in which any discrimination amongst contending claims is impossible or arbitrary). Let me briefly indicate why.

Consider first the idea that standpoint theory is supposed to give truer accounts. This appears to be an inference drawn by some of the theory's critics. Thus, for example, Jane Flax's focus of criticism is the idea of 'a feminist standpoint which is truer than previous (male) ones' (Flax 1990, p. 56). Alison Assiter clearly understands the same implication of standpoint theory even if opposing Flax's assessment: 'I disagree with her [Flax], however, in her claim that there is no feminist standpoint that is more true than previous male ones' (Assiter 1996, p. 88). Unfortunately, though, Assiter grounds her assessment in the idea that feminists have a shared set of values and that this somehow necessarily leads them on the path to truth – or at least to '"radical" insights that can be called knowledge' (1996, p. 92). Why or how, or the evidence that, this occurs remains unelaborated in Assiter's account.

It follows from the preceding discussion, however, that to dismiss standpoint theory because it is supposed to give a truer account is based on a misunderstanding of the enabling aspect of a standpoint or position. The advantage that one position may have over another is that it can facilitate the detection of different contrasts and so the pursuit of alternative lines of enquiry. In any investigation of a noted contrastive phenomenon, numerous conjectured explanations may be entertained, and the ease or difficulty with which a relevant causal mechanism is identified will depend, amongst other things, on both the context as well as the skills of the investigators involved. But this, *per se*, has nothing to do with the nature of any standpoint implicated. Specifically, the systematic advantage of the marginalised standpoint, if there is one, lies not in the truth status of the answers obtained, but in the nature of the questions that are recognised as significant and so substance of the answers arrived at.

Here my understanding seems to cohere with that of many standpoint theorists themselves, who put the emphasis on achieving alternative lines of enquiry. Consider Sandra Harding:

> the activities of those at the bottom of such social hierarchies can provide starting points for thought – for *everyone's* research and scholarship – from which humans' relations with each other and the natural world can become visible. This is because the experience and lives of marginalised peoples, as they understand them, provide particularly significant *problems to be explained* or research agendas.
>
> (Harding 1993, p. 240; emphasis in the original)

The light thrown on standpoint theory by contrastive explanation theory, then, helps dispel the idea that anyone is claiming that marginalised viewpoints are or can be privileged because they are supposed somehow to be truer. I now want to suggest that contrastive explanation theory also helps counteract the opposed inference, sometimes drawn and raised in criticism of standpoint theory, that allowing numerous, previously marginalised, voices into the conversation inevitably results in a plethora of contradictory voices. The belief that the latter must follow encourages (though clearly does not justify) the often-repeated conclusion that standpoint theorists' support for a plurality of voices betrays the acceptance of a form of judgmental relativism. Consider the reasoning of Alison Assiter once more:

> although Harding has a legitimate point in her claim that excluding representatives of certain groups cannot help the advancement of knowledge, the converse – that allowing representation to all, on grounds of democracy – leads back to the kind of [judgmental] relativism that Harding wishes to reject.
>
> (Assiter 1996, p. 86)

From the perspective of contrastive explanation theory, however, we can see that neither a plethora of contradictory voices nor a commitment to judgmental relativism is *inevitable*. The prevalence of many different voices, even if all are considering the same phenomenon, may merely reflect a focus upon different contrasts. The investigation of different contrasts can lead to a variety of causes being pursued and perhaps uncovered. For example, suppose we focus on the U.K. productivity record in the post-World War II period. Even if all of our observers are economic historians, each may note a different contrast to the others and so pursue a different cause. For example, one of our economic historians may notice that the productivity record in question is better than the prewar U.K. record and pursue the factor responsible (perhaps the postwar expansion of demand). Another may notice that the postwar productivity performance of the U.K. is below that of many otherwise comparable industrialised countries over the same period and ponder on the causal factor responsible (perhaps Britain's relatively unique system of localised industrial bargaining). And so on.

In short, it is not too farfetched to suppose that even where a similar focus is taken, on say the conditions of work or some aspect of human daily life of a specific group of people, different observers will draw contrasts reflecting their own situations (those of women, lesbians, immigrants, older people, 'unskilled' workers, etc.) and in doing so uncover different aspects of the underlying causal situation. But there is nothing in this assessment that entails that the discoveries made or causal theories formulated are *necessarily* incompatible or contradictory.

That said, it doubtless is the case that the causal explanations produced will often be in competition. But if or when this is so there need be nothing particularly problematic about this situation either, and certainly no reason to embrace a judgmental relativism. For when competing theories are produced, each must be assessed according to its relative empirical adequacy. This is a longer story I will not go into here (see Lawson 1997a, Ch. 15). But there is no reason to suppose that the problems involved are different in nature or degree than those confronting, say, a single scientist or investigator who has herself or himself formulated a set of competing hypotheses all consistent with a particular contrastive phenomenon and wishes to choose between them. Once we allow that theories can be selected according to their relative explanatory powers there is no inevitable problem in dealing with competing explanations.

Illustration 3: the possibility of human emancipation

I turn to my third and final illustration of how ontology can make a difference. Here I want to consider the feminist project of emancipation noted at the outset, and in particular the desire to empower diverse voices. Central here is the recognition by feminists that dominant values and interests need be no more than that, whereas dominant groups often presume to speak and act for, but not necessarily in the interests of, all of us. The salient fact is that in opposing the propensity of dominant groups to universalise their own perceived identity, values, interests, and customs, etc., some feminist theorists have tended to give up on the possibility of shared values and concerns altogether. Specifically, in response to the criticism of earlier feminist theorising that it marginalised differences of race, ethnicity culture, age, and so forth, there has been a tendency to suppose that there are no unifying characteristics of women or feminists at all, or indeed of any other announced grouping.

The resulting conception, in the limit, is of a world of *only* differences, of *only* unique values, interests, and experiences. Any basis for correcting ideas of shared identities, for collectively challenging the values which dominate, for progress in science, for coherent transformative projects of emancipation and so forth are undermined, and in the process any point to a feminist, or any other collective, project evaporates.[20]

This degeneration into an extreme form of individualism, with its associated near-impotency of collective expression or other form of action, is the experience of cultural theory, for example. Here the tendency in question has encouraged the suppression of all reference to feeling or to relatively persisting and transcultural forms of sensibility, grounding aesthetic judgments and accounting for their discriminations. This has culminated in a reluctance to engage with value questions in the field of cultural studies and a tendency, indeed, to collapse cultural criticism into cultural history and sociology.

Increasingly, we are witnessing the same sort of trends in economics with the emergence of injunctions to abandon normative methodology as a hopeless project and to embrace instead methodology as history or sociology of thought (see in particular E. Roy Weintraub 1989; or various contributions to Andrea Salanti and Ernesto Screpanti 1997). The result is a deconstruction of the possibility of sustaining any form of critical engagement. The culmination of the process is the validation of anything that is or happens, an undiscriminating positivism of the actual.

There is more to reality than the course of events and states of affairs

We can see, however, that such assessments serving to destabilise the feminist emancipatory project are hardly compelling once we accept that reality is structured, that it is irreducible to experience and its direct objects. I have already argued that actualism, i.e., the thesis that reality can be reduced to the actual course of events and states of affairs, is untenable, that we must recognise in addition a realm of underlying structures, powers, mechanisms, tendencies, and so forth. At least I have done so specifically in the context of considering objects of the natural sciences and society. I now want to indicate that human subjectivity is no exception, that we can and should substitute a conception of human nature as structured in place of the actual individuality espoused in (versions of) postmodernism. Once this is achieved, contributing a fuller nonactualistic conception of the individual to that already secured for society, we have a basis for seeing clearly that, even if experiences are unique in some sense, or if each human individual has a manifest nature that is unique in some way, it in no way follows thereby that all aspects of societies or of individuals need be.

There can be shared features lying at a different level. I now want to argue that the latter is indeed the case. And it is on this understanding, I also want to indicate, that the feasibility of projects of emancipatory progress mostly rests.

I have already discussed the manner in which I take society, or societies, to be so structured. Let me at this point briefly sketch something of the structure of human nature in general, as well as the distinction between human needs and wants in particular, and indicate their significance for the issues in question (for further elaboration, see Lawson 1997a, 1997b).

Human nature

I must immediately emphasise that any conception of a common human nature that is sustainable here could not be ahistorical. But equally it seems rather implausible to suppose that human beings do not possess various shared characteristics and in particular *capacities* (e.g., language capabilities – as presupposed even by the postmodernist concern with discourse), which both derive from a scientifically recognised common genetic structure and serve to differentiate us from other species. When viewed under one set of aspects, or at a high level of abstraction, then, human nature can be accepted as a common attribute, one grounded in our genetic constitution and manifest in certain species-wide needs and capacities or powers (such as language use).

Of course, even a common human nature can only ever be expressed in inherently socialised, more or less historically, geographically, and culturally specific, and very highly differentiated, forms. In other words, when human nature is viewed under a different set of aspects than the above, and specifically at a lower level of abstraction, it can be understood as an historically relatively-specific nature. Its development, at this level, has its origin at the time, place, and conditions of an individual's birth, and is subsequently influenced by the class, gender, occupational positions, and so forth, in which the individual stands, along with her or his experiences more widely. For example, we cannot just 'speak' in the abstract, we have to speak a specific geohistorically located language. To the extent that numerous people throughout their lives are subject to identical or similar forms of determination an historically quite definite nature may thus be held in common.

Now to accept any of this is not to deny that, in the limit, any individual will always be subject to a unique combination of experiences and modes of determination producing a particular personality. Thus from a third and rather more specific perspective, or a yet lower level of abstraction, the nature of any given human being must be seen as a more or less unique individuality. There is no reason to doubt that a person's individuality is primarily constituted by her or his social peculiarity. Each individual is the product of her or his actions and experiences within the social relations and other modes of determination into which he or she is born and thereafter lives. An individual's actions, or things that happen to her or him, are comprehensible in terms of the individual's socially conditioned capacities, powers, liabilities, and dispositions. The agency of each individual is thus conditioned by the relationships in which he or she stands or has stood, just as these relations, as with social structure in general, are in turn dependent upon the sum total of human doings.

Ultimately, then, an individual's manifest nature and experiences may be unique. But this is quite consistent with commonality or generality lying at a different level, an insight we can recognise only when we pass beyond an ontology of the actual and specifically of experience.

Needs

In accepting that the human subject is so structured we can also recognise a basis for common or shared real needs. And indeed it is essential to any emancipatory project that we can. The possibility of human freedom presupposes the existence of shared human objectives, i.e., real interests and motives, ultimately rooted in common needs and capabilities. If everyone's needs are merely subjective, with the possibility of being irreconcilably opposed, then projecting the goal of social emancipation is indeed likely to be question-begging from the outset. The condition of shared real interests is a presupposition of all emancipatory proposals – whether supporting (relative) change or (relative) continuity – whatever perspective is accepted. And, of course, at the very least we share in common the need to realise some or all of our capacities: to realise our potentials as human beings.

It is not difficult to see, then, that the possibility of moral theorising can, at least in part, be based on a recognised common human nature, a recognition grounded in our biological unity as a species. However, because this common nature is always historically and socially mediated, human needs will be manifest in potentially many ways. It follows, accepting the perspective on society elaborated above, that the pursuit of social goals always takes place in a context of conflicting position-related interests. It is likely, for example, that most of us most of the time need our 'own' language(s) to be spoken. Certainly, conflicts centring on the interests of class positions, age, gender, nation-states, regions, culture, and so forth, are as real and determining as anything else. Even so, different groups may cooperate allowing different, and even opposed, interests sometimes to be met. The point remains, though, that opposed, position-related interests or developed needs exist. And it may be upon our unity as a species and the more generalised features of our social and historical experience and make-up that the greater possibility of unambiguous and enduring progress rests.

Of course, there will often be practical problems of identifying human needs whatever their level of generality. Things are complicated, of course, by the irreducibility both of real needs to manifest wants and of wants to the means of their satisfaction.[21] But if real needs are thereby rendered unobservable this *per se* renders their identification no more problematic than that of other unobservables in science (such as gravitational and magnetic fields and social relationships). Indeed, this is a situation in which contrastive explanation can once more prove fruitful (although justifying this assertion will have to wait a further occasion).

Grounding the possibility of human emancipation

At this point we can see that the conception of human nature, needs, and interests that I am defending, when coupled with the social ontology elaborated in the first illustration set out above (that is, with the conception of social reality as intrinsically dynamic, highly internally related, and constituted by positions, amongst other things) allows us simultaneously to accept the relativity of knowledge, the uniqueness of experiences, *and* the possibility of progress, including emancipatory projects. For it is now clear that there is no contradiction in recognising each of us as a unique identity or individuality, resulting (in part) from our own unique paths through life, and *also* accepting that we can nevertheless possess similar needs or interests as well as stand in the same or similar positions and relations of domination to those of others around us, including gender relations. From this perspective there is no contradiction in recognising both our different individualities and experiences *as well as* the possibility of common interests in transforming certain forms of social relationships. Fundamental here is the fact that human subjectivities, human experiences, and social structure cannot be reduced one to another; they are ontologically distinct, albeit highly interdependent, modes of being.

I rush to add (or re-emphasise) that, as with processes of realising human potentials, I make no presumption that any aspects of social structure, say gender relations, are other than intrinsically dynamic or are everywhere the same. First, social structure depends upon intentional human agency for its existence. It is both condition and consequence of human practice and so is inherently dynamic, depending for its continuity on inherently transformative intentional human agency. Second, social structure is inherently geohistorical-cultural, being dependent on geohistorically rooted practices. There is no presumption that gender relations being reproduced/transformed in Cambridge in 1999 are identical to either those reproduced in Cambridge 100 years ago or those existing currently in some other parts of the U.K., Japan or wherever. It all depends. My experience is that gender relations in most places (still) serve to facilitate (localised) practices in which men can (and often do) dominate/oppress women, or appear in some way advantaged.[22] But the extent of commonality/difference across time and space is something to be determined *ex posteriori*.

This conception also allows that, for people from quite diverse backgrounds, it is feasible both that their individualities/personalities are quite different and that when they arrive in the same location they are subject to, or forced to stand within, similar, i.e. *local*, gender (and other) relations, whether or not they are aware of this, or they learn to become locally skilful. For example, it seems that currently in parts of the U.K. any (person identified as a) woman going alone to a pub in the evening is likely to meet with harassment by some 'men' whatever the former's previous experiences, realised capacities, acknowledged needs, expectations, self-perceptions, or understandings of the local gender relations, and so on.

By the same token, some 'men' in the U.K., aware that approaching a 'woman' in a dark street can cause anxiety, will purposefully cross to the other side of the road if passing or overtaking in order to minimise alarm. This can happen even if the person being overtaken does not (is sufficiently ignorant of local culture as not to) feel any alarm or anxiety, or whatever. Gender relations with a degree of space–time extension along with practices they facilitate can be *transfactually* operative irrespective of the knowledges or understandings and wishes of those affected. The existences of multiple differences in manifest identities and individual experiences is not inconsistent with this insight – any more than the unique path of each autumn leaf undermines the hypothesis that all leaves are similarly subject to the transfactual 'pull' of gravity.

In short, once a structured ontology is recognised we can see that multiplicity in the course of actuality remains coherent with a degree of uniformity at the level of underlying causes or structure. The conception defended thus secures the basis for an emancipatory politics rooted in real needs and interests. In so doing it provides grounds, in particular, for feminist projects of transforming gender relations, in an awareness that the existence of multiculturalism or of differences in general, need not in any way undermine or contradict such emancipatory practice. It also preserves, without strain, the possibility of strategies of solidarity or meaningful affiliated action between groups. In short, it transcends the sorts of tensions that currently seem to pervade much of feminist epistemology and political theory.

What seems to have happened in certain strands of feminist theorising (or in social philosophies that have been influential) is that a form of *a priori* universalising has once more been sanctioned. By correctly emphasising differences in experiences and manifest natures, but erroneously reducing reality to experience and its direct objects, the view encouraged is of a world of only uniqueness and differences. In this way, in place of the commonalities previously unquestioningly asserted by dominant groups in treating their own specific traits as though universal, we achieve only a world of universalised difference. And it seems that an essential condition for this erroneous result maintaining any credibility or ground is the neglect of explicit ontological enquiry.

Final comments

I have observed that explicit ontological analysis is conspicuously, if erroneously, downplayed in much of feminist theorising, and I have suggested that this neglect is unfortunate in that ontology matters for any would-be projects of illumination and emancipation. I have provided some illustrations to back up this claim.

Whatever the reason for the downplaying of such realist concerns, the point bears emphasising that realists are no more committed to absolutism than relativists are committed to irrealism. The relevant question, rather, is:

which realist and which relativist positions are sustainable in a given context? I have argued here, in effect, for an ontological realism and an epistemological relativism, which together amount to a rejection of a judgmental relativism in favour of a judgmental rationality.[23] In this I have defended a particular social theory that preserves and endorses, indeed itself incorporates, the impulse behind the 'deconstructive' turn in feminist theory, but which simultaneously, through its emphasis on ontology, avoids the self-subversion of *total* (including a judgmental) relativism.

The particular theory of reality defended is of a structured and open world. It is a conception that recognises that in our everyday practices, all of us, as complexly structured, socially and culturally situated, purposeful and needy individuals, knowledgeably and capably negotiate complex, shifting, only partially grasped, and contested structures of power, rules, relations, and other, possibly relatively enduring but nevertheless transient and action-dependent, social resources at our disposal. Ontological analysis provides an insight into this reality.

Thus when Deirdre McCloskey, in the manner of others, cautions against any embracing of 'material realism' on the grounds that 'What is at issue here is the philosopher's construct, Reality, a thing deeper than what is necessary for daily life' (McCloskey 1997, pp. 14–15), the primary error lies in supposing there is little depth to 'daily life', that philosophy deals (or inevitably claims to deal) with a reality apart from that continually encountered by us all. The mistaken presumption, in effect, is that social reality, and specifically 'daily life', is reducible to the actual course of social events. This reduction of reality to experience and its immediate objects is a mistake that ontological analysis allows us to rectify.

Now I am aware, finally, that the above outline is rather schematic and hurried. I suspect many will remain rather unconvinced by some or all of the sketches provided. As it happens, I do find that the broad perspective elaborated currently constitutes as sustainable (explanatorily powerful) an account as any with which I am familiar (see Lawson 1997a). But I should re-emphasise that most of the preceding discussion is provided first and foremost with the intent of being illustrative. My primary objective here is not so much to persuade others to accept precisely the conceptions developed as to suggest that such conceptions, or explicit ontological analyses of the sort grounding them, do deserve consideration by more feminists. My chief purpose here is to contribute to removing what I take to be unnecessary obstacles to a particular set of debates, with the hope of transforming or even initiating a further strand to a particular conversation. For it may just be (from where I am situated it seems likely) that if feminists, including feminist economists, allow realism, and in particular explicit ontological analysis, to come more fully out of the margin, the opportunities for advance opened up thereby will prove to be to everyone's advantage.

Notes

1 This chapter was originally published as: Lawson, T., 1999. Feminism, realism, and universalism. *Feminist Economics*, 5(2): 25–59. © IAFFE 1999, http://www.feministeconomics.org. Republished with permission.

2 Most obviously such a universalising tendency serves to exclude alternative voices and practices. In resisting it feminists have been strategic in facilitating a stage, inside and outside the academy, for otherwise marginalised or excluded voices, a contribution that has both emancipatory and enlightening dimensions (see Susan Bordo 1993).

Against this background of the opening-up of social theory in a variety of areas, feminists within economics have been endeavoring to achieve similar progress in a discipline which, over the last half-century at least, has become one of the least pluralistic of all. On the constructive side has been the creation of the journal *Feminist Economics*. Here the intention to include voices previously marginalised or excluded altogether is accepted as fundamental (see especially Diana Strassmann's opening editorial). On the more critical side feminist economists have not been slow in revealing the tendency of prominent economists, mainly white, middle-class and male, to universalise their own experiences and perspectives, and, most significantly, to use the assumed, but unestablished, universal validity of their own particular methodological and other dispositions to exclude others who might wish to do things differently (see, for example, Paula England 1993; Nancy Folbre 1993; Ulla Grapard 1995; Julie Nelson 1993, 1996; Janet Seiz 1993, 1995; Diana Strassmann 1993a, 1993b; or Diana Strassmann and Livia Polanyi 1995). Others have been concerned that implicit overgeneralising is avoided in feminist (substantive) economics itself (see, for example, M. V. Lee Badgett 1995).

3 Nussbaum writes 'By metaphysical realism I mean the view … that there is some determinate way the world is, apart from the interpretive workings of the cognitive faculties of human beings' (1995, p. 68).

4 In a reflective and critical follow-up, or response, to her own 'cyborg' paper, i.e., in her paper on 'situated knowledges', Donna Haraway acknowledges that 'feminists have both selectively and flexibly used and been trapped by two poles of a tempting dichotomy on the question of objectivity' (1988, p. 249). This dichotomy is between positions which Haraway refers to as feminist critical empiricism and radical constructionism. The empiricist wing is criticised for expecting too much in terms of knowing reality, the radical constructionist or postmodernist position for knowing too little. Haraway (1988, p. 252) formulates her resolution as follows:

> So, I think my problem, and 'our' problem, is how to have simultaneously an account of radical historical contingency for all knowledge claims and knowing subjects, a critical practice for recognising our own 'semiotic technologies' for making meanings, and a no-nonsense commitment to faithful accounts of a 'real' world, one that can be partially shared and that is friendly to earth-wide projects of finite freedom, adequate material abundance, modest meaning in suffering, and limited happiness.

5 Of course, all methods and epistemological positions generate implicit ontological claims of some kind. Hume's empiricism (as usually interpreted) is an example. By restricting knowledge to experience, (knowable) reality is itself in effect restricted to (atomistic) events given in experience. In consequence, any generalist claims are restricted to formulations of regularities in the succession and coexistence of these phenomena, to elaborations of Humean causal laws.

Just as empiricists in the Humean mode presuppose a (knowable) reality of atomistic events and states of affairs given in experience, so radical constructivists necessarily recognise a reality of the text (or the conversation or some such) and all its presuppositions. Even if discourse or conversation is thought only to be about discourse or conversation, the text being discussed in a particular discourse is at the level of ontology, it constitutes the referent of thought and knowledge, and the ongoing discourse-making reference is at the level of epistemic practice, the process of knowledge. There is nothing in philosophical realism that warrants that ontology is restricted to things immutable or known infallibly, etc. Certainly, any text is real and a potential object of knowledge. And this remains so even if someone voices disagreement with aspects of it, and even if the author changes her or his view as a result, or even if the reader has not fully understood the author's intention.

6 For an introduction to some of this literature see especially Margaret Archer et al. (1998).

7 I am not sure any contributor would want to put things quite so starkly as this. But it is a (polar) conception to which allusions appear sometimes to be made (or are easily interpreted as being made) even in the best of feminist writing. Helen Longino's important contributions provide a prominent example. In a statement about realism that is otherwise helpful she writes of 'the idea that there is one consistent, integrated or coherent, true theoretical treatment of all natural phenomena. … These ideas are part of the realist tradition in the philosophy of science'. And a few lines below she adds: 'Even more, the scientific inquirer, and we with her, become passive onlookers, victims of the truth. The idea of a value free science is integral to this view of scientific inquiry …' (Longino 1987, pp. 256–7; see also Longino 1990, p. 29).

In similar fashion Mary Tiles (employing capital letters as a distancing device, in a manner adopted in economics for example by Deirdre McCloskey 1997) writes: 'we see increasing numbers of philosophers of science rallying under the banner of Realism to defend the view of science as aiming at objective Truth and as possessed of methods of theory choice which, even if they do not guarantee truth, do at least ensure objectivity by preventing the intrusion of non-scientific interests or values into theory choice' (Tiles 1987, p. 221).

It is easy to see how influential assessments such as these (whether or not couched in terms of *scientific* realism and even allowing for their particular contexts) might encourage the view that all scientific realisms take, or at least tend towards, the narrow absolutist perspective described. My suspicion is that it is by way of universalising this very narrow version to cover the entire perspective of scientific realism, that the latter, and in particular the activity of explicit ontological elaboration closely associated with it, tends to be played down if not altogether excluded from serious discussion and debate. In this way there is a real possibility that, in feminist thinking, scientific realism is itself in effect marginalised through misrepresentation.

8 See, for example, McCloskey's (1997) "You Shouldn't Want a Realism If You Have a Rhetoric" as a recent example of attempting to play down the role of explicitly realist considerations in economics.

9 Before indicating how this constructive input might be achieved, though, I must make sure that I do not myself knowingly falsely universalise here. Specifically, I should acknowledge that there are at least some feminist theorists sensitive to, and who explicitly acknowledge, the fact that there is far more to realism than the naive or absolutist conception that some may be erroneously generalising. (See, for example, Miranda Fricker 1994; Jean Grimshaw 1986; Marnia Lazreg 1994; Martha Nussbaum 1995; Caroline New 1998; Janet Seiz 1993, 1995; Kate Soper 1991.) However, this group does seem to constitute a relatively small minority, as some of the individuals concerned themselves observe.

10 For an indication of how dominant is the practice of formalistic modelling in modern mainstream economics see Diana Strassmann's (1994) discussion.

11 A good preliminary discussion of alternative methods based on more qualitative approaches is provided by a set of contributions – by Günseli Berik, Joyce P. Jacobsen, Andrew A. Newman, Irene van Staveren, Simel Esim, and Jennifer C. Olmsted – collected together by Michèle Pujol (1997), for a 'Special Issue' of *Feminist Economics* entitled "Expanding the Methodological Boundaries of Economics."

12 A response that to some extent is already being realised. (See, for example, Esther Redmount 1995; Shelley Phipps and Peter S. Burton 1995; or Notburga Ott 1995.)

13 In their daily activities, then, human beings draw upon social structure which, in turn, is reproduced or transformed through human action taken in total. Although human acts may sometimes be performed with the intention of (1) reproducing structure (speaking to a child with the intention of imparting knowledge of language) or (2) transforming structure (collective attempts to change some feature of the current economic or legal system), it is likely that most structural reproduction and/or transformation arises as an unintended product, whether or not desired or even recognised. Of course, if the reproduction/transformation of social structure is only rarely recognised by individuals or their reason for acting in the way they do, individuals usually have some motivation for, and conception of what they are doing in, their activity. Human acts are mostly if not always intentional under some description. Even if most speakers of English, say, are not intending, in their individual speech acts, to reproduce that language, its reproduction nevertheless is the sum result of the speech acts in which English speakers engage, just as the speech acts in which individual agents engage always have their own intended objectives.

If the reproduction/transformation of social structure is rarely an intended project, it is equally the case that the individual agents are not always aware, certainly not discursively or self-consciously so, of the structures (such as language rules) upon which they are drawing. The picture that emerges, then, is one of largely unmotivated and only partially grasped social reproduction. Individuals draw upon existing social structure as a typically unacknowledged condition for acting, and through the action of all individuals taken in total, social structure is typically unintentionally reproduced. Social structure in general is neither created by, nor independent of, human agency, but rather is the unmotivated condition of all our motivated productions, the noncreated but drawn upon and reproduced/transformed condition for our daily economic/social activities. For an elaboration on all this see Lawson (1997a), especially Chapters 12 and 13.

14 Of course, both orientations are causal and have become historically associated in economics. The point is that as long as economists keep to their formalistic methods they are constrained from dealing with realistic substantive accounts even if so inclined. But the method and the theory are currently so intertwined that it is easy to support Michèle Pujol's conclusion:

> Can neoclassical economics be cleansed of its patriarchal bias so that it can open its eyes to the methodological flaws resulting from its ingrained sexism? … I want to suggest that the very logic, rhetoric and symbolism of the paradigm may be inseparable from the … sexist assumptions I have discussed here. Neoclassical economics has a *his*tory of stifling feminist approaches. We cannot wait for change. We must transcend it.
>
> (Pujol 1995, pp. 29-30)

See also Martha McDonald's (1995) assessment that 'economic theory and methodology both have to change if they are to serve feminist purposes, and the changes are interactive' (p. 191).

15 Of course, all reasoning is fallible, including ontological analysis of the sort presented here. On the pluralist/anti-dogmatic grounds of not wishing to foreclose any line of epistemic activity (in case it proves illuminating), therefore, I do not conclude that we need to reject all formalistic modelling out of hand. But I do think we must accept that there are compelling grounds for expecting the dismal record of generalised failure to continue (and for effecting a substantial reallocation of economics-research resources).

16 Contrastive explanation has been widely discussed over the last twenty years, of course (see, for example, Bas Van Fraassen 1980; Alan Garfinkel 1981; David Lewis 1986; Peter Lipton 1991). However, whilst I think it is fair to say that much of this literature has been concerned with applied explanation, with considering whether known factors can be said to constitute an (adequate) explanation, I am here concerned with the role of contrastive phenomena in the process of identifying causes that are unknown or hitherto unrecognised.

17 Perhaps this recognition lends support to Donna Haraway's remark that 'Feminist objectivity means quite simply *situated knowledges*' (Haraway 1988, p. 253).

18 These formulations, in turn, often critically built on Marx's analysis of contrasting 'class' positions in a capitalist society. A major contribution of this sort is Nancy Hartsock's (1983) "The Feminist Standpoint: Developing the Ground for a Specifically Feminist Historical Materialism."

19 This thesis does, I think, closely resonate with those of other standpoint theorists. It has close affinities, for example, with Nancy Hartsock's (1983) insistence that 'A standpoint is not simply an interested position (interpreted as bias) but is interested in the sense of being engaged' (p. 218). According to Hartsock, 'like the lives of proletarians according to Marxian theory, women's lives make available a particular and privileged vantage point on male supremacy, a vantage point which can ground a powerful critique of the phallocratic institutions and ideology which constitute the capitalist form of patriarchy' (p. 217). It also fits closely with Patricia Hill Collins's (1991) discussion of the 'outsiders within', and with Dorothy Smith's (1987, 1990) notion of 'bifurcated consciousness'.

20 All we have are different voices, interests and values, and the absence of any nonarbitrary way for distinguishing between them. Each claim is as good as anyother. There is no basis for progress, criticism, or any kind of engagement with our times. We have what we have; a situation to be described, perhaps, but not to be judged or criticised. As Susan Bordo summarises the situation:

> Assessing where we are now, it seems to me that feminism stands less in danger of the totalising tendencies of feminists than of an increasingly paralysing anxiety over falling (from what, grace?) into ethnocentrism or "essentialism." … Do we want to delegitimate *a priori* the exploration of experimental continuity and structural common ground among women? … If we wish to empower diverse voices, we would do better, I believe, to shift strategy from the methodological dictum that we foreswear talk of "male" and "female" realities … to the messier, more slippery, practical struggle to create institutions and communities that will not permit *some* groups of people to make determinations about reality for *all.*
>
> (Bordo 1993, p. 465)

Or, as Kate Soper complains:

> the logic which challenged certain kinds of identity thinking and deconstructed specific notions of truth, progress, humanism and the like, has pushed on to question the possibility of objectivity or of making reference in language to what itself is not the effect of discourse … Pushed to its uttermost, the logic of difference rules out any holistic and objective analysis of societies of a kind which allows to define them as "capitalist" or "patriarchal" or indeed totalitarian, together with the transformative projects such analyses advocate. It gives us not new identities, not a better understanding of the plural and complex nature of society, but tends rather to collapse into an out and out individualism.
>
> (Soper 1991, pp. 45, 46)

21 Clearly, needs and rights can be formulated as goals or wants or demands, and treated as legitimate or illegitimate, only under definite historical conditions. As such they may be poorly, and even misleadingly, formulated. Specifically, real needs can be manifest in a variety of historically contingent wants, which may then be met by any of perhaps a multitude of potential satisfiers. It follows that to assume either actual satisfiers (e.g., specific commodities purchased or perhaps acts of violence) or expressed objectives (such as owning more than others) are defining of human needs is to commit an ethical fallacy – to reduce needs to wants and wants to the conditions of their being satisfied or expressed.

I am not suggesting that wants as expressed in actions bear no relation to underlying needs, of course. Indeed, although certain activities sometimes appear quite undesirable from the point of view of facilitating human development and potential, it is often easy enough to see how they are nevertheless motivated by various real needs on the part of the perpetrators – for example, to obtain respect from others, inner security or simply a release of frustration. But it is important that real needs and expressed wants are not conflated (which is just what tends to happen in modern mainstream economics of course, a mistake that is encouraged by that project's continuing neglect of explicit ontological analysis). For a lengthier discussion of all this, see Lawson (1997a).

22 Consider, for example, Kate Soper's U.K.-based experience. In arguing that 'there are some concrete and universal dimensions to women's lives …' she illustrates with the case of solitude:

> I mean that women live in a kind of alertness to the possibility of attack and must to some degree organise their lives in order to minimise its threat. In particular, I think, this has constraints – from which men are free – on our capacity to enjoy solitude. As a woman, one's reaction to the sight of a male stranger approaching on a lonely road or country walk is utterly different from one's reaction to the approach of a female stranger. In the former case there is a frisson of anxiety quite absent in the latter. This anxiety, of course, is almost always confounded by the man's perfectly friendly behaviour, but the damage to the relations between the sexes has already been done – and done not by the individual man and woman – but by their culture. This female fear and the constraints it places on what women can do – particularly in the way of spending time on their own – has, of course, its negative consequences for men too, most of whom doubtless deplore its impact on their own capacities for spontaneous relations with women. … But the situation all the same is not symmetrical: resentment or regret is not as disabling as fear; and importantly it does not affect the man's capacity to go about on his own.
>
> (Soper 1990, p. 242)

23 This is a topic I explore more fully elsewhere (Lawson 1997a). It is also central to various contributions in Archer et al. (1998).

References

Archer, M., R. Bhaskar, A. Collier, T. Lawson and A. Norrie (eds.). 1998. *Critical Realism: Essential Readings*. London and New York: Routledge.

Assiter, A. 1996. *Enlightened Women: Modernist Feminism in a Postmodern Age*. London and New York: Routledge.

Badgett, M. V. L. 1995. "Gender, Sexuality, and Sexual Orientation: All in the Feminist Family?" *Feminist Economics* 1(1): 121–39.

Berik, G. 1997. "The Need for Crossing the Method Boundaries in Economics Research." *Feminist Economics* 3(2): 121–6.

Bordo, S. 1993. "Feminism, Post Modernism and Gender Scepticism," in *Unbearable Weight: Feminism, Western Culture, and the Body*. The Regents of the University of California. Reprinted in A. C. Herrmann and A. Stewart (eds.). 1994. *Theorizing Feminism: Parallel Trends in the Humanities and Social Sciences*. Boulder, CO: Westview Press (page references to the latter).

Collins, P. H. 1991. *Black Feminist Thought: Knowledge, Consciousness and the Politics of Empowerment*. London and New York: Routledge.

England, P. 1993. "The Separative Self: Androcentric Bias in Neoclassical Assumptions," in M. A. Ferber and J. A. Nelson (eds.) *Beyond Economic Man: Feminist Theory and Economics*, pp. 37–53. Chicago: University of Chicago Press.

Esim, S. 1997. "Can Feminist Methodology Reduce Power Hierarchies in Research Settings?" *Feminist Economics* 3(2): 137–40.

Ferber, M. A. and J. A. Nelson (eds.). 1993. *Beyond Economic Man: Feminist Theory and Economics*. Chicago: University of Chicago Press.

Flax, J. 1990. "Postmodernism and Gender Relations in Feminist Theory," in Linda J. Nicholson (ed.) *Feminism/Postmodernism*, pp. 39–62. London and New York: Routledge.

Folbre, N. 1993. "How Does She Know? Feminist Theories of Gender Bias in Economics." *History of Political Economy* 25(4): 167–84.

Fricker, M. 1994. "Knowledge as Construct: Theorizing the Role of Gender in Knowledge," in K. Lennon and M. Whitford (eds.) *Knowing the Difference: Feminist Perspectives in Methodology*. London and New York: Routledge.

Garfinkel, A. 1981. *Forms of Explanation*, New Haven, CT: Yale University Press.

Grapard, U. 1995. "Robinson Crusoe: The Quintessential Economic Man?" *Feminist Economics* 1(1): 33–52.

Grimshaw, J. 1986. *Feminist Philosophers: Women's Perspectives on Philosophical Traditions*. Brighton, U.K.: Wheatsheaf Books.

Haraway, D. 1985. "A Manifesto for Cyborgs: Science, Technology, and Socialist Feminism in the 1980s." *Socialist Review* 15(2): 65–108. Reprinted in D. Haraway. 1991. *Simians, Cyborgs and Women: The Reinvention of Nature*, pp. 149–81, 243–8. New York: Routledge and Chapman & Hall. Also reprinted in A. Herrmann and A. Stewart (eds.) 1994. *Theorizing Feminism: Parallel Trends in the Humanities and Social Sciences*. Boulder, CO: Westview Press.

——. 1988. "Situated Knowledges: The Science Question in Feminism and the Privilege of Partial Perspective." *Feminist Studies* 14(3): 575–99. Reprinted in E. Fox Keller and H. E. Longino (eds.) *Feminism and Science*. Oxford and New York: Oxford University Press (page references to the latter).

Harding, S. 1993. "Rethinking Standpoint Epistemology: What is 'Strong Objectivity'?" in L. Alcoff and E. Potter (eds.) *Feminist Epistemologies*. London and New York:

Routledge. Reprinted in E. Fox Keller and H. E. Longino (eds.) *Feminism and Science*. Oxford and New York: Oxford University Press (page references to the latter).

——. 1995. "Can Feminist Thought Make Economics More Objective?" *Feminist Economics* 1(1): 7–32.

Hartsock, N. C. M. 1983. "The Feminist Standpoint: Developing the Ground for a Specifically Feminist Historical Materialism," in S. Harding and M. B. Hintikka (eds.) *Discovering Reality: Feminist Perspectives on Epistemology, Metaphysics, Methodology, and Philosophy of Science*. Dordrecht: Reidel. Reprinted in (for example) L. Nicholson (ed.) *The Second Wave: A Reader in Feminist Theory*, pp. 216–40. London and New York: Routledge (page references to the latter version).

Hutchings, K. 1994. "The Personal is International: Feminist Epistemology and the Case of International Relations," in K. Lennon and M. Whitford (eds.) *Knowing the Difference: Feminist Perspectives in Methodology*. London and New York: Routledge.

Jacobsen, J. P. and A. A. Newman. 1997. "What Data Do Economists Use? The Case of Labor Economics and Industrial Relations." *Feminist Economics* 3(2): 127–30.

Lawson, T. 1997a. *Economics and Reality*. London and New York: Routledge.

——. 1997b. "Situated Rationality." *Journal of Economic Methodology* 4(1): 101–25.

Lazreg, M. 1994. "Women's Experience and Feminist Epistemology: A Critical Neo-Rationalist Approach," in K. Lennon and M. Whitford (eds.) *Knowing the Difference: Feminist Perspectives in Methodology*. London and New York: Routledge.

Lewis, D. 1986. "Causal Explanation," in *Philosophical Papers, Vol. II*, pp. 214–40. Oxford: Oxford University Press.

Lipton, P. 1991. *Inference to the Best Explanation*. London and New York: Routledge.

Longino, H. 1987. "Can There Be A Feminist Science?" *Hypatia* 2 (3)(Fall). Reprinted in A. Garry and M. Perasall (eds.). 1996. *Women, Knowledge and Reality*. London and New York: Routledge.

——. 1990. *Science as Social Knowledge: Values and Objectivity in Scientific Enquiry*. Princeton, NJ: Princeton University Press.

McCloskey, D. 1997. "You Shouldn't Want a Realism If You Have a Rhetoric." Mimeo. Erasmus University of Rotterdam and the University of Iowa.

McDonald, M. 1995. "The Empirical Challenges of Feminist Economics: The Example of Economic Restructuring," in Edith Kuiper and Jolande Sap (eds.) *Out of the Margin: Feminist Perspectives on Economics*, pp. 175–97. London and New York: Routledge.

Nelson, J. 1993. "Value-Free or Valueless? Notes on the Pursuit of Detachment in Economics." *History of Political Economy* 25(4): 121–43.

——. 1996. *Feminism, Objectivity & Economics*. London and New York: Routledge.

New, C. 1998. "Realism, Deconstruction and the Feminist Standpoint," Mimeo. Bath Spa University College.

Nussbaum, M. C. 1995. "Human Capabilities, Female Human Beings," in M. C. Nussbaum and J. Glover (eds.) *Women, Culture, and Development: A Study of Human Capabilities*. Oxford: Clarendon Press.

Olmsted, J. C. 1997. "Telling Palestinian Women's Economic Stories." *Feminist Economics* (3)2: 141–51.

Ott, N. 1995. "Fertility and Division of Work in the Family: a Game Theoretic Model of Household Decisions", in E. Kuiper and J. Sap (eds.) *Out of the Margin: Feminist Perspectives on Economics*, London and New York: Routledge.

Phipps, S. A. and P. S. Burton 1995. “Social/Institutional Variables and Behavior within Households: An Empirical Test using the Luxembourg Income Study.” *Feminist Economics* 1(1): 151–74.

Pujol, M. 1995. “Into the Margin,” in Edith Kuiper and Jolande Sap (eds.) *Out of the Margin: Feminist Perspectives on Economics*, pp. 17–35. London and New York: Routledge.

——. 1997. “Broadening Economic Data and Methods.” *Feminist Economics* 3(2):119–20.

Redmount, E. 1995. “Towards a Feminist Econometrics,” in E. Kuiper and J. Sap (eds.) *Out of the Margin: Feminist Perspectives on Economics*, pp. 216–22. London and New York: Routledge.

Salanti, A. and E. Screpanti (eds.). 1997. *Pluralism in Economics: New Perspectives in History and Methodology*. Cheltenham, U.K.: Edward Elgar.

Scheman, N. 1993. “Though This Be Method, Yet There is Madness in It: Paranoia and Liberal Epistemology,” in L. Antony and C. Witt (eds.) *A Mind of One's Own*. Boulder, CO: Westview Press. Reprinted in E. Fox Keller and H. E. Longino (eds.) *Feminism and Science*, Oxford and New York: Oxford University Press.

Seiz, J. 1993. “Feminism and the History of Economic Thought.” *History of Political Economy* 25(4): 185–201.

——. 1995. “Epistemology and the Tasks of Feminist Economics.” *Feminist Economics* 1 (3): 110–18.

Smith, D. 1987. *The Everyday World as Problematic*. Boston, MA: Northeastern University Press.

——. 1990. *The Conceptual Practices of Power*. Boston, MA: Northeastern University Press.

Soper, K. 1990. *Troubled Pleasures: Writings on Politics, Gender and Hedonism*. London and New York: Verso.

——. 1991. “Postmodernism, Critical Theory and Critical Realism,” in Roy Bhaskar (ed.) *A Meeting of Minds*. London: The Socialist Society.

Strassmann, D. 1993a. “Not a Free Market: The Rhetoric of Disciplinary Authority in Economics,” in M. A. Ferber and J. A. Nelson (eds.) *Beyond Economic Man: Feminist Theory and Economics*, pp. 54–68. Chicago: University of Chicago Press.

——. 1993b. “The Stories of Economics and the Power of the Storyteller.” *History of Political Economy* 25(4): 147–65.

——. 1994. “Feminist Thought and Economics; Or, What do the Visigoths Know?” *American Economic Review*, Papers and Proceedings 153–8.

——. 1995. “Editorial: Creating a Forum for Feminist Economic Inquiry.” *Feminist Economics* 1(1): 1–5.

——. and L. Polanyi. 1995. “The Economist as Storyteller: What Texts Reveal,” in E. Kuiper and J. Sap (eds.) *Out of the Margin: Feminist Perspectives on Economics*. London and New York: Routledge.

Tiles, M. 1987. “A Science of Mars or of Venus?” Philosophy 62. Reprinted in E. Fox Keller and H. E. Longino (eds.) *Feminism and Science*. Oxford and New York: Oxford University Press.

Van Fraassen, B. C. 1980. *The Scientific Image*. Oxford: Clarendon Press.

Van Stavern, I. 1997. “Focus Groups: Contributing to a Gender-Aware Methodology.” *Feminist Economics* 3(2): 131–7.

Weintraub, E. R. 1989. “Methodology Doesn't Matter, But the History of Thought Might.” *Scandinavian Journal of Economics* 91(2): 477–93.

2 Post-structuralist and constructivist feminism[1]

Carrie Hull

Introduction

Contemporary feminist theory has been deeply influenced by the constructivism and post-structuralism outlined in Chapter 3. Indeed, some of the most famous post-structuralist and constructivist arguments come from feminist quarters. While this form of feminism makes numerous claims, and is often loathe to be identified as a unified movement, a common denominator is its challenge to the alleged philosophical foundationalism of 'second wave' feminism. As I briefly mentioned at the beginning of this book, the feminism of the 1960s and 1970s generally used the concept *gender* to refer to the social and cultural aspects of an underlying biological male or female sex. Simone de Beauvoir's dictum, 'one is not born, but rather becomes a woman', combined with her belief that the sexed body is nonetheless a biological given, exemplified this feminist project. Biology or nature, on the one hand, and culture and society, on the other, were kept relatively distinct. The task for feminists was to unite as biological women, and confront the gender roles doled out by societies around the world.

Judith Butler is perhaps the most celebrated feminist challenging the presuppositions of her predecessors. Butler contends that biological sex itself is a social construction: '[T]he construal of "sex" [is not] … a bodily given on which the construct of gender is artificially imposed, but [is] a cultural norm which governs the materialization of bodies' (Butler 1993, pp. 2–3). It is not possible, as earlier feminists argued, to make a distinction between nature and culture, or sex and gender. There are, accordingly, no biological women outside of or before gender waiting to be liberated by feminism. Challenging gender roles alone will be inadequate to effect social change. The new goal for feminist and sexuality movements should be to defy the faith in the existence of an innate sexuality and natural sex categories.

These core arguments can be witnessed, with some variation, in much contemporary feminist and sexuality theory. Several feminists were making similar arguments even before Judith Butler popularised them. In 1978, Suzanne Kessler and Wendy McKenna – psychologists writing from a perspective informed by Harold Garfinkel's ethnomethodology – argued that 'a world of two "sexes" is a result of the socially shared, taken-for-granted methods which members [of a culture] use to construct reality' (Kessler and McKenna 1978, p. vii). They confidently use the term 'gender' to refer to 'aspects of being a woman (girl) or man (boy) that have traditionally been viewed as biological' (ibid., p. 7). Monique Wittig, also writing in the 1970s (but from a very different perspective), asserts: 'There are, not one or two sexes, but … as many sexes as there are individuals' (Wittig 1979, p. 112). This is not to detract from the force of Butler's arguments, nor to deny that there are differences amongst these feminists. It is still important to acknowledge that analogous claims emerged from disparate intellectual circles in the last thirty years.

The image of the continuum, a series of infinitesimal transformations from male to female, has recently grown popular. Thus, Ruth Hubbard speaks of the 'rainbow' or 'continuum' of biological sex, and declares that nature is no more 'immune from change' than is culture (Hubbard 1996, p. 158). Anne Fausto-Sterling states that sex is a 'vast, infinitely malleable continuum' (Fausto-Sterling 1993, p. 21) while for Alice Dreger, 'the sex spectrum is like the color spectrum; nature provides us with a range where one "type" blends imperceptibly into the next' (Dreger 2001, p. 3). According to Julie Greenberg, male and female are the end poles of a spectrum stretching between them (Greenberg 1999, p. 275).

Others focus on our apparent inability to find a failsafe determinant of biological sex. Bernice Hausman asserts: '[T]here can be no *true* sex if no single "kind of sex" (chromosomal, gonadal, hormonal, among others) can be invoked infallibly as the final indicator of sex identity' (Hausman 1995, pp. 78–9). This echoes an earlier argument in the ground-breaking work of Kessler and McKenna: 'No amount of descriptive information we could give you about [a] person would allow you to attribute gender with absolute certainty' (Kessler and McKenna 1990, p. 17). Finally, Martine Rothblatt asks rhetorically: 'If we were to separate people because different kinds of chromosomes create different kinds of reproductive capabilities, how could we account for the legitimacy of biologically or intentionally infertile persons?' (Rothblatt 1995, p. 8).

Rothblatt adds: 'Unless a characteristic … applies to all members of a group – we are just talking about generalizations …. not scientific reality' (ibid., p. xiii).

It is an easy matter to find such pronouncements in the academic literature, and increasingly, in popular publications. They are, on the one hand, strategic pleas for the release of individuals from the polar opposition male/female. Their allure is understandable, as there are certainly instances where biology is used to justify one form of social inequality or another. Most scholars and activists readily acknowledge that race is a social construction, with no basis in our biology outside of skin pigmentation. Why shouldn't sex be treated in the same fashion? The arguments that sex is a social construction sometimes appeal to the contemporary desire to be completely self-defining. Suzanne Kessler writes that gender [again, this term includes sex] is a 'responsibility and a burden' (Kessler 1998, p. 132). Why shouldn't people be free of all constraining categorisations, and pick and choose what they want to be for themselves? When expressed in this fashion, any reassertion of the sex/gender distinction can be ridiculed as somehow against freedom itself.

Yet, larger philosophical and scientific points are also being promulgated in these feminist arguments, some bearing resemblance to the theories I analysed in the previous chapter. Several of these feminists proudly invoke the logical standard of absolute certainty. Other passages show signs of the nominalism that I maintain is central to post-structuralism and constructivism. Certainty in sex determination is sought, and when it is found lacking it is concluded that sex is an individual matter, or is structured by culture rather than nature. Some of these feminists have asserted that we must locate the *single* source of a *determinate* event in order to make *any* causal claims. In many ways, this principle reflects the dominant philosophical and scientific mindset that I have been detailing since the beginning of this book, rather than a serious challenge to it. For example, as I will show in the next chapter, these feminists unintentionally echo the arguments of industrial polluters and their defenders, who typically argue that environmental harm must be traced to a single origin and lead to a very specific effect. This insistence makes it nearly impossible to prove, for example, the impact of multiple chemical contaminations, or the existence of harms less obvious than cancer. Thus, while these feminists are motivated by a desire to recognise difference and embrace biological variability, their arguments still rely on the scientific standards set by the certainty-worshiping mainstream.

Given the popularity of these arguments, and their serious implications, I want to subject them to rigorous analysis. Tony Lawson has argued that 'ontological commitments are too rarely rendered explicit' (Lawson 1999, p. 26, ch. 1 this volume, p. 16). Every philosophical claim has an ontology, and I want to make the ontological presuppositions of post-structuralist and constructivist feminism as clear as possible. I will focus primarily on Judith Butler's writings, influential as they are, but I will occasionally refer to other scholars. As was the case with Michel Foucault, Butler has occasionally argued that she belongs to no philosophical movement. More generally, she has claimed that the act of identifying a theorist in such a fashion is a 'gesture of conceptual mastery', one making the questionable Hegelian assumption that 'theories offer themselves in bundles or in organized totalities' (Butler 1992, pp. 5–6). Perhaps it is this conviction that allows Butler to ignore Kessler and McKenna's similar contribution to feminist scholarship. Regardless, as was also the case in my treatment of Foucault, I do not lose sleep over the charges of conceptual domination. Because Butler's defenders can be quite prickly, I feel compelled to engage in a lengthy exegesis to establish my claims. Thus, I will carefully proceed to illustrate the ways in which the relativism, nominalism, and behaviourism of Foucault, Goodman, and Quine unite in a novel and compelling – but, from my perspective, ultimately unsatisfactory – way in the writings of Judith Butler. Protests to the contrary, located sporadically in Butler's writings, cannot be waved as white flags to dispute this weight of evidence.

Relativism by any other name

The first level of Butler's argument deconstructing sex is her contention that there can be no access to any aspect of our world prior to its conceptualisation in thought and language. For example, Butler asks rhetorically, 'Can language simply refer to materiality, or is language also the very condition under which materiality may be said to appear?' (Butler 1993, p. 31). This premise suggests that language shapes our very thought processes (or is synonymous with them) and in effect stands between the world and our discernment of it. Our concepts bring 'materiality' into a social world always already filled with meaning. This argument is a familiar one, as it recollects the irrealism of Goodman, the ontological relativity of Quine, and Foucault's discussion of the 'already "encoded" eye' of perception (Foucault 1973, p. xxi). Butler reiterates that 'materiality [is] bound up with signification from the start' (Butler 1993, p. 13). Pretty standard fare for twentieth-century philosophy.

Butler's unique contribution to the literature is her meticulous extension of this thesis to the issue of biological sex. She draws attention to the act of sexing a baby at the moment of birth on the basis of its observed genitalia. We see the baby through the mediating categories of sex affixed to the penis or vagina, and infer that there is something in nature called girlhood or boyhood. This process of 'sexing' continues for the entire life span, producing a seemingly naturalised effect (ibid., p. 7). As I indicated above, Butler suggests that a considerable chunk of feminism since the time of Beauvoir has accepted the distinction between sex and gender, and taken the naturalness of the former for granted. '[F]or Beauvoir, sex is immutably factic, but gender acquired', Butler writes, 'and whereas sex cannot be changed – or so she thought – gender is the variable cultural construction of sex' (ibid., p. 8).[2] Butler, on the contrary, argues that men and women do not exist outside of these sex categories and that there is no definitive way to ground sex in any kind of material reality. Echoing Foucault, she proclaims that '"sex" is an ideal construct … not a simple fact or static condition of the body' (Butler 1990, pp. 1–2). The genitals to which we attach significance have meaning only insofar as humans create it.

Butler's more contentious claim is that these interpretive mediations result in the partial formation or construction of the world. She writes: 'To claim that discourse is formative … is to claim that there is no reference to a pure body which is not at the same time a further formation of that body' (Butler 1993, p. 10). The act of 'girling' is an imposition of a cultural form on the baby, readying her for a lifetime of similar directives (ibid., pp. 7–8). Like Foucault in his discussion of the criminal or the homosexual, and Goodman in his tale of emeralds, Butler adds that certain categorisations have the power to foster a specific sexual reality. The highly regulated cultural practice of sex therefore 'produces the bodies it governs' (ibid.). '[T]he regulatory norms of "sex,"' Butler continues, 'work in a performative fashion to constitute the materiality of bodies and, more specifically, to materialize the body's sex, to materialize sexual difference' (ibid., p. 2). Butler's conclusion is that girl and boy are 'performative' concepts, as individuals gradually become (albeit in a never-ending process) the sex they are christened at birth.

Trying to distance herself from philosophical idealism, Butler takes pains to reassure her readers that she is not suggesting that language has the power to make the world on its own. She occasionally accuses Foucault of this 'discursive monism' or 'linguisticism', whereby 'language effectively brings into being that which it names' (ibid., p. 35, 192). Discourse, Butler counters, always requires the material realm; it does not create the world *ex nihilo* (ibid., p. 7):

> [I]f language is not opposed to materiality, neither can materiality be summarily collapsed into an identity with language. On the one hand, the process of signification is always material; signs work *by appearing* (visibly, aurally), and appearing through material means, although what appears only signifies by virtue of those non-phenomenal relations, i.e., relations of differentiation, that tacitly structure and propel signification itself. Relations … institute and require relata, terms, phenomenal signifiers.
>
> (ibid., p. 68)

Note Butler's deliberate, and deliberately non-committal, use of language: relations 'institute and require' relata. In order to stay true to her claim that she is not a 'discursive monist', she has to make sure that she doesn't attribute any temporal priority to language. However, she is quite clear that meaning is established solely through non-phenomenal relations. Things 'signify' only because they are connected to other things through the spider's web of language, with no beginning or end to the process. The most that Butler will explicitly say about materiality is that it is 'a demand in and for language, a "that which" which prompts and occasions, … [and] calls to be explained' (ibid., p. 67). This passage borders on the supernatural, and certainly isn't very illuminating.

Furthermore, despite the occasional rhetorical flourish to the contrary, Butler cautions that effective discourses must have some type of social power supporting them. She writes:

> [Performativity] does not mean that *any* action is possible on the basis of a discursive effect. … Hence, the reading of 'performativity' as willful and arbitrary choice misses the point that the historicity of discourse and, in particular, the historicity of norms … constitute the power of discourse to enact what it names.
>
> (ibid., p. 187)

Performativity refers to a process; it cannot take place with a single utterance (ibid., p. 12). I obviously cannot say, 'I am an aardvark', and expect this to have an impact on my body, nor can an individual simply will away sexual inequality with a few strategic utterances. A specific instance of 'girling' is successful because it is embedded in a naturalised, but nonetheless historical, social norm that is reiterated time and again.

The analogy of common law creation is often used to explain the power of discourse to bring something into existence. Judicial decisions are effective because they carry the weight of precedent reaching far back in time. While one can attribute agency to the judge in the pronouncement of a sentence, post-structuralists like Butler insist that the notion of 'intent' must be qualified by this fact of social embeddedness and the resultant lack of precise origin to a law. Butler cautions that discourse becomes powerful only when it 'cites the conventions of authority' in like fashion (ibid., p. 13). If this isn't idealism *per se*, there is still a whiff of creationism, as it is absolutely forbidden to speculate on the origins of these conventions, other than through some mythical social contract in the misty reaches of time.

Regardless, the example of the little girl should again illuminate. Butler's main point is that, even at the level of more-or-less (but never entirely) raw data, the girl's sex traits only mean something because of their relationship to the boy's sex traits. Vagina means girl because penis means boy, and vice versa. Butler contends that this relationship is immaterial, or 'non-phenomenal' as she states above. Because it is the immaterial relationship that is so essential, according to Butler, it is incorrect to say that the things in themselves – here, boys and girls – have any innate meaning. The ideas 'boy' and 'girl' are connected to all of the many things it means to be a boy or a girl in our culture, defined in words, yet having real effects and requiring phenomena to signify anything at all.

Kessler and McKenna, writing twenty-five years ago, drew a similar conclusion based on an experiment they themselves designed. Individuals were presented with drawings of people featuring various combinations of sex traits. For example, one figure might have had long hair, broad hips, and a penis, while another might have had short hair, breasts and a penis (Kessler and McKenna 1990, pp. 145–6). The participants were asked whether the figures were male or female. Several interesting observations unfolded. More male attributions were made than female, even though the study was careful to represent specific gender cues equally (ibid., p. 149). Evidence of a penis was always reason enough to make a male attribution, while a masculine figure without a penis was often still judged male. Furthermore, there was no single trait that automatically caused respondents to make a female attribution. When participants were informed that a figure had a vagina, as long as there were any signs of maleness, the vagina would not necessarily lead to a female attribution. 'To be male is to "have" something', Kessler and McKenna conclude, 'and to be female is to "not have" it' (ibid., p. 153). Thus, the relationship determining the meaning of genitalia is one of presence and absence, a binary bound up with a plethora of beliefs and practices circulating around men and women that have little if anything to do with biology. Things become ever more complicated given that we seldom see the genital region of other individuals. We assume its existence on the basis of a myriad of decidedly non-genital signals, which Kessler and McKenna call 'cultural genitals' (ibid., pp. 153–5). As Kessler and McKenna quip, '[p]enises do not exist in isolation' (ibid., p. 154).

Surely these feminists have made an important argument. Our cultural understanding of the connections between masculinity and femininity influences our interpretation of something as seemingly natural as genitalia. If Butler can't find a precise acknowledgment of this relational aspect of meaning in Foucault, she should be quite at home with Quine. Quine insisted, in a concession to empiricism, that our capacity to recognise similarity and difference was a necessary starting point to the development of any science or knowledge. Analogously, Butler acknowledges that 'materiality' is indeed a force in the world, though she would never make such an explicit claim about similarity and difference. But even Quine backtracked quickly, warning that his minimalist epistemology was merely a theory. He also emphasised the intricacies of the linguistic framework growing out of the input of our senses, to the point where the precise nature of the input was impossible to determine. Furthermore, since we 'make' language (and different ones in each culture, at that) how could we expect it to miraculously reflect the world around us? Quine wrote, 'I see all objects as theoretical' (Quine 1995, p. 105) and 'we cannot know what something is without knowing how it is marked off from other things' (Quine 1969, p. 54). Butler's thesis is that the relations established in language and culture determine the meaning of the things they enmesh. Surely these are nearly identical positions. Yet, Quine quite happily acknowledged that his philosophy is indeed relativist.

Butler does have one other principle that she uses to distinguish herself from 'linguisticism', particularly as she sees it in Foucault's writings. She charges Foucault with ignoring the impact of social marginalisation on the constitution of categories and identities. The creation of a category, she notes, requires that there be some way of distinguishing its contents from everything else. Some individuals will inevitably fail to fit a particular description; in Butler's language, they will 'resist materialization' (Butler 1993, p. 35). Depending on the social significance of the category and the varying power relations in a society, Butler asserts that the elements that do not fit will be marginalised, or even more or less invisible. Again speaking rhetorically, she asks:

> Does Foucault's effort to work the notions of discourse and materiality through one another fail to account for not only what is excluded from the economies of discursive intelligibility that he describes, but what has to be excluded for those economies to function as self-sustaining systems?
> (ibid.)

For Butler, the creation of ascriptive categories means that some individuals will by necessity be excluded from their reach, and they will suffer real social consequences because of this exclusion.

For example, while girls are frequently denigrated in relation to boys, babies who are not readily classifiable throw a wrench into the sex works. Butler stresses that their birth in all likelihood silences the delivery room, and many accounts suggest that she is right. In our world, according to Butler, it is not possible to be *anything* unless you can be classified according to sex. The 'It's a girl/boy' literally brings the baby into personhood (ibid., p. 7). An ambiguous baby is not constituted in precisely the same fashion as are 'real' girls and boys. This baby, and later, adult, is instead marked by exclusion and difference, or its inability to be a perfect girl or boy (Butler 1990, p. 105). The person of indeterminate sex is culturally confusing, and will live the effects of this otherness.

However, Butler's thesis reflects more than a recognition of sexual marginalisation; it is a theory about the power of language to act as the prime force of that exclusion. While all are indeed created, as Foucault argued, all are not created equal. Yet Butler steadfastly refuses to attribute an extra-discursive status to these 'resistant' babies or any other marginalised figures. While there is 'materiality', it can never be more explicitly defined. Such an allowance would be tantamount to declaring that some individuals do indeed have access to an authentic and unmediated naturalness. Referring to Monique Wittig's work, Butler criticises the notion that there is any extra-cultural source of resistance to society's norms. Wittig claims that lesbians escape the categories of sex and sexuality and are hence no longer women (ibid., pp. 111–128). The implication is that the marginality of lesbians provides a privileged vantage point for social criticism. Butler counters that abject individuals are simply constituted in a different way: 'lesbian sexuality is no more and no less constructed than other modes of sexuality' (ibid., p. 124). Other psychoanalytically inclined theorists claim that humans are innately bisexual. Butler rejects this position for similar reasons; rather, bisexuality is 'a concrete cultural possibility that is refused and redescribed as impossible' (ibid., p. 77). Freud should have 'known better' than to posit this trait, or any other human universal (Butler 1998, n.p.). The 'other' to any particular category is therefore still constituted, albeit in a slightly different way than the dominant social group.

On this point, Butler appears to be invoking, albeit implicitly, the Hegelian critique of Kant's thing-in-itself. According to Kant, humans perceive via a combination of empirical experience and the *a priori* forms of intuition (space and time) and categories of understanding (e.g., causality) (Kant 1933, p. 65–7). Our knowledge will be limited by these forms and the information available to the senses. Kant postulates that there are indeed unknown essences, things-in-themselves, lying beyond the boundaries or limits of human knowledge. He writes:

> [W]hat we call outer objects are nothing but mere representations of our sensibility, the form of which is space. The true correlate of sensibility, the thing in itself, is not known, and cannot be known, through these representations; and in experience no question is ever asked in regard to it.
>
> (ibid., p. 74)

Similarly, Kant continues, we will never know the 'the secret of the source of our sensibility', because we have to use that faculty to know anything at all (ibid., p. 287).

Hegel replied to Kant that the mere mention of a limit to knowledge marked an attempt to say something about which you have previously declared your ignorance. 'If we take a closer look at what a limit implies', he writes, 'we see it involving a contradiction in itself' (Hegel 1975, p. 136). Hegel asserts that there is no absolute beyond of knowledge because we can only conceive of that beyond in relation to thought and language. 'We cannot therefore regard the limit as only external to being which is then and there', Hegel expands, '[i]t rather goes through and through the whole of such existence' (ibid.). The alleged 'thing-in-itself' thus influences our understanding of what we *do* know, and neither can be said to exist apart from the other.

One could be excused for thinking that Butler would be attracted to Kant's dualistic solution to the connection between thought and the world, replacing his *a priori* forms with *a posteriori* language. Indeed, constructivists and post-structuralists are sometimes said to be working within a neo-Kantian framework. Yet Butler, like Hegel, usually indicates that the mention of a realm extending beyond our capacity for knowledge is contradictory (Butler 1993, pp. 67–8). The fact that a line can be drawn implies that *something* must be known about what lies on its far side, even if it is just that 'they' are not like 'us', or that sexual difference is outside of culture. Butler revisits Hegel's argument:

> There is an 'outside' to what is constructed by discourse, but this is not an absolute 'outside', an ontological thereness that exceeds or counters the boundaries of discourse; as a constituting 'outside', it is that which can only be thought – when it can – in relation to that discourse, at and as its most tenuous borders.
>
> (ibid., p. 8)

Therefore, the setting of a limit, or a foundation, automatically puts some things on the other side of that limit. More importantly for Butler's purposes, the positing of a limit is an undeniably political act. As Butler has argued thus far, stating that the categories male and female are prior to culture sets a baseline or a limit for the effects of culture. No matter what we do, we are implying that we can't change the reality of males and females. Yet we are simultaneously saying that we can understand their deepest nature. This is a logical flaw according to Butler.

Butler also contends, surprisingly, that to posit any sort of material or natural reality outside of discourse is to negate the possibility that we could ever know what that reality is. 'To posit a materiality outside of language, where that materiality is considered ontologically distinct from language', she warns, 'is to undermine the possibility that language might be able to indicate or correspond to that domain of radical alterity' (ibid., p. 68). Butler's Hegelian roots are showing even more clearly here, as this too is Hegel's critique of the Kantian thing-in-itself. Clearly, Butler doesn't endorse this position in the 'Absolute Knowledge' sense that Hegel intended, but it is still somewhat surprising that she would invoke his language. While she does generally reject the thesis that language and the world are ontologically distinct, she does so by arguing that they are thoroughly imbricated. She steadfastly refuses to say anything definite about the extra-discursive world, other than that nebulous claim that the body is a 'demand in and for language'. Given this holism, it is hard to see how we could ever 'indicate' with language, let alone use it to 'correspond' to something.

Butler thus tries to differentiate her position, on the one hand, from Foucault's alleged linguisticism whereby all individuals are discursively constituted in exactly the same way, and on the other, with the help of Hegel, from those theorists contending that any individual or thing could somehow inhabit an extra-cultural position. But I remain unconvinced that Butler has warded off the general charge of relativism. She argues as though relativism has only one definition, and that if she makes enough vague references to materiality she has adequately refuted the charge. However, her contention that relations between things are *always* 'nonphenomenal' and that all observations are *thoroughly* contextualised within an overarching linguistic system, is central to Quinean relativism. It is the great error, in my view, of the twentieth-century philosophies emphasising language to insist that the connections between objects must be as visible as chains in order to avoid the 'nonphenomenal' tag. On this point, among others, realism fundamentally disagrees. Relations between individuals and entities are often very real, even if we cannot see them at the empirical level. I will leave my full discussion of this realist rebuttal until considerably later, in Chapter 6.

Nominalist feminism

In Butler's more specific discussions of biological sex she combines relativism with a nominalism in a fashion nearly identical to Foucault and, perhaps more surprisingly, Goodman. Before launching into this component of my argument I want to provide a brief overview of the science of sex differentiation. While most of us are aware of the basics, a refresher and news of recent discoveries will help in the remainder of our discussions.[3]

Sex differentiation involves a number of stages, unfolding in a complex cascade or network not yet fully understood. Although there is some looseness of definition in the literature, sex *determination* refers to the initial development of the gonads, and sex *differentiation* to the later growth of the phenotypic[4] sexual features, e.g., penis, seminal vesicles, prostate, vagina, clitoris, oviducts, cervix, etc. The chromosomal makeup of an embryo is determined at conception. Sex determination takes place entirely in the foetus, and is genetically controlled for the most part.[5] Sex differentiation is influenced for the most part by hormones, but chromosomes and the environment can also play a role. Sex differentiation occurs in two major phases: the first after the gonads begin developing, and the second much later in adolescence.

As indicated, the genetic makeup of an individual is determined at the instant of procreation. The embryo will typically have a pair of XX or XY sex chromosomes, along with twenty-two other pairs of autosomal or nonsex chromosomes, from day one. Every cell of an individual contains these chromosomes. For several weeks after conception, despite its genetic signature, the embryo is in a 'bipotential' state, meaning that it is more or less sexually undifferentiated and has the capacity to travel down either the male or female pathway.[6] Some hypothesise that this is a remnant of our evolution from an androgynous or hermaphroditic organism (Mittwoch 1986, pp. 103–21). Mutations or deliberate interventions can block either channel.

The gonads, one component of this relatively neutral rudiment, become either testes or ovaries. In most cases, XY chromosomes produce testes, and XX chromosomes, ovaries. Generally, the presence of a Y chromosome is adequate to lead to the growth of testes. So, for example, an XXXXY individual, though rare, will develop as a phenotypic male. Many now speculate that a single gene along the Y chromosome, known as *SRY*, is the precursor to other aspects of male sexual development (Gubbay et al. 1990, p. 240–4). If this gene is lacking, evidence suggests that the foetus will develop female gonads. For a number of years, researchers argued that female development occurred automatically, making females the default sex. Thus, the *SRY* gene, even before it was discovered, was called the 'testis determining' or even 'sex determining' factor, and no one was very interested in exploring the processes that led to the development of female gonads.

Regardless, the development of the gonads triggers further sexual differentiation. Every embryo has two sets of ducts, the Müllerian and Wolffian. In female embryos, the Wolffian ducts recede, and the Müllerian ducts become the uterus, fallopian tubes, etc. In male babies, the Müllerian ducts wither, while the Wolffian ducts differentiate into the vas deferens, seminal vesicles, etc. Famous experiments conducted by Alfred Jost showed that the removal of rabbit gonads prior to their differentiation always resulted in the development of a female phenotype – with uterus, vagina, and fallopian tubes – regardless of the rabbit's chromosomal makeup. This further contributed to the sense that the female sex was the factory model of the mammalian world. Again it was hypothesised that male sexual differentiation must require something 'extra' in those gonads (Jost 1947, pp. 271–315; 1972, pp. 38–53). Research indeed highlights the importance of several hormones, including AMH (anti-Müllerian duct factor) and testosterone, which at a certain stage converts into DHT (dihydrotestosterone). Without the presence of these hormones, female sexual differentiation will generally occur, aided by the backdrop of the estrogenic womb.

Recent studies note the extent to which hormones perform sex-specific and sex-neutral roles. For example, INSL-3 (Insulin-like hormone 3) causes the descent of the testes from the abdomen in males, and will later in life lead to follicle selection in females. In males, some testosterone is converted into oestradiol, a form of oestrogen, and influences the development of the brain. Oestrogen is so important to life itself in both sexes that defects in its synthesis are extremely rare (White 1994, p. 131–95). If anything, its receptors are too sensitive, and capable of receiving dangerous chemicals 'mimicking' oestrogen and interfering with sexual differentiation. There is also some evidence that chromosomes play a role in sex differentiation, even though hormones have long been thought to be the sole contributor. For example, XY cultures from the mid-brain of mice contain more dopamine neurons than do XX cultures. It is still possible that the influence of the chromosomes is hormonally mediated, or that it may not have a lasting effect on sexual phenotype (Arnold et al. 2004, pp. 1057–62).

The second major stage of sexual differentiation occurs during puberty, when the system integrating nervous and hormonal signals in the hypothalamus (operating at a fairly low, though not insignificant, level during childhood), is reactivated. Both sexes experience a growth spurt and weight gain influenced by oestradiol, growth hormone, and other growth factors. Full fertility is achieved as girls begin to ovulate and menstruate, and boys to produce sperm and ejaculate. Girls' breasts develop as the ovaries secrete oestrogen, while pubic and axillary hair grows as the adrenal cortex and ovaries produce androgen. Under the influence of testosterone, boys develop pubic, facial and bodily hair, the penis and testes grow, and muscles develop. Other sex-specific events also occur, such as the maturation of the vagina and uterus in girls, the deepening of the voice in boys, and oil and sweat gland development in both sexes.

Sex determination and differentiation are by no means perfect; indeed, there are occasional variations on the theme male/female. It is possible to possess a combination of male and female gonads, or to be born with ambiguous genitalia. For example, hypospadias is a condition in which the male urethra remains open along the underside of the penis, sometimes giving it the appearance of female genitalia (Paulozzi et al. 1997, pp. 831–4). Cryptorchidism is the failure of the testicles to descend from the abdomen, leaving them in an ovary-like position (Toppari et al. 1996, pp. 741–803). A number of chromosomal anomalies can also occur. There are XXY individuals, XYY individuals, XO individuals, and 'hermaphrodites' (individuals with both XX and XY gonad tissue), among others. Most interestingly, because of the apparent contradiction between genotype and phenotype, there are XX individuals with partial or full testes development, and XY individuals with either small penises, or large clitorises. In addition to these chromosomal anomalies, hormonal conditions, such as androgen insensitivity and congenital adrenal hyperplasia, may lead to some sex ambiguity, either at birth or later in life. Many but not all ambiguously sexed individuals will be infertile, and some will have physical conditions ranging from relatively minor cleft palates and hernias to more serious cancer, heart disease, or mental retardation. Others will be symptom-free, or virtually so.[7]

Judith Butler makes much of this evidence of sexual ambiguity, as do many other individuals influenced by post-structuralism and constructivism. In *Gender Trouble*, Butler uses a single genetic study revealing sex chromosome anomalies in order to question the biological indicators of maleness and femaleness. The research at issue was one of several studies leading up to the discovery of the *SRY* gene mentioned above. Led by David Page, it analysed a sample of people including XX individuals with testes who were labelled 'male', and XY individuals without testes who were called 'female'. The researchers claimed to have located the region of the Y chromosome responsible for the development of testes. Those with this region of the Y would be male, and those without, female (Butler 1990, pp. 106–11).[8] Apparently, however, the so-called male factor was also located on the X chromosome of normal females. Butler challenges Page's hypothesis that the gene is 'active' in males, and 'passive' in females, as she finds it unconvincing on one hand, and redolent of the traditionally sexist view of passive females on the other.

More importantly, according to Butler, this study provides evidence of the questionable status of biological sex, since there is apparently no known variable that allows us to predict sex with 100 percent certainty. 'Clearly there are cases', Butler writes, 'in which the component parts of sex do not add up to the recognizable coherence or unity that is usually designated by the category of sex' (ibid., p. 108). As further proof, Butler offers an undocumented (and, as I will show, simply false) statistic that 10 per cent of the population have chromosomal patterns falling outside the XX-female/XY-male categories, or secondary sex traits that do not match their chromosomal code. 'The concept of "sex" is itself troubled terrain', Butler summarises, 'formed through a series of contestations over what ought to be decisive criterion for distinguishing between the two sexes' (Butler 1993, p. 5).

Other contemporary feminists present similar arguments based on the evidence of intersexed individuals. For example, Anne Fausto-Sterling once argued that 4 per cent of all people are sexually nondimorphic (Fausto-Sterling 1993, p. 21). She has now revised this figure to 1.728 per cent, an estimate intended to include 'any individual who deviates from the Platonic ideal of physical dimorphism at the chromosomal, genital, gonadal, or hormonal levels' (Blackless et al. 2000, p. 161). Fausto-Sterling uses this data to argue that '[s]ince intersexuals quite literally embody both sexes they weaken claims about sexual difference' (Fausto-Sterling 2000, p. 8). Suzanne Kessler takes the information and declares: 'A world populated with flat-chested, hairy women with penis-sized clitorises and largebreasted, hairless men with micropenises would be a world of blended gender and eventually, blended gender is no gender' (Kessler 1998, p. 117). Others argue that the existence of sexual ambiguity is adequate to eradicate the distinction between sex determination and sex differentiation, since some people have phenotypic traits that conflict with their sex chromosomes. '[T]he division between genital surface and depth is at least "constructed" and at worst utterly bogus' (Morland 2001, p. 543), writes Iain Morland, at the same time that he recommends calling all males and females '*intra*sex' (ibid., p. 544).

These arguments are presently quite popular, with a number of mainstream magazines and newspapers picking up on the high estimates of intersexuality. University professors tell their students that one in twenty to twenty-five of their classmates is intersexed,[9] while an open-minded Presbyterian tells her flock that their small congregation alone must have four or five intersexed worshipers.[10] I have had graduate students earnestly inform me that men, too, have breasts. Unfortunately, any expression of doubt about the figures or the leap in logic is enough to land the sceptic in the camp of the reactionaries.

Feminists, and all social scientists, are on difficult terrain when we place so much reliance on a single scientific study or piece of data. Butler's dabbling in genetics means that she missed the progression of the research looking for the gene(s) on the Y chromosome responsible for testicular development, and, by the time her next book came out, she had apparently lost interest. Her estimate that 10 percent of the population expresses some degree of sexual nondimorphism shows even less interest in the biological sciences, untroubled by evidence as it is. Fausto-Sterling is no dabbler, as she is a respected scientist. But she draws massive conclusions based on her estimates of intersexed individuals.

As someone who formerly relied on Fausto-Sterling's 4 per cent estimate of intersex without much thought, I decided to study her recent survey article reducing the figure to 1.728 percent with greater care. I found numerous errors and oversights, ranging from minor to substantial. Decimal points are in the wrong place. The incidence of two anomalies, Turner Syndrome (XO) and vaginal atresia, both specific to females, are represented as the incidence across both sexes, effectively doubling their frequency. Findings of zero cases of certain conditions in several studies are treated as blanks in the data, whereas a '0' would have the effect of lowering the average incidence of the conditions. Studies with above-average incidences of anomalies are sometimes used to create the impression that were we more open to the possibility of intersex we would see that it is more common than we think. In reality, some of these studies should have been excluded, as they involved non-random samples of high-risk populations. The condition that contributes the lion's share to Fausto-Sterling's figure – 1.5 of the 1.728 intersexed per 100 live births, or a full 87 per cent – is a form of congenital adrenal hyperplasia (non-classic CAH). This is an inherited metabolic disease leading in some cases to excess production of androgen. Frustratingly, Fausto-Sterling's team fails to disclose that the statistic they use is from a patient population, and that experts in the field typically cite an overall incidence of 0.1 percent, or one in 1000, for the condition.

My analysis therefore indicates that Fausto-Sterling's reduced estimate of the incidence of intersex is still a dramatic overstatement (Hull 2003, pp. 112–15), and that a more realistic figure is 0.373 per 100 live births. My figure includes a generous allowance for missed cases and several chromosomal variants that do not result in genital ambiguity. I use the most frequently cited incidence of non-classic CAH (0.1 percent). Even if this figure were to double or triple with further research, the condition does not produce sexual ambiguity in males, and often goes unrecognised even in females. In other words, I have not questioned Fausto-Sterling's inclusion of conditions that some specialists do not consider intersex; I simply correct the math and use more representative studies. For these reasons, Leonard Sax has suggested that 0.018 percent is a fairer estimate of intersex incidence (Sax 2002, pp. 174–8).

I am also disturbed that Fausto-Sterling and her co-authors permit their numbers to stand uncorrected. Furthermore, many feminists and activists unquestioningly cite these results – some even as 'meticulous' (Kessler 1998, p. 135)[11] –

while ignoring the lower estimates in other studies. Deciding between my figure and the one calculated by Sax is a matter of debate and probably some hair-splitting. Yet in her response to my corrections, Fausto-Sterling implies that our differing conclusions are simply part of the intellectual conversation raising awareness of intersexuality. She explicitly leaves it to readers to 'judge for themselves' between the competing numbers (Fausto-Sterling 2003, pp. 115–16). Post-structuralism and constructivism prove convenient here, as Fausto-Sterling seems unwilling to make a distinction between statistical errors and differences in judgment. Andrew Sayer cautions against such a stance, as it is tantamount to saying, 'all science is ideological, only we admit it, and we will not let the facts get in the way of our favored stories' (Sayer 2000, p. 59). While Fausto-Sterling has done an admirable job in drawing our attention to the sometimes unnecessary and disabling surgical interventions faced by intersexed children and adults, her philosophy is too deeply vested in uncovering relatively high rates of sexual nondimorphism.[12]

Butler, despite her limited contact with the scientific literature, did make some helpful observations about sex determination and differentiation research, as has Fausto-Sterling on other occasions (Fausto-Sterling 1989, pp. 319–31). Both note that the implied assumption of sex determination and differentiation research is that male development is interesting and active, whereas female development is unremarkable and passive. Butler writes 'active ovarian contributions to sex differentiation have never been strongly considered'. (Butler 1990, pp. 109, 197–8). Eva Eicher and Linda Washburn, prominent geneticists, have argued that it is highly unlikely that female development happens spontaneously and passively. They challenged the scientific mainstream for its monofocus on the male sex, and its equation of *testis* determination with sex determination (Eicher and Washburn 1986, pp. 328–9). Recent research has corrected this imbalance somewhat, and it is now far more common to see discussions of 'ovary determination' too. Indeed, there is now evidence that specific genes, *DAX1* and *WNT4*, are necessary for female development (Vainio et al 1999, pp. 405–9). Certainly, the oestrogen hormones of the mother and the placenta (and possibly the gonads, when they aren't excised by a scientist) contribute to female sexual differentiation (Wilson et al. 1981, pp. 1283). Female development is perhaps not so automatic as previously thought. Current research also suggests that male development requires positive *and* negative signals, as male processes need to be initiated, and female processes repressed. Thus, there is perhaps an element of 'passivity' in male development as well (McElreavey and Fellous 1999, pp. 176–85).

However, though both sexes require specific genetic activity to produce their respective gonads, the notion that the Y chromosome determines sex and that females are the default sex was not solely the product of sexist dogma. Two distinct hypotheses regarding sex determination were at one time available to scientists. The first was that human sex is decided by the dosage of the X gene: if you have two Xs, you are going to be female, and one X, male. When it was discovered that the ratio of X chromosomes to autosomes determined sex in fruit flies, scientists adopted this model for humans as well (Painter 1923, pp. 291–321). Years later, when researchers were able to observe that XO humans developed as phenotypic females, while XXY and XXXY developed as males, the original hypothesis was rejected and the second option chosen (Ford et al. 1959, pp. 302–3). This second hypothesis was that something on the Y chromosome must counteract the genetic directions on the X, which all mammals share, in order for male sexual determination to occur. The scenario is quite different in birds, where females have ZW chromosomes and males ZZ, and the removal of embryonic gonads leads to male sexual differentiation. Over twenty years ago, one of the major figures in the field of sex determination and differentiation could therefore write: '"Defeminization" is produced by the testes in male mammals, and 'demasculinization' is produced by the ovary in female birds' (Jost 1983, p. 183).

Furthermore, the study of genetics is filled with talk of up-regulation and down-regulation, and activity and passivity. This is in part the by-product of a physicalist science that initially contended (and, in some quarters, still believes) that genes could be in one of only two positions: on or off, the convenient Boolean logic of 1s and 0s. Butler falls for the same either/or logic, as she seems to agree that genes are either operative or inoperative. However, there is adequate proof that the simple presence of the same variable in both sexes need not mean that it will have the same effect on each. Quite obviously, *all* male mammals have an X chromosome (there are indeed no exceptions to this thesis), yet most develop distinguishing male features all the same. There is now evidence that *SRY*, the 'testis-determining gene', is inhibited or down-regulated in females by the active presence of another gene, *DAX1*. Thus, females with the *SRY* gene do not necessarily develop testes. '[T]he same signalling molecule', one group of geneticists notes, 'can act on two different cell types to coordinate sex development' (Jeays-Ward et al. 2003, p. 3663). Geneticists now conclude that dosage level, timing, and background tissue of gene expression are all capable of influencing the pathways of male and female development (and indeed, all other types of development).

Butler is correct that there was a rush to locate the *single* determinant of male sex, and a desire to squeeze apparent exceptions to the male/female binary into one of the two permitted slots, even when there was evidence that these goals would be impossible. Genetics is at times an overconfident field, given the early stages of its development. Scientists are in a rush to be the first to discover the next big gene. Geneticists are also prone to dogmatism about the role of genes in all developmental processes. In the specific case of sex determination, they conveniently ignore the fact that, for example, temperature controls sex in some reptile species. But again, Butler simply overturns the original thesis: if a single gene cannot be located, sex must be indeterminant. Today, however, geneticists recognise that a number of genes are vital for complete sex determination and differentiation. *SRY* – perhaps along with *SOX9* and even *DAX1*[13] – is necessary, though again perhaps not sufficient, for the development of testes (MacLaughlin and Donahoe 2004, pp. 367–78). If these genes are not expressed at the right levels in the early foetal development of an XY foetus, it will *not* develop testes. If it has these genes, it generally will develop testes, greatly increasing the likelihood of further male differentiation. Yet other genes are necessary for the development of functioning sperm. As indicated above, several genes have also been linked to ovary development. Indeed, the idea that a single gene could do all of these things is now discredited. Sex is, after all, quite complex.

However, once the genetic choice has been made, other factors pile up to reinforce the decision:

> The primary decision between male and female pathways seems to be finely balanced, so that allelic differences [alternative forms of the same gene] that result in minor differences in the expression of key genes might have a significant impact at the pivotal point of sex determination. Once the balance is tipped one way or the other, male or female development is strongly canalised by secondary feedback regulation (Brennan and Capel 2004, p. 514).

Dosage thresholds and limits are an important component of many biological processes. Once a line is crossed, other processes combine to promote development along that path. Some genes might even be redundant – functionally substituting for one another – and serving to increase or decrease the likelihood a particular event will occur (ibid., p. 514). Even though there is sexual variability, and even though we have less than a full understanding of these events, some fairly fundamental processes must explain why most mammals are either male or female.

I will have yet more to say about biological sex in the next chapter. For now, I need to step back a bit, and look at this issue of sex determination and the phenomenon of intersex from the philosophical perspective of my overarching argument. In all of the post-structuralist and constructivist treatments of intersex presented thus far, I have shown that the logic that informs the hunt for the single, determinate cause of sex leads the critics of that logic to the inverse conclusion. When the physicalist standard of absolute certainty is inevitably proved impossible to attain, these feminists – like Foucault, Quine, and Goodman before them in their own illustrations – conclude that the biological sex binary is a construction or a continuum, and that there are no mechanisms tending to divide bodies into two types. This is not simply relativism, it is relativism informed by a nominalist ontology. These philosophers all conclude that similarity, if it were truly to exist, would have to operate with logical definitiveness. Any sign of variation is viewed as adequate proof that a category or kind is not in operation.

Butler herself entertains several alternative theories about the ontology of biological sex. She generally poses the options rhetorically as she discusses the works of other authors, and tries to avoid endorsing any one in particular. Regardless, it is clear that she holds to the key nominalist premise that intersex individuals negate the possibility of a general binary pattern to biological sex (Butler 1990, pp. 108–10). On first considering the Page study discussed above, she speculates:

One might argue that the discontinuities in these instances [unexplained cases of intersex] cannot be resolved through recourse to a single determinant, and that sex, as a category that comprises a variety of elements, functions, and chromosomal and hormonal dimensions, no longer operates within the binary framework that we take for granted (ibid., pp. 109–10).

Through the lenses of Monique Wittig's ideas, Butler continues this train of thought. 'Sex', she writes, 'imposes an artificial unity on an otherwise discontinuous set of attributes' (ibid., p. 114). Butler seems to play with two ideas here: first, that sex is more complex than the male/female dichotomy permits; second, that chromosomes, gonads, hormones, and genitalia have *nothing* to do with each other.

Butler continues with her speculations, pushing them further and further down the nominalist road. As I noted above, Wittig eventually argues that there are as many sexes as there are individuals. Kessler and McKenna make a similar argument, contending that every individual has a unique – because slightly different – mix of each of the sex hormones androgen, oestrogen, and progesterone, further breaking the link between bodies and binary logic (ibid., p. 74). They propose, in a suggestion reminiscent of Foucault's advocacy of strict empiricism, that scientific studies correlating hormone levels and behaviour could be conducted *without* the superimposition of the sex categories (ibid., p. 72). Butler simply points out that such arguments would entail the negation of sex, as 'one's sex would be a radically singular property and would no longer be able to operate as a useful or descriptive generalization' (ibid., pp. 118–19). But I think it is fair to say that this is close to Butler's final position, given that her only criticism of it seems to be that it isn't quite anti-foundationalist enough:

> Is there a 'physical' body prior to the perceptually perceived body? An impossible question to decide. Not only is the gathering of attributes under the category of sex suspect, but so is the very discrimination of the 'features' themselves.
>
> (ibid., p. 114)

Thus, Wittig's argument that each person is a unique sex, and her earlier argument that lesbians are somehow outside of culture, commits the cardinal sin of claiming to know something about the extra-discursive. Even the category 'body' is still a category, as it entails a grouping of traits. Butler accuses Foucault of this same foundationalism, writing disparagingly of his positive references to 'bodies and pleasures'. This, too, reflects an ontologisation of individuals and subindividuals, no different, philosophically speaking, than one of sex (Butler 1993, p. 33).

Thus, underneath a number of Butler's arguments about biological sex lurks the easiest of the post-structuralist and constructivist premises: how could we ever know, with certainty, what exists outside of language and culture ('an impossible question to decide')? This is a fairly safe philosophical warrant, and an extremely useful conversation-stopper. In one of the public lectures I have heard Butler deliver, she boasted that she used this principle as a trump card whenever an opponent made an ontological claim. 'Ahh, but how can you *know* for certain?' she told her audience, as they laughed knowingly at the hapless naïf still dedicated to making affirmative statements (Butler 1998, n.p.).

But if it were really the case that we cannot know anything with certainty, we must entertain all prospects equally, including those stating that there are two sexes, or that everybody-is-their-own-sex. To make things interesting, Butler occasionally pretends to this catholic openness. At one point in her lengthy analysis of intersex, she argues:

> [N]ot that valid and demonstrable claims cannot be made about sex-determination, but rather that cultural assumptions regarding the relative status of men and women and the binary relation of gender itself frame and focus the research into sex-determination.
>
> (Butler 1990, p. 109)

I doubt that any thoughtful individual would challenge this proposition. Similarly, in *Bodies That Matter*, Butler writes that it must be possible to 'concede' the reality of biology, anatomy, and the like. In the same breath, she adds, 'But the undeniability of these "materialities" in no way implies what it means to affirm them' (Butler 1993, pp. 66–7).

This appears to be the point of Butler's exercise: neither to condemn nor condone, in any absolute sense, efforts to find a biological basis for the sex categories. Temporary bodily truths can be affirmed (although Butler does not engage in such plebeian declarations on her own), but these should never be fixed into permanent categories. We cannot state with definitiveness that there are bodies and pleasures, or an innate bisexuality, but nor can we reject the possibilities out of hand. From this perspective, one should encourage and heed scientific studies of sex and the body, while acknowledging the social constitution of knowledge, and remaining wary of attempts to cement human nature. Once again, this reads like sound feminist and philosophical advice.

In *Bodies That Matter*, Butler insists that the philosophy she is advocating escapes the traps of both idealism and materialism (ibid., p. 12). In the essay 'Contingent Foundations', she further avows that her principles cannot be traced to any traditional philosophical position. She claims that her feminism is neither foundationalist nor anti-foundationalist. Furthermore,

> [t]he point is not to do away with foundations, or even to champion a position that goes under the name of antifoundationalism. Both of those positions belong together as different versions of foundationalism and the skeptical problematic it engenders.
>
> (Butler 1992, p. 7)

Foundationalism and anti-foundationalism are two sides of the same coin because each meta-philosophy ultimately claims to prove something: that there either is or is not objective knowledge. Butler's assertion obviously resembles my claim that the drive to ground knowledge in the absolute certainty of foundationalism can only result in failure and lead to relativism. Butler is agreeing that each of these philosophies results in the formulation of untenable absolutes.

Yet I do not think Butler can fairly claim that her project, as presented, is so different from earlier, well-established philosophies. In particular, Butler's 'contingent foundations' calls to mind Goodman's nominalistic 'judicious vacillations' between competing world-views (Goodman 1982, p. 32). As Butler both encourages and rejects the experimental results of science, Goodman advocates alternating between various versions of the world. 'We are monists, pluralists, or nihilists', he wrote, 'not quite as the wind blows but as befits the context' (ibid.). Butler has stated that we can make tentative affirmative statements, but we can never grant them any objective truth. She has never provided the means by which such tentative statements can be formulated or evaluated against one another. She has repeatedly rejected the claim that any statement about what lies beyond culture can be defended objectively; in particular, she denounces all efforts to posit any sort of natural sex or sexuality. The most that Butler has said about the body is that it is 'a demand in and for language', hardly a foot in the door for further philosophical or biological study (Butler 1993, p. 67). Without such an effort at conceptual clarification, Butler is stalled at the thesis that all knowledge is equally mediated and equally defensible/indefensible. Her philosophy can thus be connected to Goodman's nominalist ontology and relativist epistemology. He explicitly calls his project by these names. Butler should similarly concede the nominalism and relativism inherent in her position, or explain precisely how her philosophy differs from Goodman's, or from that of other individuals openly avowing their positions on the basis of similar principles.

Behaviourist agency

There is one last component to my analysis of Butler's philosophical presuppositions. Butler's contention that sex is a construction and that there is no 'outside' of culture has implications for our understanding of human agency and theories of social change. Indeed, Butler claims to be providing a rationale for the repudiation, or at least a drastic rethinking, of the political strategies of feminist and sexuality movements. However, in this last section I will demonstrate that this rethinking of political strategies ends up being profoundly behaviourist, despite Butler's protestations to the contrary. It is not my goal merely to accuse her of covert behaviourism. Rather, I will ultimately argue that behaviourism provides an incomplete understanding of human agency and the possibilities for social change.

Once again, Butler tries to position herself between what she sees as two untenable extremes. If Foucault nearly rules out the possibility of agency when he ascribes a monolithic power to discourse, in Butler's eyes, Wittig and others overestimate the utopian potential of alternative forms of sexuality. Butler has argued that the creation of a category necessitates the making of a distinction between members of that class and all other individuals. She suggests that agency lies not in some body or identity outside of or before power, but in the possibility for change implicit in this relationship between a category and its limits. She expands:

> The paradox of subjectivation … is precisely that the subject who would resist such norms is itself enabled, if not produced, by such norms. Although this constitutive constraint does not foreclose the possibility of agency, it does locate agency as a reiterative or rearticulatory practice, immanent to power, and not a relation of external opposition to power.
>
> (ibid., p. 15)

For example, the individual who resists the norms of heterosexuality via homosexual or bisexual practice is indeed rebelling, but this rebellion is defined in terms of heterosexuality. There is no natural homosexual force or drive upon which the individual draws, as there is nothing external to the operations of culture. There is only the possibility for behaving differently raised through the example of other behaviour. The establishment of the category 'normal sex' immediately introduces the possibility of 'abnormal sex'. Homosexuality and bisexuality, Butler suggests, would be literally meaningless without this connection to their socially superior cousin.

Butler continues that the identity and social status of 'normal' individuals are similarly dependent on the relationship between a category and its margins. Even though the 'abnormal' individuals are rejected by their culture, they provide a continual challenge to the 'normal' individuals as reminders of a different way to be and think. Thus, the existence of a sexually ambiguous baby or adult threatens the supposedly solid ground of the 'real' boys and girls, or the 'true' heterosexuals, of the world. '[T]his disavowed abjection …' writes Butler, 'threaten[s] to expose the self-grounding presumptions of the sexed subject, grounded as that subject is in a repudiation whose consequences it cannot fully control' (ibid., p. 3). We believe that our sex is an expression of some fundamental inner truth, yet it turns out that it depends on a *relationship*, the rejection of those individuals unlike ourselves. In other words, our sex depends on a nonphenomenal connection to other sexes and sexualities, not on a natural drive external to culture (ibid., p. 68).

For Butler, the naturalness of the category 'woman' is questioned when a man convincingly presents himself as a woman. One person's confusing status could force others to rethink the sex and sexuality previously taken for granted. If sex can be contrived or performed, what could be so essential about it? Other feminist and queer theorists have expressed related arguments.

Kessler and McKenna summarise the literature on *berdache*, individuals in certain aboriginal populations who lived as members of the opposite sex (Kessler and McKenna, 1990, pp. 21–9). A son might reject traditional male chores and demonstrate an interest in female tasks, and accordingly be raised as a daughter. A family with several daughters but no sons might 'decide to make [a] child a son' (ibid., p. 21). In all likelihood, write Kessler and McKenna, the *berdache* were biologically normal (ibid., p. 26). The traditional interpretation of the *berdache* is that the individuals are merely 'treated like' the opposite sex (ibid., p. 28). Kessler and McKenna instead contend that in some cultures, the criterion for determining sex is 'the role one performed', rather than the genitals one possessed (ibid., p. 38).

Even amongst supposedly 'normal' males and females in our culture, Kessler and McKenna insist that sex is an accomplishment, the meeting of an externally set standard rather than the fulfilment of an internally driven programme (ibid., p. 163). Here they are partly influenced by John Money's theory of 'gender neutrality' (Money et al 1957, pp. 333–6). Money, a well-known psychologist, had long argued that gender identity (the sense one has about one's sex) was not established until the age of three, and was accordingly malleable up until that time. Thus, when an infant had his penis ablated (the clinical term for removed) after it was horribly burnt in a botched circumcision, Money convinced the parents to raise the child as a girl. For many years, Money argued that the experiment was a complete success.[14] So confident were Kessler and McKenna of Money's general premise, and their own research, that they issued a blanket proclamation: 'Research clearly indicates that there are no causal links between gender identity or gender role and gonads, internal reproductive organs, or genitals' (Kessler and McKenna 1990, p. 70). Readers may already know how Money's experiment ended, as it became evident that it was an abject failure.[15] Surely, years of feminist theory have shown us the extent to which gender is a highly variable phenomenon. However, Butler, Kessler, and McKenna go much further to argue that biological sex, gender identity, and sexuality could become completely delinked if sex ambiguity became widespread.

Butler continues that even the limits of socially approved identities function as the basis for agency and change. A performance of womanhood, for example, is a citation of the norms of womanhood. The ongoing repetition of all such norms entails the inevitability that 'real' girls and boys and 'perfect' heterosexuals will fail to live up to the requirements of these ideals. Each citation or performance, Butler writes, 'will be at once an interpretation of the norm and an occasion to expose the norm itself as a privileged interpretation' (Butler 1993, p. 108). The copy will deviate from the original, in effect. If every performance involves a variation – however slight – it can highlight the inauthenticity of the norm, and reveal that the norms themselves are ultimately cultural interpretations. Without a secure origin, no identity is stable. Butler summarises: 'Identifications are never simply or definitively *made* or *achieved*, they are insistently constituted, contested, and negotiated' (ibid., p. 76; emphasis in original). Although our sense of self is dependent on our interpretation of and relation to the identity of others, in mimicry and reaction there is inevitable, gradual, mutation. This argument provides a window for social change, and offers a possible explanation for the slow evolution of culture over time.

Because of Butler's insistence that the sexed subject's materiality is always within culture, she cautions that her political openings are emphatically not those provided by a voluntarist subject. Sex is not assumed in the way that one picks out clothes. The ways in which we become our sex are many, complex, and difficult to comprehend fully. Sensitive to criticisms that she anticipates the massive de-sexing of individuals in the wake of her writings, Butler clarifies that 'it would be a mistake to associate "constructivism" with "the freedom of a subject to form her/his sexuality as s/he pleases"' (ibid., p. 94). Furthermore, she recognises that gender parody is not an adequate strategy for the displacement of the dominant norms of sex. Gender parody also puts the heretical performer at the risk of violence or even death (ibid., p. 125, p. 133). Thus, it is no easy matter to dissimulate one's sex or sexuality. However, de-sexing *is* a theoretical possibility for Butler, for to be constituted is not to be determined (Butler 1990, p. 143; 1993, p. 10). Because constitution is a never-ending process dependent on the citation, and hence variation, of social norms, the opportunity for change does exist. Butler consistently maintains, however, that any resultant variations in identity will always be thoroughly social, as the choices available to individuals are meaningful only in relationship to items already inscribed on the cultural menu.

Implicit in the above paragraphs, and indeed the gist of Butler's entire analysis to this point, is the thesis that there are no natural women outside of or before gender waiting to be liberated by feminism. Just as the lesbian or bisexual is constituted, so are women in general. Butler suggests that it is counterproductive to the agendas of feminism and other social movements to make ontological claims regarding the distinctness and priority of any body or identity, including that of women. If women are discursively constituted in relation to men, defending a movement on the basis of 'women's rights' further fixes an identity that is the effect of a hierarchical discourse. Furthermore, if the establishment of any category necessitates the creation of an abject realm, all statements on the behalf of 'women' will entail the marginalisation of some individuals. Butler writes:

> [T]here is some risk that in making the articulation of a subject-position into the political task, some of the strategies of abjection wielded through and by hegemonic subject-positions have come to structure and contain the articulatory struggles of those in subordinate or erased positionalities.
>
> (Butler 1993, p. 112)

A supposedly liberatory movement can duplicate the patterns of the dominant culture in establishing *the* feminist identity. The exclusion of minority women from the hegemonic projects of white, middle-class feminists is perhaps the best-known example.

Correspondingly, Butler continues, if individuals are constituted by a variety of discourses, the foundation of a movement on the basis of a single identity is a limitation of potential for all involved. 'To prescribe an exclusive identification for a multiply constituted subject', she writes, 'is to enforce a reduction and a paralysis' (ibid., p. 116). This dilemma does not spell the end of emancipatory movements, however, and Butler denies that all categories are equally exclusionary and limiting (ibid., p. 207). It may on occasion be desirable to refer to some sort of collective subject grounded in a category, even that of sex. In fact, it is necessary to use such categories if one is to gain political recognition within our current system (ibid., pp. 114–123). Butler concedes that normative judgments need to be made in the establishment of political goals (Butler 1995, p. 141).

However, as I suggested above, Butler herself never offers such normative judgments, nor does she furnish the means by which any could be made. She simply asserts that the resulting norms must remain indeterminate and tentative, even as they employ such established monikers as 'women' or 'lesbians'. Butler hopes that, in the process, we can begin conceiving of ourselves in a way that would not absolutely exclude whatever it is that is allegedly different from us. New political identities would no longer entail fixedness or stasis along with the corresponding rejection of otherness (Butler 1993, p. 118). This goal effectively marks the political adaptation of Butler's 'contingent foundationalism' and nominalist/irrealist ontology. Although few details are presented, Butler suggests that heterosexuals could see that the belief in their 'naturalness' literally requires the existence of the 'unnatural' alternatives, homosexuality and bisexuality. Men would discover that masculinity entails the abnegation of the feminine, and femininity, too, the rejection of certain possibilities. All could recognise the limitations inherent in a static identification, and awaken to the liberatory possibility of a more diffuse sense of self (ibid., p. 119). This aspect of post-structuralism is perhaps its most optimistic proposal, and it is justifiably lauded. Rigid senses of identity are undoubtedly responsible for considerable personal unhappiness at one end of the scale, and atrocities at the other. Perhaps in recognition of this uncharacteristic hopefulness, Butler immediately warns, 'I invest no ultimate political hope in the possibility of avowing identifications that have conventionally been disavowed' (ibid., p. 115).

Hate speech

Butler further elaborates her understanding of agency in *Excitable Speech*, her analysis of hate speech. She now accepts the distinction between two kinds of performative utterances: illocutions and perlocutions. The former enact a deed as soon as they are uttered, as do the ceremonial statements 'I now pronounce you man and wife', and 'guilty' (Butler 1997, pp. 3, 17, 44). The latter aid in the performance of a deed, but do not enact the deed in and of themselves.

The speech act and its consequences are 'temporally distinct' (ibid., p. 17). As a consequence, a gap opens up between word and event.

This distinction permits Butler to distance herself from those who advocate censorship because of the harmful impact of hate speech. One might have expected that her philosophy, emphasising the marginalising potential of linguistic labels, would have been sympathetic to censorship. However, Butler suggests that hate speech is an example of a perlocutionary utterance. Epithets do not immediately constitute the things they name. The political strategy of censoring hate speech assumes, mistakenly, the illocutionary approach, contending that slurs by definition take instant effect. Butler cautions against censorship laws while granting that slurs and epithets *do* harm.[16] In the way that cultural norms of sex define our identities as men and women, we depend in general on being named (ibid., p. 26). Thus, when someone calls us by a slur, the word sticks and stings. Butler asks rhetorically: 'Why should a merely linguistic address produce such a response of fear? Is it not, in part, because the contemporary address recalls and re-enacts the formative ones that gave and give existence?' (ibid., p. 5). Our social existence is brought into being through language; thus, it is natural that words can hurt.

Yet Butler's preferred strategy for challenging hate speech is to take the words that hurt us and mimic them in a slightly different context. As gender norms are challenged through ironic parody, the best way to target hate speech is the 'restaging and resignifying' of hate words (ibid., p. 13). Similarly, pornography proliferating derogatory images of women is best challenged through the resignification of its content (ibid., p. 69). Women can make pornography that defies the meanings of most sexually explicit material. If we use hate speech or pornography in a positive or amusing ironic fashion, it can gradually lose most of its power to hurt. It will become so recontextualised that its original meaning will be almost (although not ever completely) lost (ibid., pp. 15, 150, 161). '[S]peech is … vulnerable to failure' (ibid., p. 12) Butler writes, because, '[it] is finally constrained neither by its specific speaker nor its originating context' (ibid., p. 40). Were we to censor speech and porn – insisting that their meaning is fixed in the foundational intent of the speaker, or in a specific referent in the world – they would forever maintain their capacity to injure (ibid., pp. 15, 38).

Butler contends that much political action in the past several decades has been a form of this redefinition. Rosa Parks was reiterating the actions of whites when she sat at the front of the bus (ibid., p. 147). The attempts by various social movements to be granted equality, freedom, and justice are performative and rearticulatory, as the definition of these words is challenged and rewritten (ibid., pp. 157–9). Butler periodically indicates that rearticulation is the only form of struggle possible. While she does not explicitly rule out other types of political action, her statements about the potential of recontextualisation are quite dramatic. '[T]he logic of iterability … governs the possibility of social transformation', she insists (ibid., p. 147). She cites Pierre Bourdieu favourably when he writes, 'The body believes in what it plays at: it weeps if it mimes grief' (ibid., p. 154). If grief can be so constructed, the implication is that we can effectively change people if we alter what we say about them and, eventually, what they say about us. Butler closes *Excitable Speech* with the following declaration: 'Insurrectionary speech becomes the necessary response to injurious language, a risk taken in response to being put at risk, a repetition in language that forces change' (ibid., p. 163). The claims Butler makes here for performative politics are thus substantial.

Despite the use of a different language, I am convinced that this analysis shows many signs of influence by twentieth-century behaviourism, Quinean and otherwise. Seyla Benhabib has similarly noted the connection (Benhabib 1995, p. 21), which Butler has explicitly and adamantly rejected (Butler 1993, p. 2). Certainly, Butler wants no part of the reductivist physicalism that inspired the behaviourist rejection of consciousness, instinct, and emotion as explanatory variables. Yet she redefines these variables in comparable fashion. For Butler, Quine, and behaviourism, there are no extra-linguistic or extra-cultural dimensions to anything, either in the world or in our minds. The linguistic community mediates which aspects of the environment will be discriminated, and which aspects of the person will become the self. Behaviour or speech is either mimicry (albeit inexact) or reaction. Interestingly enough, the concept 'performance' that Butler champions (or her preferred variant, performativity, to note the ongoing nature of the process) was often used by behaviourists to describe the actions of their experimental subjects. 'Performance' supposedly captured the notion that subjects were behaving as scripted, rather than expressing internal states or capacities.[17] Clearly this is a key principle for Butler as well.

There is, all the same, considerable truth to Butler's thesis of 'rearticulation', as she calls it. Most serious thinkers acknowledge that the individual is not the purely self-constituting origin of his or her thoughts, utterances, and actions. Behaviourism surely explains some aspects of linguistic acquisition and transmission. Regardless, Noam Chomsky's famous reply to Skinner years ago mounts important criticisms of Butler's theory as well (Chomsky 1959, pp. 26–58). Consider these simple examples from Chomsky's criticism. When individuals see a painting and some respond with the word 'tilted', some with 'beautiful', and others with 'clashes with the wallpaper', Chomsky insists that Skinner can only conclude that each response is under the control of different physical stimuli (ibid., p. 31). Butler replaces the notion of physical stimuli with discursive stimuli. If individuals are heterosexual or homosexual, racist or egalitarian, this signifies only that each person is constituted within a slightly different discursive regime.

Chomsky locates two difficulties with this general approach. It either makes implicit reference to internal qualities of the individual in question (why that person chose the response they did), or, failing these covert references, it turns to an empty notion of reinforcement. In the first case, there is agency, in that the individual somehow focuses on different stimuli or different discursive regimes. But how or why these differences occur is left unexplored. The notion that individuals could *choose* one alternative over another is apparently dismissed. Chomsky argues that the behaviourist rejection of reasoned choice as a variable leads to the absurdity that torturing someone to say that the earth is motionless is the same as changing his or her opinion (Chomsky 1971, p. 21). Both are apparently conditioned responses. While we must continue to challenge the notion that the individual is fully self-constituting, the *a priori* alternative that people are simply determined or constituted into their social roles must be avoided. As Chomsky put it, to assume otherwise is to insinuate that 'people have wills, impulses, feelings, purposes, and the like no more than rocks do' (ibid.).

This leads to the second difficulty. Butler would surely deny that she is reducing people to rocks. Instead, she turns our attention away from inner factors to constitutive discourses, whereas Skinner emphasises reinforcing physical stimuli. Chomsky asserts that these forces are so vague as to be completely non-explanatory:

> Skinner's claim that all verbal behavior is acquired and maintained … through reinforcement is quite empty, because his notion of reinforcement has no clear content, functioning only as a cover term for any factor, detectable or not, related to acquisition or maintenance of verbal behaviour.
>
> (Chomsky 1959, p. 38)

I suggest that this is a valid, and perhaps the most important, criticism of Butler's notion of discursive constitution. It functions as a cover term for any and every fact related to the acquisition or maintenance of behaviour, verbal and otherwise. As Chomsky concludes, we know no more about the process of learning, or the role of agency, than we did before, when we were naïve voluntarists (ibid.). In a way, the theory of discursive constitution reminds me of the rational actor model. Both are totalising. If every action is rational, or discursively constituted, it becomes difficult to explain why people behave differently in similar circumstances. Butler's rejoinder that these defectors are constituted in reaction to the discursive norm may open up the explanatory door somewhat, but it is still extremely unhelpful in its generality.

I thus question whether Skinnerian conditioning or Butlerian resignification adds sufficiently to our knowledge of human motivation and behaviour. In the example of Rosa Parks, Butler's argument that she was 'rearticulating' the concepts of freedom and equality tells us nothing more about Rosa Parks, racism, or the fight against it. Why was it Rosa Parks that was able to engage in her brave act? Why did she refuse to give up her seat in 1955, and not 1950? Butler can only reply that Parks was somehow able to tap into a relationship between the discourse of racism and another discursive network. The reference to the individual is thus thrown back to discourse, in an apparent loop with no origin other than the whole of language, culture, and the individuals inhabiting their domains. If the regress is ever to be terminated, behaviourism and now post-structuralism seem to adhere to the view that human behaviour is random, and only fixed as it is selected and reinforced by the community. Such a solution to the very difficult problem of explaining human behaviour appears to be a covert retreat into either metaphysics or, perhaps, even the mathematical concept of chance.

There are certainly other ways in which Butler's project is remote from Quine's and Skinner's behaviourism. Yet she has primarily defended herself against the charge of behaviourism by arguing that her 'subject' of discourse is never final or fixed. As I have summarised, the capacity for intention or agency is located in either the individual's inexact mimicry of norms, or the reaction made possible by relationships between two or more norms. Butler writes:

> To be constituted by language is to be produced within a given network of power/discourse which is open to resignification, redeployment, subversive citation from within, and interruption and inadvertent convergences with other such networks. 'Agency' is to be found precisely at such junctures where discourse is renewed.
>
> (Butler 1995, p. 135)

Every single woman will perform a slightly different version of womanhood. A lesbian woman's actions are constituted in relation to the sanctioned norms of heterosexuality. A constituted identity is never *fully* determined, and thus the thesis of rearticulation is allegedly not behaviourist (ibid., and 1993, p. 2).

Yet it was no part of Skinner's doctrine to argue that human behaviour was inalterable, or that identities were fixed. For both Butler and Skinner, as we are always already conditioned, social change is the result of reconditioning. Butler has argued that hate speech can be recontextualised and hence redefined because it has no fixed links to either the hateful speaker's intent or to a condition in the world. The only thing cementing the meaning of a word – and this is a relative cementing – is its repeated association with a particular context. Individuals have thus been conditioned into these word–context linkages. Because context varies, it becomes possible to orchestrate the variation to the advantage of individuals injured by hate speech. When minority members accept an epithet, but insist that its 'meaning' is now altered, individuals who originally utter the word with hateful intentions will be reconditioned. The target of the hate speech apparently accepts the designation ironically, thwarting the original speaker's goal. The original speaker has, in Skinner's language, been punished. The best chance for a more equal society, for both Skinner and Butler, depends on getting people to associate old words with new contexts; in effect, reconditioning people in the expectation that this will change behaviour.

I do not think Butler's refutation gets to the heart of the allegation: it is the rejection of instincts, natural capacities, and the like, that is the hallmark of behaviourism. Butler has consistently maintained one of two things. Either we have no means of *knowing* whether there is any innate sex or sexuality because discourse mediates all of our knowledge, or there *are no* such inner forces because these are either overridden by or intertwined with cultural forces. She has now articulated a more general theory of agency in which reference to spontaneous instincts or a capacity to reason existing prior to culture or language is similarly forbidden. Agency, as I just summarised, is a cultural 'rearticulation', not an expression of innate tendencies, urges, potentials, or reason. Agency is either inexact mimicry or reaction. Butler's overall philosophy is extremely close to Quine's and Goodman's in its relativism and nominalism; her political analysis is not as far from Skinnerian and Watsonian behaviourism as she has proclaimed.

Notes

1 This chapter was originally published as: Hull, C., 2006, 'Poststructuralist and constructivist feminism', in Hull, C. *The Ontology of Sex*. Routledge, pp. 54–82. Republished by permission of the publisher.

2 While it may be fair to generalise Beauvoir's argument in this fashion, we should note that there are exceptions in her work. The early pages of *The Second Sex* raise the possibility that procreation could be asexual, or that bodies could be hermaphroditic. Beauvoir writes:

> [W]e can regard the phenomenon of reproduction as founded in the very nature of being. But we must stop there. The perpetuation of the species does not necessitate sexual differentiation. True enough, this differentiation is characteristic of existents to such an extent that it belongs in any realistic definition of existence. But it nevertheless remains true that both a mind without a body and an immortal man are strictly inconceivable, whereas we can imagine a parthenogenetic or hermaphroditic society.
>
> (S. de Beauvoir, *The Second Sex*, trans. H.M. Parshley, New York: Vintage Books, 1989, p. 7)

3 For general overviews on sexual development I relied on the following articles (studies are cited separately when a more specific finding is discussed): J.D. Wilson, F.W. George, and J.E. Griffin, "The Hormonal Control of Sexual Development," *Science* 211, 1981, 1278–84; J.W. Gordon and F.H. Ruddle, "Mammalian Gonadal Determination and Gametogenesis," Science 211, 1981, 1265–71; E.M. Eicher and L.L. Washburn, "Genetic Control of Primary Sex Determination in Mice," *Annual Review of Genetics* 20, 1986, 327–60; C.M. Haqq and P.K. Donahoe, "Regulation of Sexual Dimorphism in Mammals", *Physiological Reviews* 78, 1998, 1–33; B.C. Morrish and A.H. Sinclair, "Vertebrate Sex Determination: Many Means to an End," *Reproduction* 124, 2002, 447–57; D.T. MacLaughlin and P.K. Donahoe, "Sex Determination and Differentiation," *New England Journal of Medicine* 350, 2004, 367–78; and J. Brennan and B. Capel, "One Tissue, Two Fates: Molecular Genetic Events that Underlie Testis Versus Ovary Development," *Nature Reviews* 5, 2004, 509–21.

4 The genotype of an organism is its genetic makeup; the phenotype is virtually everything else – its entire constellation of observable traits.

5 Ursula Mittwoch has argued that under exceptional circumstances, environmental factors may play a role in the etiology of true hermaphroditism (presence of ovarian and testicular tissue in the same individual). She speculates that this may be a remnant of the role played by temperature in the sex determination of our reptilian ancestors. However, Mittwoch still insists "[t]his is of no consequence in normal sexual differentiation, which is firmly controlled by the sex chromosomes." See Mittwoch, "Genetics of Sex Determination: Exceptions that Prove the Rule," *Molecular Genetics and Metabolism* 71, 2000, 407.

6 Ursula Mittwoch also challenges the hypothesis that the embryo goes through this bipotential phase. She argues that male embryos have higher rates of metabolism even prior to testis determination, and that this increased metabolism may play a greater role in the processes of determination and differentiation than is generally acknowledged. See "The Elusive Action of Sex-Determining Genes: Mitochondria to the Rescue?," *Journal of Theoretical Biology* 228, 2004, 359–65.

7 For overviews of the various chromosomal and hormonal combinations possible in human beings, see: M. Blackless, A. Charuvastra, A. Derryck, A. Fausto-Sterling, K. Lauzanne, and E. Lee, "How Sexually Dimorphic Are We? Review and Synthesis," *American Journal of Human Biology* 12, 2000, 151–66 (although some of their figures are inaccurate, this review provides a good summary of the various conditions).

8 The study to which she refers is D.C. Page, R. Mosher, E. Simpson, E.M.C. Fisher, G. Mardon, J. Pollack, B. Mcgillivray, A. de la Chapelle, and L.G. Brown, "The Sex Determining Region of the Human Y Chromosome Encodes a Finger Protein," *Cell* 51, 1987, 1091–104.

9 See the following websites: ShiPS Resource Center, Philosophy of Sex, Available online at: www1.umn.edu/ships/gender/phil'sex.htm (accessed 11 December 2004); and Gail Bederman, Intersex: Questions for Discussion, Available online at: www.nd.edu/~gbederma/core/discintersex.html (accessed 12 December 2004).

10 E. Swenson and S. Craig, "More Light on Bisexuality and Transgender," 156 Notes Available online at: www.mlp.org/resources/MLOBiTran.pdf (accessed 11 December 2004).

11 Kessler apparently had access to the 2000 Fausto-Sterling manuscript prior to its publication.

12 Infants with below regulation-sized penises and above-average clitorises have been surgically reassigned to the other sex or merely "downsized," rendering them inorgasmic and often horrifically scarred in the process. The Intersex Society of North America (ISNA) estimates that five baby girls are subjected to clitoral reduction every day. Encouraged by Fausto-Sterling's work in particular, the ISNA has advocated that medically unnecessary genital surgery on infants be halted.

13 There is controversy about whether DAX1 suppresses or promotes testicular determination in XY tissue. See J.J. Meeks, J. Weiss, and J.L. Jameson, "Dax1 is Required for Testis Determination," *Nature Genetics* 34, 2003, 32–3; Morrish and Sinclair, "Vertebrate Sex Determination," pp. 447–57; and L.M. Ludbrook and V.R. Harley, "Sex Determination: A 'Window' of DAX1 Activity," *Trends in Endocrinology & Metabolism* 15, 2004, 116–21.

14 For details of this story, and similar case studies, see J. Money, "Ablatio Penis: Normal Male Infant Sex-Reassignment as a Girl," *Archives of Sexual Behavior* 4, 1975, 65–71.

15 As is now known, the experiment proved a disaster. Always sensing that something was amiss, the boy was eventually told the truth about his biological sex. He underwent further surgery and hormone therapy, and tried to live his life as a male. Unfortunately, David Reimer killed himself in 2004. See M. Diamond and H.K. Sigmundson, "Sex Reassignment at Birth: Long-term Review and Clinical Implications," *Archives of Pediatrics and Adolescent Medicine* 151, 1997, 298–304.

16 However, at one point in *Excitable Speech* (p. 50), Butler indicates that there are 'probably occasions' on which individuals should be prosecuted for hate speech.

17 For example, see B.F. Skinner and W.H. Morse, "Sustained Performance During Very Long Experimental Sessions," *Journal of the Experimental Analysis of Behavior* 1, 1958, 235–44.

References

Arnold, A. P., J. Xu, W. Grisham, X. Chen, Y. H. Kim and Y. Itoh. 2004. "Minireview: Sex Chromosomes and Brain Sexual Differentiation." *Endocrinology* 145(3): 1057–1062.

Benhabib, S. 1995. "Feminism and Postmodernism," in S. Benhabib, J. Butler, D. Cornell, N. Fraser. *Feminist Contentions: A Philosophical Exchange*, pp. 17–34. New York: Routledge.

Blackless, M., A. Charuvastra, A. Derryck, A. Fausto-Sterling, K. Lauzanne and E. Lee. 2000. "How Sexually Dimorphic Are We? Review and Synthesis." *American Journal of Human Biology* 12: 151–166.

Brennan, J. and B. Capel. 2004. "One Tissue, Two Fates: Molecular Genetic Events that Underlie Testis Versus Ovary Development." *Nature Reviews* 5: 509–521.

Butler, J. 1990. *Gender Trouble: Feminism and the Subversion of Identity.* New York: Routledge.

———. 1992. "Contingent Foundations: Feminism and the Question of 'Postmodernism,'" in J. Butler and J. Scott (eds.) *Feminists Theorize the Political.* New York: Routledge.

———. 1993. *Bodies That Matter: On the Discursive Limits of Sex.* New York: Routledge.

———. 1995. "For A Careful Reading," in S. Benhabib, J. Butler, D. Cornell and N. Fraser (eds.) *Feminist Contentions: A Philosophical Exchange*, pp. 127–144. New York: Routledge.

———. 1997. *Excitable Speech: A Politics of the Performative.* New York: Routledge.

———. 1998. Antigone's Claim. Public Lecture, University of Toronto, 15 April 1998.

Chomsky, N. 1959. "A Review of B.F. Skinner's Verbal Behavior." *Language* 35(1): 26–58.

———. 1971. "The Case Against B.F. Skinner." *The New York Review of Books* 17, 30 December 1971.

Dreger, A. D. 2001. *Top Ten Myths About Intersex*, ISNA News, February: 3–5. Available online at: https://isna.org/files/hwa/feb2001.pdf

Eicher, E. M. and L. L. Washburn. 1986. "Genetic Control of Primary Sex Determination in Mice." *Annual Review of Genetics* 20: 327–360.

Fausto-Sterling, A. 1989. "Life in the XY Corral." *Women's Studies International Forum* 12(3): 319–331.

———. 2000. *Sexing the Body: Gender Politics and the Construction of Sexuality.* New York: Basic Books.

———. 1993. "The Five Sexes: Why Male and Female are Not Enough." *The Sciences* March/April: 20–25.

———. 2003. "Response." *American Journal of Human Biology* 15: 115–116.

Ford, C. E., K. W. Jones, P. Polani, J. C. De Almeida and J. H. Briggs. 1959. "A Sex-Chromosome Anomaly in a Case of Gonadal Dysgenesis (Turner's Syndrome)." *Lancet* 4(1): 711–713.

Foucault, M. 1973. *The Order of Things: An Archaeology of the Human Sciences.* New York: Vintage Books.

Goodman, N. 1982. "Notes on the Well-Made World," in W. Leinfellner, E. Kraemer and J. Schank (eds.) *Language and Ontology: Proceedings of the Sixth International Wittgenstein Symposium*, Wien, Austria: Hölder-Pichler-Tempsky.

Greenberg, J. A. 1999. "Defining Male and Female: Intersexuality and the Collision between Law and Biology." *Arizona Law Review* 41: 265.

Gubbay, J., Collignon, J., Koopman, P., Capel, B., Economou, A., Munsterberg, A., Vivian, N., Goodfellow, P. and Lovell-Badge, R. 1990. "A Gene Mapping to the Sex-Determining Region of the Mouse Y Chromosome is a Member of a Novel Family of Embryonically Expressed Genes." *Nature* 346(6281): 245–250.

Hausman, B. L. 1995. *Changing Sex: Transsexualism, Technology, and the Idea of Gender.* Durham, NC: Duke University Press.

Hegel, G. F. W. 1975. *Logic*, trans. W. Wallace. Oxford: Oxford University Press.

Hubbard, R. 1996. "Gender and Genitals: Constructs of Sex and Gender." *Social Text* 46/47: 157–165.

Hull, C. L. 2003. "Letter: Comment on Fausto-Sterling *et al.*'s 'How Sexually Dimorphic Are We?.'" *American Journal of Human Biology* 15: 112–115.

Jacobs P. A. and J. A. Strong. 1959. "A Case of Human Intersexuality Having a Possible XXY Sex-determining Mechanism." *Nature* 183: 302–303.

Jeays-Ward, K., C. Hoyle, J. Brennan, M. Dandonneau, G. Alldus, B. Capel and A. Swain. 2003. "Endothelian and Steroidogenic Cell Migration are Regulated by WNT4 in the Developing Mammalian Gonad." *Development* 130(16): 3663–3370.

Jost, A. 1947. "Recherches sur la differenciation sexuelle de l'embryon de lapin." *Archives Anatomie Microscopique & Morphologie Expérimentale* 36(2): 242–270.

———. 1972. "A New Look at the Mechanisms Controlling Sex Differentiation in Mammals." *Johns Hopkins Medical Journal* 130(1): 38–53.

———. 1983. "Genetic and Hormonal Factors in Sex Differentiation of the Brain." *Psychoneuroendocrinology* 8(2): 183–193.

Kant, I. 1933. *Critique of Pure Reason*, trans. N. K. Smith, London: Macmillan.

Kessler, S. J. and W. McKenna. 1978. *Gender: An Ethnomethodological Approach.* Chicago, IL: University of Chicago Press.

Kessler, S. 1998. *Lessons from the Intersexed.* New Brunswick, NJ: Rutgers.

Lawson, T. 1999. "Feminism, Realism, and Universalism." *Feminist Economics* 5(2): 25–29.

MacLaughlin, D. T. and P. K. Donahoe. 2004. "Sex Determination and Differentiation." *New England Journal of Medicine* 350: 367–378.

McElreavey K. and M. Fellous. 1999. "Sex Determination and the Y Chromosome." *American Journal of Medical Genetics* 89(4): 176–185.

Mittwoch, U. 1986. "Males, Females and Hermaphrodites." *Annals of Human Genetics* 50(2): 103–121.

Money, J., J. G. Hampson and J. L. Hampson. 1957. "Imprinting and the Establishment of Gender Role." *Archives of Neurology and Psychiatry* 77(3): 333–336.

Morland, I. 2001. "Is Intersexuality Real?" *Textual Practice* 15(3): 527–547.

Painter, T. S. 1923. "Studies in Mammalian Spermatogenesis, II: The Spermatogenesis of Man." *Journal of Experimental Zoology* 37(3): 291–336.

Paulozzi, L. J., J. D. Erickson and R. J. Jackson. 1997. "Hypospadias Trends in Two US Surveillance Systems." *Pediatrics* 100(5):831–834.

Quine, W. V. O. 1969. "Ontological Relativity," in W. V. O. Quine. *Ontological Relativity and Other Essays*, pp. 26–68. New York: Columbia University Press.

———. 1995. "Things and Their Place in Theories," in P. K. Moser and J. D. Trout (eds.) *Contemporary Materialism*, pp. 193–208. New York: Routledge.

Rothblatt, M. 1995. *The Apartheid of Sex: A Manifesto on the Freedom of Gender.* New York: Crown Publishers.

Sax, L. 2002. "How Common is Intersex? A Reply to Anne Fausto-Sterling." *The Journal of Sex Research* 39(3): 174–178.

Sayer, A. 2000. *Realism and Social Science*. London: Sage.

Sinclair, A. H., P. Berta, M. S. Palmer, J. R. Hawkins, B. L. Griffiths, M. J. Smith, J. W. Foster, A. M. Frischauf, R. Lovell-Badge and P. N. Goodfellow. 1990. "A Gene from the Human Sex-Determining Region Encodes a Protein with Homology to a Conserved DNA-Binding Motif." *Nature* 346(6281): 240–244.

Swenson, E. and S. Craig. "More Light on Bisexuality and Transgender." Available online at: https://mlp.org/more-light-on-series/

Toppari J., J. C. Larsen, P. Christiansen, A. Giwercman, P. Grandjean, L. J. Guillette jr., B. Jégou, T. K. Jensen, P. Jouannet, N. Keiding, H. Leffers, J. A. McLachlan, O. Meyer, J. Müller, E. Rajpert-De Meys, T. Scheike, R. Sharpe, J. Sumpter and N. E. Skakkebaek. 1996. "Male Reproductive Health and Environmental Xenoestrogens." *Environmental Health Perspectives* 104(Suppl. 4): 741–803.

Vainio, S., M. Heikkila, A. Kispert, N. Chin and A. P. McMahon. 1999. "Female Development in Mammals is Regulated by Wnt-4 Signaling." *Nature* 397(6718): 405–409.

White, P. C. 1994. "Genetic Diseases of Steroid Metabolism." *Vitamins and Hormones* 49: 131–195.

Wilson, J. D., F. W. George and J. E. Griffin. 1981. "The Hormonal Control of Sexual Development." *Science* 211(4488): 1278–1284.

Wittig, M. 1979. "Paradigm," in E. Marks and G. Stambolian (eds.) *Homosexualities and French Literature: Cultural Contexts/Critical Texts*, Ithaca, NY: Cornell University Press.

3 Sex and gender

A critical realist approach[1]

Caroline New

Introduction

In this essay I introduce some key concepts of critical realism, then go on to use them to defend the second wave feminist distinction between 'sex' and 'gender'. I shall argue that sexual difference is real, an extra-discursive property of human beings, and that male and female bodies have different causal powers. Since reproduction is always socially salient, complex gender orders have emerged which regulate sex and gender, rendering them culturally intelligible. These gender regimes condition the embodied agents positioned within them, who, collectively and severally, reproduce, modify and over time transform the gender orders.

Second wave feminism was implicitly realist. The arguments it deployed fall into the category which, in critical realism, are known as 'explanatory critiques' (Collier 1994). Such critiques take two main forms. (1) They criticise some particular representation(s) of social relations and of human (or of women's) nature, offering evidence that this version of reality is untrue; they explain how the untrue account came to be accepted, and whose interests it served; and they put forward an alternative account which they claim is truer. Explanatory critiques allow us to move from claims about how the world *is* to statements about what *should* be done or brought about. Since truth is a good, social relations that systematically give rise to illusions *should* be transformed (Bhaskar 1989). Thus second wave feminists exposed the falsity and the interested nature of employers' arguments that women were paid less because they merely worked for 'pin money', and advocated equal pay legislation. Feminist standpoint theory was also a source of explanatory critique (Hartsock 1983, pp. 283–310; Hekman 1997, pp. 341–364; New 1998, pp. 349–372). It argued that women's social positioning offers them epistemological advantage (potentially better access to knowledge of oppressive social relations – what *is*), and that both social scientists and activists should therefore pay attention to the experiences of women, to gain insight into the systematic illusions produced by male dominated societies. (2) A second type of explanatory critique argues from the exposure of unmet human needs to the need for change, on the grounds that, *ceteris paribus*, human needs should be met (Collier op. cit. New 2003, pp.

57–74). Feminists criticised the gender order on the grounds that it harmed women and prevented their flourishing. Sexual objectification through pornography, for instance, came under attack as harmful to women. The harm identified included the gendered construction of false selves, of women who apparently loved their bondage (for example, the 'painted birds' of Mary Daly's *Gyn/ecology*, 1978).

The sex/gender distinction, elaborated by 1970s feminists, was also realist, and central to feminist explanatory critiques of the period. Sexist defences of the gender order (for instance, functionalist sociology and its everyday versions) described it as a social expression of the real natures of men and women. Most feminists counter-argued that sexual difference was real but relatively trivial; it could in no way account for the dichotomous traits of 'masculinity' and 'femininity'. However, 'radical' or 'revolutionary' feminists did see women's oppression as resulting from real, enduring differences between women and men, that is from men's desire for power over women: their account thus reversed the conventional one. Liberal, Marxist and socialist feminists understood women's oppression as resulting from a motivated refusal to acknowledge that women and men were in most respects similar.

All second stage feminists saw womanhood as a real basis for solidarity, grounded in women's common interests (if not in their similar natures), at least while the oppression of women persisted. To end women's oppression, different approaches called for different sources of power to be mobilised. For radical feminism, the power of women, united across all differences to refuse co-operation with the patriarchy, could bring about a cultural revalorisation of the subordinate terms in the repeated dualisms of Western thought: man, woman; culture, nature; human, animal; reason, emotion. For liberal feminism, women united had to harness the power of the state to render its laws and practices consistent and gender-equal. For Marxists and socialists, women had to unite with men to seize the state, and at the same time use female solidarity to ensure that the interests of half of the working class did not get forgotten. These different strategies were rooted in accounts of sexed human nature and social relations, in analyses of human social possibilities.

From the 1980s, feminist critics of second stage feminism argued that the call to 'sisterhood' obscured the differences *between* women, making middle-class white Western womanhood the default position, and membership of other oppressed groups mere 'add-ons' (Spelman 1992). This was still a realist critique. 'Universalism' and 'essentialism' were opposed on the grounds that they were inaccurate and misleading. If 'woman' was a fragmented identity, not a unitary one, because so many oppressive relationships took place between women themselves, womanhood could not be a usable basis for political solidarity. Feminist politics became increasingly fragmented, with single-issue campaigns and coalitions replacing the broad sweep of a movement. The politics of 'recognition' (of subordinated identities) became increasingly important, and with them the idea of struggle as situated primarily in the discursive realm (Fraser and Honneth 1998).

'Woman' was first deconstructed into fragmentary identities, and then, as we know, postmodern thinking challenged the very gender categories 'woman' and 'man'. As strong social constructivism became increasingly fashionable, many scholars, including feminists, came to identify the social world with the cultural realm, with discourse or 'text'. The discursive was seen as the primary source of power, 'exercised through the constitution of subjectivity within discourse and the production of social agents' (Weedon 1997, p. 163), and therefore as the effective locus for action. Much gender theorising shifted attention from material forms of gender oppression to the categories in terms of which gender relations are described, and to the possibility of becoming free from their power by processes of 'disidentification'. This was not simply a question of a change of tactics and strategy, but a sea change in feminist politics. Thoroughgoing perspectivalism had made explanatory critiques problematic, since they are realist in form. Arguments from unmet needs had also become suspect, since they involved an implicit reference to human nature, which was rejected on methodological grounds as 'the basis for causal, deterministic (as opposed to interpretative) explanations of human behaviour or culture' (Flax 2002, pp. 1042–1055).

There are certain difficulties, however, in the projects of postmodern feminist politics, including theory-practice inconsistencies (New 1998, pp. 349–372; 2003, pp. 57–74). Without going into these here, I offer an alternative way forward in this paper: a more sophisticated, nuanced version of realism that recognises the power and importance of discourse, is epistemologically relativist, yet insists, in Haraway's phrase, on 'a no-nonsense commitment to faithful accounts of a "real" world', accounts in which 'the object of knowledge ... [is] pictured as an actor and agent, not as a screen or a ground or a resource ... Indeed, coming to terms with the agency of the "objects" studied is the only way to avoid gross error and false knowledge of many kinds in these [social] sciences (Haraway 1997, pp. 56 and 66).

Haraway does not believe her vision of 'situated knowledges' is a version of realism, but I think in this respect she is wrong. Critical realism, I shall argue, offers feminism a way forward that is realist, but neither foundationalist or determinist. For readers unfamiliar with critical realism, I begin by explaining some of the basic concepts which I go on to apply to sex and gender.

Transitive and intransitive dimensions

A key distinction in critical realism is between the 'transitive' and 'intransitive' dimensions, between our (always partial and 'situated') knowledge of the world, and the world that is the object of our knowledge. Things and processes exist in the world, 'active independently of their identification by human beings' (Bhaskar 1989, p. 11). The transitive realm, the realm of concepts, ideas and theories, is historical, value-laden, and perspectival. But, like Haraway and Harding (I am thinking of her concept of 'strong objectivity') (Haraway op. cit. Harding 1991), realists regard the necessity of knowing *from a particular place* as enabling knowledge rather than hindering it. We differ from strong social constructionists in our insistence that the world which our concepts and theories are *about*, their referent – the intransitive dimension – is not entirely constituted by the processes of reference. The world is *already* differentiated, complex and stratified, in ways which our concepts may or may not adequately express, and when our concepts are inadequate this has practical consequences (Sayer 1992). True, many phenomena are affected by, or even partially constructed by, the ways in which we think about them, but the structures of the world cannot be reduced to our knowledge of them.

If we exemplify this with reference to sex, we can say that human beings are (almost all) sexually dimorphic, female and male, whether and however this difference is conceptualised. This dimorphic structuring is *active*, causally powerful, enabling (in certain contexts) different reproductive roles and certain (hetero and homo) sexual possibilities and pleasures, while rendering others less likely (elbow as erogenous zone) and ruling others out (male parturition). The characteristics of bodies are part of the intransitive realm. We categorise them as male, female or intersexed, and these categories are part of the transitive realm. Dichotomous sex is highly valued in most societies. Judith Butler describes how babies with ambiguous genitalia are surgically adjusted to fit the social requirement that all citizens be readily identifiable as either male or female (Butler 2001, pp. 523–556). But such interventions do not justify Butler's further conclusion that sexual difference is merely conceptual. The categories of sex (which are in the transitive dimension) have causal power to motivate these social practices, but if bodies did not have particular characteristics (in the intransitive dimension) such surgical alteration would not be possible. Butler collapses the intransitive into the transitive dimension. For her, although bodies may in some sense exist outside of discourse, attempts to discover or describe their characteristics are constructing what they claim to represent.

Conceptual work takes place within the transitive dimension, and constantly reproduces or modifies its structures and contents. Although produced by human subjects, the transitive dimension is also external to us, and constrains and enables what we can think and therefore do. The contents of the transitive dimension – ideas, taxonomies, theories, ways of seeing the world, discourses – are therefore real and causally powerful, and both they and their effects on human action can themselves become objects of knowledge. So for critical realists, the transitive dimension has an intransitive aspect. We would agree with social constructionists in their emphasis on the causal power of discourse, but in our view adequately to describe this power requires a realist distinction between the transitive and intransitive realms.

Stratification and generative mechanisms

The intransitive dimension is not flat: reality is stratified. It is the twin ideas of 'levels' and 'emergent properties' that give critical realism its 'depth'. Most frequently cited is Bhaskar's distinction between the actual, the empirical and the real, although this is just a beginning way of characterising the complexity of ontological stratification (Collier 1994, p. 44). The 'actual' refers to things and events in their concrete historicity, only some of which will ever beknown or experienced by human beings (there must have been events on the other side of the moon which no human being ever experienced). The empirical is a subset of the actual, consisting of those phenomena which are experienced. 'Experience' must here be understood not as given but as socially produced, whether from the concepts of science or those of everyday life: 'in this sense it is the end, not the beginning of a journey' writes Bhaskar, in a passage that exemplifies the social constructionist aspect of critical realism (Bhaskar 1998, p. 43).

The actual and the empirical are, of course, both *real*, and as such are contained within the third domain. But the domain of the real also includes mechanisms, powers and tendencies. 'A generative mechanism ... is that aspect of the structure of a thing by virtue of which it has a certain power' (Collier 1994, p. 62). An army, for instance, by virtue of its structure (its organisation and resources, and the rules which govern their use), has emergent properties and powers irreducible to those of the soldiers and other personnel who make it up. An army can besiege and take over a city, an unorganised crowd could not do so. Changing the organisation will change the properties of the mechanisms – as I write, the British Army is merging some of its smaller regiments because it believes that bigger units have greater power to evoke loyalty in the soldiers who belong to them, which would in turn change what these units could do in war. However, generative mechanisms only operate when set into motion. The army has to be mobilised and set into action for its military powers to be realised, though its powers to evoke loyalty to its regiments could operate in its peacetime barracks. Even when a mechanism is operating, its effects depend on the co-acting of other generative mechanisms – sometimes referred to, by Pawson for instance, as 'context' (Pawson 2004). Outcomes at the level of events are 'complexly co-determined' (Collier 1994, p. 62).

The term 'generative mechanism', then, does not imply that the relationship between cause and effect is 'mechanical' in the sense of predictable and automatic (indeed, some realists prefer to talk of 'causal configurations' and 'causal powers', and those who use the term 'mechanism' do not do so in exactly the same way) (Carter and New 2004). A mechanism could be working without any apparent effects, or with effects which are unexpected or seem paradoxical – because of the existence of other, counter-acting and interacting mechanisms.

> [T]here are many mechanisms concurrently active. The outcome of this – that is the events – is therefore a complex compound effect of influences drawn from different mechanisms, where some mechanisms reinforce each other and others frustrate the manifestations of each other ... there are countless combinations of accidental circumstances ... which may influence whether a specific causal power will manifest itself or not ...
>
> (Danermark et al. 2002, p. 56)

For this reason critical realists talk about 'tendencies'. A tendency is the working of a mechanism (always in conjunction with others) which usually, but not always, gives rise to a specifiable range of outcomes recognisable as the effects of that mechanism. The continual injunction to boys that they should not cry (in order to be distinguishable from girls), and contempt directed at those who do, may or may not have the effect of inhibiting crying. When the mechanism is operating, it *tends* to reduce frequency of crying in boys. (Nowadays there are counteracting cultural messages to the effect that boys have the right to cry – at least a bit.) If we were to analyse in detail how boys respond to the wealth of messages and practices aimed at preventing them expressing feelings by crying, we would find some cases where the boy went on crying, but felt bad about himself and compromised in his gender identity because of this. Thus a tendency always makes a difference to what actually happens, even when the outcome is not obviously affected by its operation, or when it is 'counterfactual' – in other words the outcomes are distinctly not what the mechanism is supposed to bring about.

Causal explanation

Critical realism aims to explain how things are and what they do by mapping the causal relations within and between them, by identifying relevant mechanisms and tendencies. (This approach is not as much at odds with 'interpretivist' explanations as might be thought, since it can subsume them as a form of causal explanation – since the emergent powers of humans include the power to act on the grounds of reasons; our understandings, states of mind, perceptions can bring about, and therefore cause, our doings.) In everyday parlance, a cause is what Aristotelians call an 'efficient' cause. In an approximation of Hume's 'constant conjunction', an event A precedes, and is more or less reliably followed by, another event B, which we understand A as, in some unspecified sense, 'bringing about'. In the toilets at work, Tracy tells a friend how annoyed she is that her manager has asked her to stay late, so that she will not be able to go out with her friends as she'd intended. In everyday explanation the manager's requirement (A) is enough to explain her outburst of annoyance (B), 'Tracy's pissed off again: Rob made her stay late'. However, in social science, to 'explain' events in terms of other events is to presuppose causal mechanisms without illuminating them. Thus 'actualism' accepts the reality of things and events, but denies that there are 'underlying structures which determine how the things come to have their effects, and instead locates the succession of cause and effect at the level of *events*: every time A happens, B happens' (Collier 1994, p. 7). An actualist explanation of worker absenteeism would be satisfied with establishing a correlation with other 'variables' such as length of employment, age of worker, or management style, while a realist explanation would consider in some detail such possible mechanisms as gendered power relations within the organisation.

To get going, both attempts at explanation would begin by subsuming these particular concrete events under some more general description, but while the actualist grouping of variables tends to focus on outcomes or superficial descriptors, the critical realist would be attempting a causal taxonomy from the beginning (with the obvious risk of getting it wrong and having to revise the initial abstractions). A critical realist investigation might look at relations between managers and subordinates, men and women, and older and younger people, in the context of this organisation. Whichever focus it took, it would aim to identify some of the causal conditions which made this particular interaction possible: perhaps the mechanism of gender training as a result of which women tend to accept male authority, perhaps counteracting psychological mechanisms of seeking autonomy in small things when constrained in large. To 'explain' is to identify what is going on at deeper levels than events; to discover the mechanisms and resulting tendencies which, in their intricate combination, bring about actual events.

Mechanisms are themselves stratified, as are the sciences which study their workings (ibid.). (But disciplinary stratification, being part of the transitive realm, is a fallible representation of the real stratification of the objects addressed by those disciplines.) The powers of objects in the higher strata, such as those of social structures, are rooted in the mechanisms of lower levels, such as the biological properties of human beings. For Tracy to be able to tell her friend how annoyed she was, she had to use some means of communication, and unless some other means is mentioned it is assumed that Tracy can speak and her friend can hear, but we take these mechanisms so for granted that we would be unlikely to include them as causal conditions in any account of the event.

Events and things cannot be attributed to one particular level of reality, while mechanisms may be. People, for instance, are themselves structures with emergent properties. People cannot sensibly be characterised as 'physical' or 'chemical' or 'biological' or 'psychological' or 'social': the fact that we are always embodied is crucial to our agency (Shilling 2005). However, some of our emergent properties (not necessarily instantiated in any one individual) could be characterised in this way – you might call the capacity for empathy a psychological property, and the capacity to produce eggs a biological property, and the causal powers emerging from membership of a particular group social properties. All of these mechanisms exist simultaneously and in non-additive interactions, enabling and constraining and otherwise affecting each other.

Footbinding can be used to illustrate the interaction and stratification of mechanisms. This practice was experienced by millions of women in China between the mid-tenth and early twentieth centuries (Feng 1994). It is sometimes explained in terms of *events*: 'The emperor Li Yu ordered his concubine to bind her feet' at one point in history, while at another 'Mao Tse Tung forbade the practice'. No doubt the emperor's original order (if it really happened) was preceded by other happenings in his personal life which might shed light on his sexual predilections, but even these cannot be explained by stringing events on a Humean chain without reference to underlying mechanisms. For one man's demand to give rise to a fashion, and that fashion to become a widespread and long lasting institution, many things had to be the case. At the level of biological mechanisms, sexual dimorphism had to be such that women tend to be smaller than men (or there would have had to be some other contingent origin of the practice's symbolic significance). Human feet had to have certain powers and liabilities, such that if most of the toes were broken and bound under when the child was about three, the foot would remain small. Yet although the properties of the human foot are presupposed by the practice, footbinding cannot be accounted for by reference to biological mechanisms alone – those can only make it possible. Any explanation would have to address higher psychological, cultural and social levels. At the psychological level, human sexuality, in particular male sexuality, had to be culturally malleable, so that a mincing gait could become imbued with erotic meaning. In particular, differences expressing or symbolising sexual and gender difference (such as the exaggeration of the relatively small size of women's feet) had to have a tendency to excite. At the cultural level, beliefs about sexual difference had to legitimise such a practice, and symbolic associations had to make it intelligible and capable of being sexually charged. At the social level, the class structure, including the emperor's power, authority and symbolic role, had to enable him to set fashions. Power relations between men and women, and adults and children, had to be such that the female relatives would carry out the initial act ('otherwise no good man will want her') and the girl child and the various witnesses would permit it. The economy had to allow the disabling of most middle and upper class women. These and many other mechanisms at various levels had to exercise their emergent powers in particular ways and particular relationships to each other for this institution to develop and to endure.

Biological mechanisms are basic in relation to the social, which always presupposes that they are already working. The relationship between the psychological and the social is harder to characterise. Collier believes the social gives rise to the psychological, and here he is in agreement with postmodern discursive psychology (Collier, op. cit., Harre and Gillett 1994). However, he recognises that ontologically speaking, society, language and mind must all have emerged together. In my view, ontological stratification is not simply hierarchical, and the mechanisms relevant to the social sciences do not invariably fit within the disciplinary boundaries of the academy. Some psychological mechanisms emerge directly from the structuring of human brains. Examples would be the capacity to recognise human faces, turn-taking in conversation (prefigured in infant babbling), the tendency to empathy and theory of mind, the power to perceive, and the capacity for language. However, some of these mechanisms cannot be exercised unless they are triggered in developing children by certain social contexts. Children who are not loved may never develop empathy. The power to generate language emerges from the organisation of the human brain, but the actual ability to speak depends on the social context. Some other psychological mechanisms are at a higher level, depending both on lower level psychological mechanisms, and on the symbolic systems of human cultures. These might include processes of acquiring gender identity, the cultural specificities of the formation of ingroups and out-groups, the 'cognitive scripts' of cognitive behaviour therapy, and so on. It is probably these that Collier is thinking of as emerging from the social, since they are far more affected by language and culture than the more basic psychological capacities.

The reality of sex

Having introduced and illustrated some critical realist concepts and distinctions, I can now go on to sketch a critical realist theory of gender. The much criticised 'second stage' feminist distinction between sex and gender is a good place to begin.

The sex-gender distinction has been criticised as 'caught within a surface/depth opposition' (Felski 1997, p. 17) akin to that of the much disputed base/superstructure distinction. From a critical realist perspective, however, the stratified nature of the sex-gender distinction is a strength. A critical realist theory of sex and gender would indeed identify structures at lower levels (the 'base' or 'depth'), and, in a non-reductionist way, would seek to explain how these lower-level structures condition possibilities at higher levels (the 'superstructure' or 'surface'). It would *not* make the mistake of assuming that the second terms were mere expressions of the first, or that the causal relationship was invariably one way. Let us see how this could work for sex and gender.

Sexual dimorphism is a necessary aspect of sexual reproduction, which is in turn an evolved characteristic of the human species. Through the process of sexual dimorphism, foetuses which initially have the same morphology differentiate, resulting in differently sexed bodies with different causal powers. Our human bodies enable different reproductive roles for females and for males, different sexual possibilities (famously, multiple orgasms for females), and by the same token limit what we can do. Little boys discover that they have no wombs in which to grow babies, that they will never have breasts with which to feed them. Little girls discover they cannot urinate standing up without getting wet legs.

Sexual difference in humans is therefore real, and largely extra-discursive. The sex categories are 'good abstractions', bringing together characteristics that are internally (not just nominally or formally) connected (Danermark et al. 2002). Of course, social mechanisms play a role in the allocation of sex categories and thus in the resultant social divisions into maleness and femaleness. Since categorisation is a social process, social mechanisms must always be crucially involved. Where the natural kinds of the world have fuzzy edges (or where there are no natural kinds) there is more scope for the social construction of boundaries. Sexual difference in humans is not entirely dichotomous (more of that in a moment), but nearly so. The division into maleness and has some slight cultural variability, depending on local theories about sexual difference. The reality of sexual difference, however, is a different question from the social processes through which sex categories are allocated.

In humans, as in other mammals, the features of biological sex – chromosonal and hormonal differences affecting development, genital formation, and the 'secondary' bodily differences that develop from puberty – almost always fall into two clusters, female and male, with a very small percentage of ambiguous or mixed cases in between (Rogers 2001). Within each group there is, indeed, more variation than most human societies like to admit. Most of the variation within the groups of males and females is not attributable to intersexuality. The size and shape of sexual parts, the amount and distribution of hair, body fat, muscles, and tone of voice, all vary just as nose shapes and hair colours vary, but the social pressure to exaggerate sexual dimorphism leads us to underestimate the ranges of variation. A woman whose voice is deeper than many men's voices is not therefore intersexual. Intersexuality implies either chromosomal difference, or that the developmental process of differentiation was for some reason compromised or incomplete. The process through which foetus, and then infant and child, develop as male or female (or intersexed) is only very loosely related to the socio-psychological process of the construction of a gendered self.

Human sexes, then, are 'natural kinds', categories so-called because they tell us something about the causal structures of the world. While the causal properties of a natural kind are contingently clustered (for example breasts which can lactate, soft skin, a certain vocal range, a womb, little and fine facial hair), the presence of some of these properties renders the presence of others more likely – because there are common underlying properties that tend to maintain the clusters of features (Keil 1989, p. 43).

These underlying properties continue to exist even in those cases which do not readily fit into male and female clusters. In fact, ambiguous cases are only explicable in terms of the evolved norm of dimorphism, as Hull explains:

> Approximately 99.6% … of all humans are born biologically male or female. Because several processes are involved in the sexual development, the laws do not operate with one hundred percent predictability … hypospadias, the condition in which the male urethral opening extends along the underside of the penis, is … made explicable when the common tissue origin of all genitalia is acknowledged. The condition reflects a shortage of the hormones necessary to convert the bipotential foetal genitalia into a male penis; in other words, hypospadias is a penis with a female urethra… Thus, the phenomenon of intersexuality *is a reflection of the causal structure of sex*, a real structure that intimately links male and female bodies while explaining differences. It is not the effect of a 'resistance' to discourse or a lawless chaos or even a continuum.
>
> (pre-publication version of Hull 2006)

Hull goes on to point out that a male adult who wants to grow breasts, for whatever reason, *must* ingest large quantities of oestrogen. The mechanism on which he must draw to produce a form of intersexuality are also those which produce sexual dimorphism.

To sum up, sexual difference – the differentiation of most humans into males and females, and of a minority into intelligible intersexed forms of human beings – is *basic* in two senses. First, there are real differences between the emergent properties of male and female bodies, their physical capacities and vulnerabilities. For fear of being misunderstood, let me repeat that we are talking about *tendencies* here, not inevitabilities – the tendency of males to be more muscular, of females to menstruate and lactate in certain circumstances, the greater average vulnerability of the male foetus and so on. Other mechanisms, such as gendered differences in the distribution of nourishment or amount of physical exercise, can stop these tendencies resulting in the outcomes mentioned. Second, sexual difference is the referent for the many ways of conceptualising sexed bodies, representations which legitimise various gender orders.

From sex to gender

Sexual difference is, indeed, a natural mechanism, in that the different but related causal powers of female and male sexed bodies, when brought into interaction in specific ways have emergent powers – to reproduce. If impregnated through penetrative sex with male humans, female humans may give birth to children and feed them from their bodies (and in technologically advanced societies may have children in other ways too, which are also related to sexual difference and its properties). The meanings and implications of this depend on social and cultural context, but they will always be socially significant in human societies. 'Gender' refers to the social representations of sexual difference: the beliefs, values and expectations attached to sex categories, and the social relations and ordered practices which they legitimate.

Sexual difference can be understood in many different ways. Women's bodies can be seen as similar to men's bodies (but with inverted genitals), or as completely different (Helliwell 2000, pp. 789–815). Rape can be seen as the inevitable result of sexual difference, or as unthinkable (New 2003). Same-sex sexual relations can be seen as an unfortunate twist in normal psychological development, as a normal genetic variation, or as a liberating escape from oppressive gender orders (Hawkes 2003). All these different representations are social constructions, but

> we should take the metaphor of construction seriously: attempts at construction are only successful if they take adequate account of the properties of the materials that they use … these properties are at any particular time relatively independent of the constructors: they are not merely a product of wishful thinking … Social constructions may fail or be only partially successful.
>
> (Sayer 2004, p. 17)

The 'relatively independent' properties in this case are those of sexed bodies, and the relationships between them. Bodies are malleable, but only up to a point.

Gender orders cannot be read off from the real causal powers of differently sexed bodies (powers which are, of course, affected by gendered practices). Sexual difference is just one among many mechanisms co-acting to produce the many varied gender orders, and probably best seen as a kind of 'background mechanism' or causal condition. In the Humean 'constant conjunction' sense of cause, sexual difference does not 'cause' the institution of marriage or any particular historical form of it, nor does it 'cause' sexual regulations forbidding or permitting homosexuality. But in a critical realist sense, sexual (reproductive) difference *is* one of the mechanisms contributing to the development of such institutions and such rules. Just because it is a 'basic', lower level mechanism, its workings are compatible with many different ways of regulating reproduction and sexuality.

The 'higher' level of gender orders is evident in their extraordinary richness, if such a term can be used to refer to regimes which so often channel the possibilities for human flourishing into narrow and restrictive courses, which make women sick, legitimise homophobic attacks, result in millions of 'missing girls' and in millions of corpses of obedient soldiers. Nevertheless, sociologically speaking, they are rich, far richer than the sexual differences to which they refer. In sum, sex is ontologically prior to gender, and is one of the many mechanisms the workings of which shape gender orders. Gender *is* necessarily linked to sex, but not in the sense that it expresses sex, or is reducible to sex, or is determined by sex. Gender is linked to sex because sex is its referent and its basis, the powers and properties which gender ideas and gender orders make meaningful.

Objections

In the remainder of this essay I will discuss likely objections to my sketch of a critical realist approach to sex and gender.

First the question of stratification. Connell is a broadly realist writer on gender, yet, influenced in some ways by post-structuralism, he rejects ontological stratification.

> Gender refers to the bodily structures and processes of human reproduction. These structures and processes do not constitute a 'biological base', a natural mechanism that has social effects. Rather, they constitute an *arena*, a bodily site where something social happens. Among the things that happen is the creation of the cultural categories 'women' and 'men' (and any other gender categories that a particular society marks out).
>
> (Connell 2002, p. 48)

I find it hard to understand categorisation as taking place in or at 'a bodily site' rather than as referring to it. I suspect that, like post-structuralists, Connell is wary of stratified accounts because he (rightly) fears biological determinism. In fact, recognising sexual difference as a 'natural mechanism' need not be determinist or reductionist. Accounts which see gender as an expression or reflection of sexual dimorphism are obviously wrong, for the reasons Connell and many others have given. Gender arrangements are eminently culturally variable. But what they retain (and Connell himself insists on this, against the radical contingency asserted by post-structuralists such as Butler) is that they *refer* to sexual difference. 'What makes a symbolic structure a gender structure, rather than some other kind, is the fact that its signs refer, directly or indirectly, to the reproductive relationship between women and men' (ibid., p. 38). It seems that Connell does not want to see the symbolic system as a 'social effect' of its referent, presumably because reproductive difference and sexual dimorphism are compatible with many different forms of the gender order. And yet, as I have argued, this does not preclude sexual dimorphism being a *causal condition* – one among many, the most basic but not therefore the most powerful in forming outcomes – of all and any gender orders.

Most postmodern writers would take issue with Connell as well as with me, rejecting our shared view of sexual difference as a referent of gender discourses. For Braidotti, 'as soon as the categories of the social and the natural are dichotomised, the sexes likewise are polarised in a situation of dialectical confrontation' (Braidotti 1994, p. 129). The way out of this sterile impasse is to recognise that 'the notions of nature and culture can only be formulated inside an *already established* cultural order … if one believes that the nature/culture opposition is *real*, one must be blind to the role of language …' (ibid.). There are important differences among postmodern feminists, but they share the view that since we 'have no direct, innocent or unconstructed view of our bodies', sex, like gender, has to be understood as categorical and situated at the same level – that of discourse (Bordo 1993, p. 289). This does not mean (though it often seems to) that postmodern feminists are irrealist in relation to the body. It means rather that they are unwilling to accord the extra-discursive body any causal powers. From a critical realist point of view, this is an instance of the epistemic fallacy: 'the view that statements about being can be reduced to or analysed in terms of statements about knowledge' (Bhaskar 1998, p. 27). The impossibility (which I cheerfully admit) of any unmediated knowledge of the body is wrongly taken to mean that its powers are limited to those we simultaneously recognise and construct.

There is no space to do justice here to probable postmodern objections to what I have written, so I can only offer three placeholders. First, I briefly discuss what I shall call the 'radical contingency view', which seeks to deconstruct both sex and gender to contingent fragmented phenomena. Second, I mention Butler's strong social constructionism, and lastly, I touch on 'sexual difference theorists'. My aim is simply to indicate to readers some elements of a critical realist response to these positions. From a 'radical contingency' perspective, bodies are indeed differentiated. They vary in the amount of subcutaneous fat, width of the pelvis, distribution of hair, shape of internal and external genitalia, number of X and Y chromosomes and so on. Such differences are not stratified, nor otherwise theorised. The categorisation of such attributes into 'male' and 'female' is seen as arbitrary, comparable to dividing humanity according to whether they have attached or unattached ear lobes, ignoring or operating on ambiguous cases, and organising society around this distinction. Since there is no dimension on which these two groups can be *reliably* distinguished, the distinction between 'males' and 'females' is seen as entirely socially constructed. Women have moustaches, men get breast cancer, and the plethora of supposed expressions have no essence behind them. Gender narratives, then, are 'totalising fictions that create a false unity out of heterogeneous elements' and have 'little to offer in a postmodern world that understands the body, sex and sexuality as socially constructed' (Hawkesworth 1997, pp. 653–85, 651–2).

This is a realist conception, but a reductive, actualist one, in which phenomena all have the same status and theorising is seen as something humans do to satisfy themselves by making meaning, rather than as a process of discovery of real relations. Hawkesworth maintains that females and males are not 'natural kinds' because there is no set of properties possessed by every member of each of these groups. Biological kinds can never meet the essentialist criteria she implicitly requires (Boyd 1992). Biology is messy and complex, and its regularities take the form of tendencies rather than laws. In the case of sexual difference, these tendencies are strong, 'the genotypic and phenotypic division of bodies into two sexes crosses species and millennia' (Hull 2006, p. 105).

Postmodern writers have massively exaggerated intersexuality (Fausto-Sterling 2000; Sax 2002). Beyond the numbers debate, many believe sexual attributes form a continuum, rather than a dimorphic distribution into two clear, though internally variable and fuzzy edged, groups with a small minority of intersexed people in between. Their concern to document and expose the conventionality and cruelty of the processes of sexual allocation is completely appropriate (Kessler 2002). I would agree that both variations within the bodily shapes and sizes of females and males, and intersexuality, should be accepted as something ordinary and unthreatening that does not affect the human value of the people concerned. But this is a battle against oppressive gender orders: it cannot best be fought by misrepresenting sexual difference as a question of reaching a certain conventional threshold of enough contingently gendered bodily features.

Sex and 'race'

In arguing that gender narratives are 'totalising fictions', postmodern thinkers are claiming that sex is like 'race', and should similarly be embellished with scare quotes. 'Race' has been exposed as a series of constructions from disparate elements with no intrinsic significance. In social realist terms, 'race' is a bad abstraction, theoretically misleading (Sayer 1992; Danermark et al. 2002). Differences in skin pigment are real enough, and so are the other markers of 'race' at the level of the empirical. However, at a deeper, structural level, discrete races do not exist. The genotypical differences between them are less significant than the differences within these groups, counter to scientific racism. 'Race categories have far more to do with politics than they have to do with science' (Carter 2000, p. 3). The argument against the ontological validity of race classifications is that they *do* impose a spurious unity on groups of humans who are actually diverse – and do so for the worst of reasons.

Carter, a social realist, argues that because there are no such things as races, the sociological use of the term to refer to beliefs in and discourse about races, and social relations and practices understood in terms of race, is highly misleading; preventing analysis and explanation of what is going on (Carter 2000). Analogously, post-structuralists argue that all talk about gender should be detached from ideas about sex, or alternatively that sex should be seen as a creation of gender. 'What is really going on' is entirely within discourse.

However, as Linda Alcoff also argues, sex is *not* like 'race' (Alcoff 2005). Unlike racial groups, males and females are natural kinds. Sexual difference is also socially significant. This significance is an emergent property of human societies, given the sorts of (sexed, mortal) beings humans are. Means of reproduction will probably always be a salient feature of human societies, variously institutionalised but always deeply meaningful in their symbolic orders. While 'race' could be exploded and lose its credibility as a means of classification, this could not happen to sexual difference. It is relatively easy to imagine a world without 'races' and racism, but very hard to imagine a world where sex difference was socially so insignificant that there was no sex-gender order. Perhaps if humans lived to be two hundred, and their adult sexual and reproductive life lasted for only one eighth of that life span, gender arrangements might become far less significant and gender identity a temporary phenomenon, to be shrugged off at the end of the reproductive period as some workers seem to shrug off their occupational identities on retirement. It might even happen that sexual difference remained of some importance in the second hundred years because it affected vulnerability to different illnesses, but otherwise had no effect on social practices. But even such far-fetched thought experiments do not make credible a social world without sex (and therefore gender) as a partial basis for social organisation.

Judith Butler

Butler is famous for rejecting the sex-gender distinction, on the grounds that the naturalness of sex is constructed through gender. In *Gender Trouble* Butler argued that gender is 'a *corporeal style*, an act, as it were, which is both intentional and performative, where "performative" suggests a dramatic and contingent construction of meaning' (Butler 1990, p. 139). Such performance is generally 'a strategy of survival within compulsory systems' (ibid.), but could also become liberatory through parody and 'strategies of subversive repetition' (ibid., p. 147). Concerned lest she had been taken as too voluntarist, in *Bodies that Matter* she took up the theme of the (constructed) materiality of sex: '"Sex" is part of a regulatory practice which produces the bodies it governs' (Butler 1993, p. 1). In an interview in *Radical Philosophy*, she explained: 'I wanted to work out how … we might understand the materiality of the body to be not only invested with a norm, but in some sense animated by a norm, or contoured by a norm' (Butler 1994, p. 32). The norm here is reproductive. Butler is not denying the reality of sexual dimorphism, but is arguing that its framing in terms of 'the problematic of reproduction' is a social construction emanating from heterosexual dominance. Although in her later work she admits the materiality of the body, its powers to constrain are seen as socially constructed. For instance, in the *Radical Philosophy* interview, she remarks in passing that maybe a woman could not get pregnant 'for biological reasons', but sees her as 'struggling with a norm that is regulating [her] sex' because of the difficulty of avoiding feelings of failure and of finding any other ways of taking part in child-rearing. From a critical realist point of view, I would say that Butler chooses to downplay the causal powers of sexed bodies and to focus on the co-acting social and linguistic mechanisms which affect outcomes.

Difference feminism

All social constructionist accounts which stress the contingency of sexual difference invite the question as to why, in that case, discourses about it produce such surprisingly constant dualisms. Where did our dichotomous gendered spectacles come from? In Lacan's work this question is answered: the 'law of the father' operates as an unacknowledged 'base' which makes the repudiation of the feminine, and therefore the subordination of women, inevitable. Post-Lacanian difference feminists believe it is possible to 'recover the feminine within sexual difference, to generate an autonomous female imaginary beyond existing stereotypes of women ... outside the binary structures of patriarchal thought, including, paradoxically, the very distinction between masculine and feminine' (Felski 1997, p. 5).

Difference feminism does recognise the reality of sexual difference. This is a stratified account, one which is reluctant to attribute causal powers to bodies (the phallus is not the penis), but at the same time suggests that genital shape carries enormous psychological/discursive significance. This is puzzling to those of us who see the body as a real thing, 'that cannot be dissolved into discourse, possessed of causally generative properties' (Shilling 2005, p. 12). Instead, the body is seen 'as an inter-face, a threshold, a field of intersection of material and symbolic forces' (Braidotti 1994, p. 218) The trouble is that this deliberate muddling of mechanisms makes it impossible to describe the relationship between the material and the symbolic, as Shilling shows in his discussion of Elisabeth Grosz, a difference feminist who 'is determined to hold on to a view of the materially sexed body' and who describes how the 'morphology of the male and female body exerts an inevitable effect on how individuals psychically perceive their embodied selves' (Shilling 2005, p. 67). He views her as a structuration theorist, because she sees the sexed body as simultaneously constituting and constituted. Her insistence on these as two analytically inseparable aspects prevents her offering criteria for when the body is causing and when being moulded. Shilling argues that she falls into 'central conflation' and loses explanatory purchase (Archer 1995).

To sum up, my sketch of a critical realist account of sex and gender depends on a stratified and causal theory which would be objectionable to postmodern feminists on various grounds. To the radical contingency actualists, to insist on the reality of sexual difference is to ontologise discursively produced collections of phenomena and attribute a spurious facticity to them. To Judith Butler, this account accepts and perpetuates a reproductive heterosexist norm, without recognising its source in established power relations. To sexual difference theorists, the critical realist approach puts the 'base' in the wrong place: in the sexed body rather than in the unconscious mind.

Conclusion

I have argued that sexual difference is an inescapable part of human embodiment, and thus of our agency. In this sense, it is basic, and among the background causal conditions for *every* form of the sexual division of labour, whether egalitarian or oppressive, segregated or gender-flexible. To explain the particular forms taken by gender orders we have to look to the many other mechanisms involved – but that does not mean that sexual difference just drops out, as a 'tedious universal'. To ignore its role as a referent and its powers to constrain and enable is to reject old forms of reductionism in favour of new ones.

Just because sexual difference is basic, it does not constitute automatic grounds for solidarity between males or between females – here critical realists would entirely agree with postmodern feminists. Sexual difference has no political implications in itself: those emerge from organisation at higher levels. However, for those who want change, some changes are possible (while others are not) at each of the levels I have discussed, including the relatively enduring one of biological sexual difference. This is not the place to argue about different sorts of feminist strategies and tactics, from mimesis and subversive performance to women's peace camps or lobbying for legal change. All activists have to ask themselves what they want and attempt to identify what changes are possible. The power to bring about changes that are both wanted and possible depends on an adequate understanding of real causal relationships. Claims to knowledge are always fallible, and therefore inevitably risky, but if we refuse to strive for them we surrender a key dimension of agency.

Note

1 This chapter was originally published as New, C., 2005. Sex and gender: a critical realist approach. *New Formations*, *56*, p. 54. © Lawrence and Wishart. Reproduced with permission of the Licensor through PLSclear.

References

Alcoff, L. 2005. *Visible Identities: Race and Gender*. Oxford, Oxford University Press.

Archer, M. 1995. *Realist Social Theory: The Morphogenetic Approach*. Cambridge: Cambridge University Press.

Bhaskar, R. 1989. *The Possibility of Naturalism*. Hemel Hempstead: Harvester Wheatsheaf.

———. 1998. "Philosophy and Scientific Realism," in M. Archer, R. Bhaskar, A. Collier, T. Lawson and A. Norrie (eds.) *Critical Realism: Essential Readings*, pp. 16–47. London: Routledge.

Bordo, S. 1993. *Unbearable Weight: Feminism, Western Culture and the Body*. Berkeley: University of California Press.

Boyd, R. 1992. "Constructivism, Realism and Philosophical Method," in J. Earman (ed.) *Inference, Explanation and Other Frustrations*, pp. 131–198. Berkeley: University of California Press.

Braidotti, R. 1994. *Nomadic Subjects: Embodiment and Sexual Difference in Contemporary Feminist Theory*. New York: Columbia University Press.

Butler, J. 2001. "Gender as Performance: An Interview with Judith Butler.", interviewed by Peter Osborne and Lynne Segal. *Radical Philosophy*, 67: 32–39.

Butler, J., with P. Osborne and L. Segal. 1994. "Extracts from Gender as performance: An Interview with Judith Butler." *Radical Philosophy* 67, Summer. https://www.radicalphilosophyarchive.com/issue-files/rp67_interview_butler.pdf

———. 1993. *Bodies That Matter: On the Discursive Limits of Sex*. New York: Routledge.

———. 1990. *Gender Trouble: Feminism and the Subversion of Identity*. New York: Routledge.

Carter, B. 2000. *Realism and Racism: Concepts of Race in Sociological Research*. London: Routledge.

———. 2003. "What Race Means to Realists," in J. Cruickshank (ed.) *Critical Realism: The Difference it Makes*, pp. 149–160. London: Routledge.

——— and C. New. 2004. "Introduction," in B. Carter and C. New (eds.) *Making Realism Work: Realist Social Theory and Empirical Research*. Abingdon, Oxfordshire: Routledge.

Collier, A. 1994. *Critical Realism: An Introduction to Roy Bhaskar's Philosophy*. London: Verso.

Connell, B. 2002. *Gender*. Cambridge: Polity.

Daly, M. 1978. *Gyn/Ecology: the Metaethics of Radical Feminism*. Boston: Beacon Press.

Danermark, B., M. Ekstrom, L. Jakobsen, J. C. Karlsson. 2002. *Explaining Society: Critical Realism in the Social Sciences*. London: Routledge.

Fausto-Sterling, A. 2000. *Sexing the Body: Gender Politics and the Construction of Sexuality*. New York, Basic Books.

Felski, R. 1997. "The Doxa of Difference." *Signs: Journal of Women in Culture and Society*. 23(1): 1–21.

Feng, J. 1994. *The Three-Inch Golden Lotus*. Honolulu: University of Hawaii Press.

Flax, J. 2002. "Reentering the Labyrinth: Revisiting Dorothy Dinnerstein's The Mermaid and the Minotaur." *Signs: Journal of Women in Culture and Society* 27(4): 1037–1055.

Fraser, N. and A. Honneth. 1998. *Redistribution or Recognition? A Political-Philosophical Exchange*. London: Verso.

Haraway, D. 1997. "Situated Knowledges: The Science Question in Feminism and the Privilege of Partial Perspective," in *Simians, Cyborgs and Women: The Reinvention of Nature*. London: Free Association Books.

Harding, S. 1991. *Whose Science? Whose Knowledge? Thinking from Women's Lives*. Buckingham: Open University Press.

Harre R. and G. Gillett. 1994. *The Discursive Mind*. London: Sage.

Hartsock, N. 1983. "The Feminist Standpoint: Developing the Ground for a Specifically Feminist Historical Materialism," in S. Harding and M. B. Hinkikka (eds.) *Discovering Reality*, pp. 283–310. Dordrecht: D. Reidel.

Hawkes, G. 2003. *A Sociology of Sex and Sexuality*. London: Open University Press.

Hawkesworth M. 1997. "Confounding Gender." *Signs: Journal of Women in Culture and Society* 22(3): 649–685.

Hekman, S. 1997. "Truth and Method: Feminist Standpoint Theory Revisited." *Signs: Journal of Women in Culture and Society* 22(2): 341–365.

Helliwell, C. 2000. "'It's Only a Penis": Rape, Feminism and Difference." *Signs: Journal of Women in Culture and Society* 25(3): 789–816.

Hull, C. 2006. *The Ontology of Sex: A Critical Inquiry into the Deconstruction and Reconstruction of Categories*. London: Routledge.

Keil, F. C. 1989. *Concepts, Kinds and Cognitive Development*. Cambridge, Mass.: MIT Press.

Kessler, S. J. 2002. "Defining and Producing Genitals," in S. Jackson and S. Scott (eds.) *Gender: A Sociological Reader*, pp. 447–456. London: Routledge.

Mohanty, C. 1992. "Feminist Encounters: Locating the Politics of Experience," in M. Barrett and A. Phillips (eds.) *Destabilising Theory: Contemporary Feminist Debates*, pp. 74–92. Cambridge: Polity.

New, C. 2003. "Feminism, Critical Realism and the Linguistic Turn," in J. Cruickshank (ed.) *Critical Realism: The Difference it Makes*, pp. 57–74. London: Routledge.

———.1998. "Realism, Deconstruction and the Feminist Standpoint." *Journal for the Theory of Social Behaviour* 28(4): 349–372.

Pawson, R. 2004. "Evidence-based policy: a realist perspective," in B. Carter and C. New (eds.) *Making Realism Work: Realist social theory and empirical research*, pp. 26–49. London: Routledge.

Preves. S. E. 2001. "Sexing the Intersexed: An Analysis of Sociocultural Responses to Intersexuality." *Signs: Journal of Women in Culture and Society* 27(2): 523–556.

Rogers, L. 2001. *Sexing the Brain*. New York: Columbia University Press.

Sax, L. 2002. "How Common is Intersex? A response to Anne Fausto-Sterling." *Journal of Sex Research* 39(2): 174–178.

Sayer, A. 1992. *Method in Social Science*. London: Routledge.

———. 2004. "Restoring the Moral Dimension: Acknowledging Lay Normativity." Paper delivered at the British Sociological Association Conference, York, April 2004, available at: https://www.lancaster.ac.uk/fass/resources/sociology-online-papers/papers/sayer-restoring-moral-dimension.pdf

Shilling, C. 2005. *The Body in Culture, Technology and Society*. London: Sage.

Spelman, E. 1988. *Inessential Woman: Problems of Exclusion in Feminist Thought*. Boston, Mass.: Beacon Press.

Weedon, C. 1997. *Feminist Practice and Poststructuralist Theory*. Oxford: Blackwell.

4 A defence of the category 'women'[1]

Lena Gunnarsson

Introduction

In the closing session of a recent feminist conference,[2] the moderator asked about what it is about feminist theory that makes it feminist. One of the conference participants offered an elaborate answer, without ever mentioning the words 'women' or 'men' or anything representing specifically gendered relations. Instead, the fabric of the answer was general assumptions about power and resistance. Slightly disturbed, yet not very surprised by this, I asked what made this answer apply specifically to feminist theory, when actually it could pertain to all theoretical frameworks somehow occupied with issues of power and resistance. Interestingly enough, my question seemed to take the individual by surprise, who then answered that he 'had not thought about that'.

How can this be? Is it not the very point of departure of feminist theorising that women are oppressed/exploited/discriminated/excluded by virtue of their being women? And is it not the case, as Iris Marion Young states, that 'without some sense in which "woman" is the name of a social collective, there is nothing specific about feminist politics' (1994, p. 714), nor about feminist theory? For any feminist theorist before the deconstructionist turn, the answer to these questions would indisputably be in the affirmative. However, my opening anecdote shows that within contemporary feminist academia there is no unanimity about this question; on the contrary, the stigmatisation of the category 'women' has become such a taken-for-granted element in feminist discussions that the conference participant who excluded 'women' from his feminist vocabulary had never even been compelled to reflect upon the tensions such an exclusion implies, until confronted by my rather basic question. Another illustration of this taken-for-grantedness is the way that Clare Hemmings defends the feminists of the 1970s against the charge of essentialism, by invoking that they too 'challeng[ed] "woman" as the ground for feminist politics and knowledge production' (2005, p. 116). This cognitive structure, wherein intrinsic links are held to exist between essentialism and appeals to the category 'woman'/'women', helps explain why I felt somewhat awkward about posing my unanticipated question in the conference plenary. 'Women', as Susan Gubar states, has become 'an invalid word' (1998, p. 886).

As I agree with Young that the category 'women' is absolutely indispensable to the feminist project, in this article I lay bare some conceptual confusions underpinning the widespread tendency to write it off. I show that the category 'women' is vital since it relates to something real, and that this statement implies neither essentialism nor homogenisation. Firstly, I examine the characteristic ways that feminist theorists have influentially argued against the use of 'women' as a category of analysis on the grounds that it implies ethnocentrism, essentialism et cetera. I scrutinise the meta-theoretical assumptions underpinning these arguments, which can be said to emerge from specific versions of what I call the intersectional and constructionist paradigms. The theorists I examine do not reject the category 'women' in any wholehearted way, but acknowledge the analytical and political problems implied by such a rejection. Prescribing parodic (Butler 1999) or strategic (Spivak 2006) uses of identity categories like 'women' are solutions that have been offered to the dilemma produced by this acknowledgement. Still, what remains throughout all these ambivalences is a deep scepticism against any positive (as opposed to deconstructive) theoretical validity, not to say realness of the category 'women'. It is this scepticism that I confront by demonstrating that it rests on implicit meta-theoretical premises that are highly disputable. Secondly, informed by the philosophical framework of critical realism, I present an argument about how we can think about the category 'women' in more fruitful and consistent ways. In this endeavour the method of abstraction plays a crucial role.

The intersectional challenge: women are not only women

Intersectionality is a theoretical perspective, method and concept that has recently gained an immense influence among feminist theorists (see Davis 2008; Lykke 2007; McCall 2005; Zack 2005). It refers to the intersection of different social relations in every concrete subject, so that studying gender through an intersectional lens means emphasising that women are not only women, but also black, white, rich, poor, heterosexual, homosexual, etc. I here use the term in an unusually broad sense so as to include postcolonial feminism and black feminism, the common denominator being that they all highlight the complexities stemming from women's different positioning in power relations other than gender. Although theoretical attention to people's multiple positioning might seem a rather unspectacular undertaking, intersectionality has, as Kathy Davis puts it, 'been heralded as one of the most important contributions to feminist scholarship', even as 'a feminist success story' (2008, p. 67). What is it about intersectionality and its propagation that rendered/renders it such an allegedly indispensable challenge to other feminist perspectives? I will show that, while intersectionality in its most basic terms does not need to define itself against feminist theory in a more traditional sense, the intersectionality paradigm as a whole harbours two moves, one rhetorical and one theoretical, which largely account for its pioneer status.

The background of the rhetorical move is that intersectional feminism emerged out of a disappointment among feminist women of colour with what they saw as ethnocentric and homogenising modes of feminist thinking about women. Non-white and non-Western feminist scholars (see, for example, Collins 1990; Crenshaw 1991; hooks 1981; Mohanty 1988, 2003) brought to light that, contrary to what many feminist theorists seemed to believe, unless other power relations than gender are taken into account some women's experiences will be invalidated and power relations among women made invisible. It was, for example, emphasised that for women who do not enjoy racial and class-based privileges, womanhood was not necessarily the most salient factor of oppression, and that ways of referring to 'women' and 'blacks' actually tended to include only white women and black men respectively, while ignoring the specific experience of black women (Crenshaw 1991; hooks 1981; McCall 2005; Spelman 1990). As well as calling attention to these modes of neglecting the specificities of non-white women's lives, intersectional feminists also pointed to modes of distortion, wherein non-white and non-Western women tend to be represented as a homogenised whole, defined as the victimised Other (e.g. Mohanty 1988, 2003).

This scrutiny of assumptions about 'women's experiences' has been crucial to the project of revealing ethnocentric biases and generally simplifying tendencies. Many feminist theorists, indeed, have made untenable generalisations about what it means to be a woman, obscuring the complexity and diversity caused not only by women's different positions in racial, class and sexual relations, but by the multi-levelledness of power and being itself. However, these legitimate grounds for criticism aside, the sharp dichotomy between a universalising before and an intersectional after has been questioned by, for example, Davis, who emphasises that Kimberlé Crenshaw, known for having introduced the concept of intersectionality, 'was by no means the first to address the issue of how black women's experiences have been marginalised and distorted within feminist discourse. Nor was she making a particularly new argument when she claimed that their experiences had to be understood as multiply shaped by race and gender' (2008, pp. 72–73). For example, in 1977 the black US feminist lesbian group Combahee River Collective gave out their influential manifesto making the case for a feminist analysis including issues of race, class, and sexuality along with gender.

Much of the rhetorical force of intersectional arguments has come to depend upon caricature-like representations of 'earlier', 'Western' or 'hegemonic' feminist theories. For example, although Chandra Talpade Mohanty, widely praised for her seminal work on Western feminists' ethnocentric intellectual practices, does seek to qualify her use of the term 'Western feminism' – a term she repeatedly invokes as the subject guilty of homogenisation and objectification of non-Western women (2003, p. 18) – the end result is nevertheless that 'Western feminism' appears as much a homogeneous entity in her account as the 'Third World women' in the writings she confronts. Anna G. Jónasdóttir and Kathleen B. Jones point to the tendency among post-structuralist feminists to simplify and obscure the theoretical past in order to make their own argument appear as 'a necessary remedy' (2009, p. 34) and, in a similar vein, Hemmings highlights the frequent mode of unreflectedly contrasting oneself against the 'naïve, essentialist seventies' (2005, p. 116). Perhaps Leslie McCall is right when stating that 'the social construction of all new knowledge tends to have a particular structure to it. In this structure the development of a new field is celebrated on the tomb of the old' (2005, pp. 1783–1784). The framing of intersectional feminism as a fundamental challenge to other kinds of feminism is partially due to the rhetorical strategy of contrasting oneself against 'invented targets', to borrow Andrew Sayer's expression (2000, p. 68).

Besides this rhetorical element, there are also theoretical tendencies accounting for the sometimes antithetical relation between intersectional and 'regular' feminism. McCall highlights that intersectionality can be based on different meta-theoretical assumptions, ranging from simple attention to the complex interplay between different axes of power (Crenshaw 1991) to more radical perspectives 'that completely reject the separability of analytical and identity categories' (McCall 2005, p. 1771). In the most elaborate versions of the latter approach, which McCall labels 'anticategorical', the rejection of the category 'women' comes logically from the general theoretical framework that denies categories any analytical validity by virtue of their empirical inseparability. It is this version of intersectionality that I take issue with here. Judith Butler summarises the foundational principles of this approach, when stating that 'because gender intersects with racial, class, ethnic, sexual, and regional modalities of discursively constituted identities … it becomes impossible to separate out "gender"' (1999, p. 6). Although this way of arguing may seem plausible at first sight, it suffers from self-contradiction. As Jónasdóttir and Jones highlight, Butler's statement that 'gender intersects with racial, class, ethnic, sexual, and regional modalities' becomes absurd if it is impossible to distinguish gender analytically from other categories, 'since intersection logically implies the coming together of "parts" that are conceptually distinct from each other in some identifiable way' (2009, p. 41).

Some anticategorical feminists like Wendy Brown are aware of this contradiction and, in the name of consistency, sceptical of the concept of intersectionality itself. Few wish, however, to completely reject concepts like race, class and gender: the awareness of the dangers of individualism and voluntarism is too strong. Brown is concerned to find ways of theoretically recognising that power relations, like race, gender and class are different in kind and that therefore they must be attributed some kind of separate analytical existence. However, she does not embrace this need for analytical distinctions and make it an integral part of her theoretical framework. Instead, the necessity of distinction, albeit recognised, is conceived as fundamentally at odds with the fact that 'we are not fabricated as subjects in discrete units by these various powers: they do not operate on and through us independently, or linearly, or cumulatively [and] are not separable in the subject itself' (1997, p. 86). For Brown, the need for categorisations on the one hand, and the empirical inseparability of categories on the other, seems to be a theoretical enigma that she can only think of in terms of a 'paradoxical moment' (1997, p. 93).

Elizabeth Spelman also displays a largely unresolved ambivalence about her generally disapproving approach to categorisations. She concedes that she has no trouble sorting herself out as woman and white. 'What gender are you?' and 'What race are you?' 'appear to be two separate questions, which I can answer separately' (1990, p. 133). However, like Brown, she feels a need to emphasise that there are no 'discrete units' (Brown 1997, p. 86) of gender, race et cetera; Spelman is careful to stress that it is impossible to distinguish the 'woman part' from the 'white part' of herself.

> If there is a 'woman part' of me, it doesn't seem to be the kind of thing I could point to – not because etiquette demands that nice people don't point to their private or covered parts, but because even if I broke a social rule and did so, nothing I might point to would meet the requirements of being a 'part' of me that was a 'woman part' that was not also a 'white part'. Any part of my body is part of a body that is, by prevailing criteria, female and white.
>
> (1990, pp. 133–134)

In Brown's and Spelman's theoretical universes, the possibility of thinking about women as women is conditioned on the possibility of pointing out specific 'women parts' or 'units' – that is, we must be able to separate out the 'womanness' on the concrete level of existence. However, if we distance ourselves from an empiricist fixation with physical appearances and directly accessible entities, we can avoid being caught by irresolvable paradoxical moments.

Before outlining how we can think of 'womanness' in other terms than an empirical entity, I want to call attention to a somewhat different mode of dismissing the category 'women' than the one offered by proponents of the anticategorical approach. Mohanty, for example, explicitly distances herself from postmodernist approaches that fail to take into account the structural reality of the power relations which categories represent. Still, she sees the specific category 'women' as inherently problematic, asserting that '[t]he phrase "women as a category of analysis" refers to the crucial assumption that all women, across classes and cultures, are somehow socially constituted as a *homogeneous* group' (2003, p. 22; emphasis added). This, indeed, is a radical contention, which would need an elaborate theoretical justification, since the awareness that women are different far from necessitates a rejection of 'women' as an analytical category. Sayer reminds us that the search for commonalities actually presupposes diversity, which in turn becomes meaningful only from the perspective of some kind of sameness. He points out that '[t]he nature of the difference between various groups of people is more interesting than the difference between people and toothpaste partly because the former have some things in common' (1997, p. 457). Developing this point in relation to gender, Naomi Zack emphasises that 'commonality … does not ignore or suppress differences because it is the basis on which difference exists, and what we implicitly refer to whenever we say that women are different' (2005, p. 9). We must question the very dualism between sameness and difference that rejections of commonality are so often premised upon.[3]

Mohanty does not offer any theoretical defence of her categorical dismissal of 'women' as a category of analysis, considering it enough to show that some feminists have used the category in homogenising ways. It is my contention that this kind of slide is indicative of a lot of contemporary feminist scepticism towards talking about 'women'. Mohanty has no problem invoking other categories as highly meaningful analytical devices; notably, she addresses the 'common social identity of Third World women workers' (2003, p. 163). Might not the category 'Third World women workers', just as much as 'women', be deemed inherently homogenising according to the theoretical standards she applies to dismiss the latter? After all, differences related to, for example, sexuality and nationality risk being made invisible when the women are categorised in these terms. Ann Ferguson is critical of how Mohanty's discriminatory way of dealing with categories gives analytical (and political) priority to work-related structures while neglecting the more gender-specific 'sex-affective relations' (2011, p. 248). Similarly, Nina Lykke notes that some intersectional feminists are 'so absorbed by feminist-bashing' and by questioning the 'primacy of gender' that they tend to emphasise class and race at the cost of gender (2007, p. 138).[4] This kind of discriminatory anticategoricalism, in which the category 'women' has become something of a particular minefield, can only be understood in the light of the rhetorical tendencies highlighted above.

The constructedness of women/'women'

The assumption that gender is socially constructed is an all-pervasive fundament of feminist theory and gender studies, although there is no consensus as to how gender is socially constructed or whether there is any pre-social ground at all for the process of construction. For example, Carrie Hull (2006) and Caroline New (2005, ch. 3 this volume) emphasise that there is a fundamental biological base to sexual difference, while theorists like Butler (1993, 1999) and Judith Halberstam (1994) view such biological conceptions as themselves altogether discursive constructions. Disagreements aside, the assumption that gendered relations and identities are historical/social products rather than universal or 'natural' givens constitutes a necessary condition for occupying the feminist philosophical position. The important point, though, is that whether one believes that a world without sex/gender is possible or not, it is still a fact that women and men exist as categories pervasively structuring the world.

In the theoretical landscape of queer-oriented feminists like Butler, the notion that gender is constructed entails that it is a fiction. Butler asserts that, since there is no 'univocity of sex' or 'internal coherence of gender', these are 'regulatory fictions' (1999, pp. 43–44).[5] Furthermore, she holds the category 'women' to be fictive and arbitrary on the grounds that it is not 'a stable signifier that commands the assent of those whom it purports to describe and present' (1999, p. 6), that there is no 'substance' of gendered identities (1999, p. 25), and that 'a good ten percent of the population has chromosomal variations that do not fit neatly into the XX-female and XY-male set of categories'

(1999, p. 137). In addition to implying that some unnamed other feminists consider 'women' to be a stable signifier and gender identities to have a substance, Butler also makes some presuppositions about what can be considered to be real and about what categories are for. Reality can only be conceived of in terms of coherent substances, and categories are held to be valid only if they reflect concrete reality in all its singularities. Jónasdóttir and Jones rightly contend that Butler 'conflates feminists' efforts to formulate concepts of gender and complex theories of gender systems' (2009, p. 39) with the 'development of a language that fully or adequately represented women' (Butler 1999, p. 4).[6]

Sayer has coined the term 'pomo flip' to describe this phenomenon in which theorists, in their efforts to break with positivist and empiricist assumptions, tend to invert the theoretical structure and thereby 'retain ... the problematic structures which generated the problem in the first place' (2000, p. 67). Hull similarly highlights the continuities between post-structuralism and positivism, to the extent that they both tend to presuppose that 'theories are verified only when 100 percent accurate predictions of empirical events can be obtained, and categories or kinds are considered legitimate only when every individual within them is identical' (2006, p. 87). The radicality of the insight that gender is socially constructed lies exactly in the element that our experiences as women, men, transsexuals and queers, although real, are not pre-given, static entities but products of historically determined human activity and thus subject to change. The radicality does not lie in refuting the reality of that which is socially constructed; that only retains the positivist assumptions of what reality is, assumptions that feminists have found crucial to dismiss since gendered power structures could not possibly be proved to exist according to such standards. Although gender categories are socially constructed, they are not mere nominal categories only arbitrarily related to the world. Women and men may be social constructs, but nevertheless, as Jónasdóttir puts it, 'women and men are the kinds of people they are, historically, at present' (1994, p. 220; emphasis in original). Feminists have long been aware of the political dilemma constituted by the fact that when we invoke the word 'women' in order to describe, explain and challenge gendered power, this also risks reproducing patriarchal notions of the significance of sexual difference. But instead of seeking to erase this contradiction by simplified emphasis on one of its poles, we should seek to develop theoretical frameworks that can contain it – because the dilemma is real and must therefore be lived through and solved through practical struggle.

Butler and her followers have carried out an important task in highlighting how the very subjects that we struggle to liberate are themselves products of relations of power sustained by certain significatory systems that make some identities intelligible at the expense of others. The ways that we use categories like 'women' and 'men', 'feminine' and masculine' will never be innocent but part of determining how possibilities and vulnerabilities are distributed in the world. However, gendered identities cannot be reduced to the significatory processes through which they are produced, even if we see them as produced entirely through such significatory processes. However produced they may be, as products they possess a relative stability, autonomy and causal efficacy of their own. It is in this sense that gender categories are not only conceptual in character but also real groupings in the world. The crucial import of this is that not only do symbolic gender categories structure our perception of human beings; also, the real groupings of women and men act back upon our systems of meaning so that these categories are necessary if we are to make sense of – and effectively change – the world.

Butler and others have acknowledged the political problems that their philosophical framework can cause. What, after all, as Linda Martín Alcoff puts it, 'can we demand in the name of women if "women" do not exist and demands in their name simply reinforce the myth that they do?' (2006, p. 143). Strategic essentialism has been suggested as a way of enabling political claims in the name of groups, with the ontological existence of such groups nevertheless interrogated (Spivak 2006). Butler, for her part, emphasises that

> [although] "gender" only exists in the service of heterosexism, [that] does not entail that we ought never make use of such terms … On the contrary, precisely because such terms have been produced and constrained within such regimes, they ought to be repeated in directions that reverse and displace their originating aims.
>
> (1993, p. 123)

However, so long as women and men are denied an unequivocally real existence, we will have neither reliable nor credible criteria for judging when it is appropriate and strategic to invoke their names and not. As Alcoff argues, 'a claim can only be taken seriously – and thus have its strategic effect – when it is taken as truth in a real and not merely strategic sense' (2001, p. 323). In the following I draw on the philosophical framework of critical realism[7] in order to show how we might think of the category 'women' as real without the implications of essentialism, homogenisation or ethnocentrism.

The concrete and the abstract

Sayer, a critical realist sociologist, notes that, in popular usage, the adjective 'abstract' often refers to something vague, esoteric and 'removed from reality' (1992, p. 87). However, besides being essential to theoretical activity in the qualified sense, abstractions are actually an inevitable part of our most mundane dealings with the everyday world. What, then, is an abstraction? It may be illuminating to have a close look at a passage in Spelman's Inessential Woman. Aimed at revealing the absurdity of talking about women simply as women, Spelman invokes a line by the American author Gwendolyn Brooks: 'The juice from tomatoes is not called merely *juice*. It is always called *tomato* juice' (cited in Spelman, 1990, p. 186; emphasis in the original). Now, little effort is needed to disqualify this statement, for it is certainly not the case that we always call tomato juice 'tomato juice'. Sometimes – and appropriately so – we call it 'juice', sometimes 'drink', and occasionally even 'liquid'. One might also hold that it is utterly important to distinguish between a branded and boxed tomato juice and freshly made tomato juice, arguing that subsuming these under the same category would be a serious simplification of reality. The simple truth is that all these words are valid ways of calling attention to the qualities of the concrete object 'tomato juice', but that they all operate on different levels of abstraction, which place the tomato juice in different categories. As Bertell Ollman puts it, abstraction operates 'like a microscope that can be set at different degrees of magnification' (2001, p. 292). Which level of abstraction we choose depends on which aspect of reality we wish to call attention to, in turn depending on the reasons for the calling of this attention.[8]

Neither in everyday life nor in scientific practice can the truth about something be simply translated into one concept or the other, for our conceptualisations are always determined by the problem that made us approach a thing in the first place. As Ollman emphasises, 'it is essential, in order to understand any particular problem, to abstract to a level of generality that brings the characteristics chiefly responsible for the problem into focus' (2001, p. 293). If we want to explain, for example, a person's experience of discrimination, we normally do not draw attention to the fact that the discriminated person is a mammal or a Libra, while the fact that she is a woman and an immigrant will probably be held to be more significant. This judgement depends on our theories – academic or intuitive, explicit or implicit – about the nature of zoological, astrological, gendered and racial structures, which operate relatively autonomously from each other in spite of their unification in the specific person and situation at hand.

The word 'concrete' stems from the Latin concrescere, meaning 'grow together'. Sayer notes that this etymology 'draws attention to the fact that objects are usually constituted by a combination of diverse elements or forces' (1992, p. 87). Karl Marx puts it in a similar way: '[t]he concrete is concrete because it is the concentration of many determinations, hence unity in the diverse' (1993, p. 101). The term 'abstract', for its part, originates from the Latin abstrahere, meaning 'draw away', referring to the activity of 'drawing away' certain aspects from the concrete whole. As Sayer puts it:

> an abstract concept, or an abstraction, isolates in thought a one-sided or partial aspect of an object. What we abstract from are the many other aspects which together constitute concrete objects such as people, economics, nations, institutions, activities and so on.
>
> (1992, p. 87)

If tomato juice is a composite matter, people are even more complex, not the least since they have the capacity to reflect upon and change the conditions of their own being. However, recognising that people are continuously constituted by a range of diverse determinations, which themselves constantly change and which people's self-reflective agency can counteract, is not valid grounds for disqualifying efforts to sort out these determinations. We can talk about 'women' without thereby assuming that 'women' is the only thing that these persons are, or that 'woman' is a fixed category. By its very definition, the method of abstracting presumes that the concrete totality from which one abstracts is not exhausted by the abstracted element. Berth Danermark et al. emphasise that 'abstractions are not there in order to *cover* complexity and variation in life; they are there in order to *deal* with just that' (2002, p. 42; emphasis in original).

If we acknowledge that abstract concepts, such as 'women', are qualitatively different from lived reality, we can seek to use them effectively without any expectation that they will correspond to this lived reality in any clear-cut sense. As Sayer (1992) stresses, abstractions are not problematic as such; the danger lies in making false abstractions (such as 'woman is goodness') or in not taking abstractions for what they are (that is, treating them as if they gave a total picture). Nira Yuval-Davis (2006) points out the crucial fact that differences between people cannot be understood simply as a matter of identity, since they are based in social structures which are autonomous from each other and reside on a level distinct from that of our concrete embodiment and experience. Spelman and Brown are right that there are no discrete racial, gender and class parts at the level of concrete identity; nevertheless, the structures of race, gender and class have distinct existences in so far as they exercise their causal force on our lives in ways relatively independent from each other. One of the great merits of abstraction is that it is an indispensable tool for identifying structures of this kind. Indeed, we can obtain knowledge of structures only in so far as we experience their effects on an empirical level. Yet, the intellectual recognition of a gender-specific power structure was not based on any kind of straightforward discovery of an empirical entity called patriarchy, but on the creative development of new modes of abstracting certain invisible but pervasive features from the concrete reality that we could measure, observe and feel. No matter how different women's lives were, what feminists put their fingers on was that there was something quite disadvantageous about all women's lives and that this something had to do with their being women.

Structures, positions and people

If womanhood is typically thought of as a reified property contained in each female individual, the tools of critical realism allow for a radically different understanding. According to the critical realist perspective, people exist only by virtue of the relations and forces that constitute them, through the medium of structural positions. For Douglas Porpora,

> [s]ocial structures are systems of human relationships among social positions which shape certain structured interests, resources, powers, constraints and predicaments that are built into each position by the web of relationships and which comprise the material circumstances in which people must act and which motivate them to act in certain ways.
>
> (1998, pp. 343–344)

Because of their enabling, constraining and motivating power, our structural positions make us able and inclined to act in specific ways and likely to suffer certain things. The position as woman will make its occupant apt to act in ways commonly understood as feminine and experience things that males do not tend to experience. She will tend to earn less than her male colleagues, since those who decide her wages are in positions motivating them to discriminate against women, and in order to promote her short-term interests she will be motivated to dress in feminine clothes. Breaking with these structural tendencies is likely to cause suffering in the short run (Porpora 1998).

However, and importantly, people's actions and experiences are not predetermined by or reducible to the tendencies inherent in their positions. Thus, stating that women share a common position as women is not the same as maintaining that women are the same. The reason is twofold. Firstly, people have a certain amount of freedom vis-à-vis their positions in virtue of their reflexivity: 'we can interpret the same material conditions and statements in different ways and hence learn new ways of responding, so that effectively we become different kinds of people' (Sayer 1992, p. 123). This is what makes it possible for us to act back upon and change the constellation of relations of which we are made up. Secondly, as intersectional theorists point out, women and men as concrete individuals are never simply women and men. We exist only by virtue of our positions in an array of overlapping structures on different levels of reality. It is through these multiple determinations that we become unique and complex individuals. The important and simple point that I want to make is that this multiple positioning is not the same as no positioning. Although women and men are more than women and men, they are still women and men.[9]

Conceptualising women as those who occupy the position as woman is thus very different from reifying, homogenising and essentialising accounts of women. From this perspective, instead,

> [t]o speak of what women and men are is … actually to speak about the social conditions in and on which they act. Thus, the attempt to conceptualise what women and men are does not necessarily imply any kind of mysterious essentialism or biological reductionism.
>
> (Jónasdóttir 1994, p. 220)

It is crucial to note, however, that although the identity and experience of a woman cannot be reduced to her position as woman, the relation between the gendered position and its occupant is not one of disconnection and arbitrariness, as Mohanty suggests (2003, p. 19). The womanhood or 'womanness' emerging from the position as woman is a real feature of women, whether they wish it or not. This is because people are what they are by virtue of the assembly of relations – biological, economic, cultural – that constitute them. In this sense, as put by Mikael Carleheden, '[t]o find one's identity is to be able to relate to one's historical situatedness' (2003, p. 57). Although I have not chosen my position as woman, I can only be the one I am by means of this position (amongst others). This is why it is so problematic not to recognise the reality of women's 'womanness', however much we disapprove politically of the gendered structure by virtue of which we emerge as women. Through collective struggle we may be able to change the very structure of which our position as women is part, but without a category that can take this positioning into account, such a struggle will not be possible. The problem with the post-structuralist tendency to downplay the realness of 'women' as collective category is that it rules out conceptualisations of the material relation between a woman's life and her structural gender position. As opposed to Mohanty, who distinguishes between '"women"' as a discursively constructed group and "women" as material subjects of their own history' (2003, pp. 22–23; emphasis added), from the critical realist point of view the group of women has just as material an existence as individual women, in so far as the people belonging to the group are intrinsically tied to a common position in a materially (and discursively) constituted gender structure.

Conclusion

As many intersectional feminists have pointed out, understanding the life of a particular person is not a mechanical matter of 'adding' the 'contents' of the different positions that constitute her. Theorising is a messy and never clear-cut project, taking place in the dialectic between the concrete and the abstract, the subjective and the objective, the specific and the general, and not the least between the fundamentally processual character of concrete reality and the irredeemably static quality of the words and signs which we employ to understand and explain it. We can never single out gender from, for example, race and class in any neat and absolute way, since these structures are in constant transformation and only relatively autonomous from each other. Gender is not a global monolith, but must be studied and theorised in all its local variations. Nevertheless, it is possible to think of women as a group on a global level, because although the gender structure looks different in different locations, it possesses so much internal coherence so as to deserve to be thought of as one (differentiated) whole.[10] As Jónasdóttir puts it, women's commonality has to be thought of as very 'thin' and cannot be transferred to the empirical level in any direct sense. This thin commonality implies neither a common experience nor a unified struggle, but it entails 'a common *basis* for experience and thus a common *basis* for struggle' (1994, p. 41; emphasis added). The reason why it would be fatal to leave 'women' behind as a feminist category of analysis is that we need it to denote women's specific relation to a gender structure the properties of which we may only then struggle to define. We should, indeed, continue to deconstruct deterministic and essentialist notions of what it means to be man or woman, but such negative relating to gendered categories can never be exhaustive of feminist theorising.

Notes

1 This chapter was originally published as Lena Gunnarsson, "A defence of the category 'women'", *Feminist Theory* (12, no. 1) pp. 23–27. © 2011, Sage. DOI: 10.1177/1464700110390604
2 Gender, Sexuality, and Global Change, Conference of Workshops arranged by GEXcel Centre of Gender EXcellence, Örebro University, Sweden, 22–25 May 2008.
3 While my focus here is the tendency to emphasise difference at the cost of similarity, Carolyn Pedwell draws attention to the equally questionable 'temptation to substitute problematic "difference" with problematic "sameness"' (2008, p. 91) which is at work in some feminists' cross-cultural comparisons between, for example, female genital cutting and cosmetic surgery.
4 My translation.
5 Butler makes no distinction between sex and gender, since she refutes the claim that there is a biological reality relatively autonomous from discourse.
6 Jónasdóttir and Jones also point out how post-structuralist rhetoric uses 'a politically charged language to establish that feminist theoretical concepts were not only analytic heuristics but also were ideologically constructed ontological categories defining an "essential" being of woman/women' (2009, p. 34).
7 Critical realism is a philosophical framework, developed by Roy Bhaskar, which is critical of both positivism and postmodernism. One of its crucial tenets is the distinction between ontological and epistemological questions. Another important feature is the stratified and differentiated view of reality wherein entities, aspects and levels of reality are seen as distinct and irreducible albeit co-constitutive of each other (Archer et al., 1998; Danermark et al., 2002).
8 For example, if I have walked through a desert for ten hours without drinking, the most significant aspect of the tomato juice would probably be that it is a drink. An expert on tomato juice who is searching for the best tomato juice in the country, however, would most likely feel motivated to set the microscope at a much larger degree of magnification.
9 By this I do not mean that all people are either men or women in any unambiguous sense; what I claim is that those who are, are so in spite of the fact that there being men or women is not exhaustive of what they are and although these identities are not fixed.
10 The notions of 'differentiated totalities' and 'unity in difference' are crucial for critical realism (Bhaskar, 2008).

References

Alcoff, L. M. 2001. "Who's afraid of identity politics?," in P. M. L. Moya and M. R. Hames-García (eds.) *Reclaiming Identity: Realist Theory and the Predicament of Postmodernism*, pp. 312–344. Hyderabad: Orient Longman.

Alcoff, L. M. 2006. *Visible Identities: Race, Gender and the Self.* London: Oxford University Press.

Archer, M., R. Bhaskar, A. Collier, T. Lawson and A. Norrie (eds.). 1998. *Critical Realism: Essential Readings*. London: Routledge.

Bhaskar, R. 2008 *Dialectic: The Pulse of Freedom*, 2nd edition. London and New York: Routledge.

Brown, W. 1997. "The impossibility of women's studies." *Differences: A Journal of Feminist Cultural Studies* 9(3): 79–101.

Butler, J. 1993. *Bodies that Matter: On the Discursive Limits of 'Sex'.* New York: Routledge.

———.1999. *Gender Trouble: Feminism and the Subversion of Identity*, 2nd edition. New York: Routledge.

Carleheden, M. 2003. "The emancipation from gender: A critique of the utopias of postmodern gender theory," in: S. Ervø and T. Johansson (eds.) *Among Men: Moulding Masculinities*. Vol. 1, pp. 44–56. Aldershot: Ashgate.

Collins, P. H. 1990. *Black Feminist Thought: Knowledge, Consciousness, and the Politics of Empowerment*. Boston: Unwin Hyman.

Crenshaw, K. 1991. "Mapping the margins: Intersectionality, identity politics, and violence against women of color." *Stanford Law Review* 43(6): 1241–1279.

Danermark, B., M. Ekström, L. Jacobsen and J. C. H. Karlsson. 2002. *Explaining Society: Critical Realism in the Social Sciences*. London: Routledge.

Davis, K. 2008. "Intersectionality as buzzword: A sociology of science perspective on what makes a feminist theory successful." *Feminist Theory* 9(1): 67–85.

Ferguson, A. 2011. "How is global gender solidarity possible?," in: A. G. Jónasdóttir, K. B. Jones and V. Bryson (eds) *Sexuality, Gender and Power: Intersectional and Transnational Perspectives*. New York: Routledge, 243–258.

Gubar, S. 1998. "What ails feminist criticism?" *Critical Inquiry* 24(4): 878–902.

Halberstam, J. 1994. "F2M: The making of female masculinity," in: L. Doan (ed.) *The Lesbian Postmodern*, pp. 210–228. New York: Columbia University Press.

Hemmings, C. 2005. "Telling feminist stories." *Feminist Theory* 6(2): 115–139.

hooks, b. 1981. *Ain't I a Woman? Black Women and Feminism*. Boston, MA: South End Press.

Hull, C. 2006. *The Ontology of Sex: A Critical Inquiry into the Deconstruction and Reconstruction of Categories*. London: Routledge.

Jónasdóttir, A. G. 1994. *Why Women are Oppressed*. Philadelphia: Temple University Press.

Jónasdóttir, A. G. and Jones K. B. 2009. "Out of epistemology: Feminist theory in the 1980s and beyond," in A. G. Jónasdóttir and K. B. Jones (eds.) *The Political Interests of Gender Revisited*, pp. 17–57. Manchester: Manchester University Press.

Lykke, N. 2007. "Intersektionalitet pa svenska," in: B. Axelsson and J. Fornäs (eds.) *Kulturstudier i Sverige*, pp. 131–148. Lund: Studentlitteratur.

McCall, L. 2005. "The complexity of intersectionality." *Signs: Journal of Women in Culture and Society* 39(3): 1771–1800.

Marx, K. 1993. *Grundrisse: Foundations of the Critique of Political Economy*. Harmondsworth: Penguin.

Mohanty, C. T. 1988. "Under western eyes: Feminist scholarship and colonial discourses." *Feminist Review* 30 (Autumn): 61–88.

———.2003. *Feminism without Borders: Decolonizing Theory, Practicing Solidarity*. Durham, NC: Duke University Press.

New, C. 2005. "Sex and gender: A critical realist approach." *New Formations* 56(Autumn): 54–70.

Ollman, B. 2001. "Critical realism in light of Marx's process of abstraction," in J. López and G. Potter (eds.) *After Postmodernism: An Introduction to Critical Realism*, pp. 285–298. New York: Athlone Press.

Pedwell, C. 2008. "Weaving relational webs: Theorizing cultural difference and embodied practice." *Feminist Theory* 9(1): 87–107.

Porpora, D. 1998. "Four concepts of social structure," in M. Archer, R. Bhaskar, A. Collier, T. Lawson and A. Norrie (eds.) *Critical Realism: Essential Readings*, pp. 339–355. London: Routledge.

Sayer, A. 1992. *Method in Social Science: A Realist Approach*. London: Routledge.

———.1997. "Essentialism, social constructionism, and beyond." *Sociological Review* 45(3): 453–487.

———.2000. *Realism and Social Science*. London: SAGE.

Spelman, E. 1990. *Inessential Woman: Problems of Exclusion in Feminist Thought*. London: Women's Press.

Spivak, G. C. 2006. *In Other Worlds: Essays in Cultural Politics, new edition*. London: Routledge.

Young, I. M. 1994. "Gender as seriality: Thinking about women as a social collective." *Signs: Journal of Women in Culture and Society* 19(3): 713–738.

Yuval-Davis, N. 2006. "Intersectionality and feminist politics." *European Journal of Women's Studies* 13(3): 193–209.

Zack, N. 2005. *Inclusive Feminism: A Third Wave Theory of Women's Commonality*. Lanham, MD: Rowman & Littlefield.

5 Gender theory non-conforming

Critical realist feminism, trans politics, and affordance theory

Angela Martinez Dy

Introduction

Over the course of the twentieth century, several different waves of feminism have conceptualised gender and defined womanhood in divergent ways. They thereby created tensions that are still at the core of political controversies over gender today. Pioneering feminist theory engaged with historical materialism to conceptualise gender – or, as it was called at the time, sex roles – as a systemic function of patriarchal oppression in which biology functioned as the origin of inequality between the sexes (Davis 1981; de Beauvoir 1989; Firestone 1979). Female biology, prior to birth control, was understood as maintaining women's subordination to, and dependency upon, men (Firestone 1979). This structuralist view, echoed in science that focused on biological contributions to sex difference – sex hormones and their effects on the mammalian brain in particular (Risman and Davis 2013) – was followed by a move towards post-structuralist feminism, which rejected normative assumptions about the body and explicitly rejected ontology and materiality. Contemporary feminism and gender studies are dominated by such post-structuralist perspectives (Gunnarsson et al. 2016). Both structuralist and post-structural feminism constituted, in their time, radical and reasonable responses to the ways in which hegemonic notions of nature, biology and sexual difference have been used to dominate and suppress women (New 2005, ch. 3 this volume), as well as queer sexualities (Butler 1990), throughout history. The outcome of this theoretical trajectory was an interactionist framework that still holds today, in which the structural, systemic aspects of gender have moved to the background, and gender is understood primarily as an individualised, enacted performance that is constantly 'done' (Lorber 1994; West and Zimmerman 1987).

This process of arriving at a methodologically individualistic view of gender was arguably facilitated by Judith Butler's seminal post-structuralist work on gender performativity (1986, 1990, 1993). Butler persuasively deconstructed both sex and gender by questioning the epistemology of sex (1986, p. 39) by asserting that the biological foundations upon which it was assumed to be based were gendered from the outset, and highlighting the primacy of self-situation within discourses in the formation and maintenance of gender (1990).

Furthermore, her 'queering' (Honeychurch 1996) of feminist theory called important attention to the ways in which non-heterosexual forms of sexuality are suppressed through heteronormativity, and how normative expectations for both gender and sexuality are discursively constructed and socially enforced to serve existing political and economic structures (Butler 1997). Although substantive critiques have tackled her underdeveloped engagement with trans issues (Namaste 1996) and elision of the material aspects of human nature (Gunnarsson 2014), Butler's claim that 'gender … promises to proliferate into a multiple phenomenon for which new terms must be found' (1986, p. 47) – later echoed by trans activist Kate Bornstein (1995) – arguably set the theoretical scene for contemporary gender politics, trans theory, and the myriad gender identities that are in use today (Sparkes 2014).

I note that a key point of intersection for feminist and trans theory and politics (Heyes 2003; Kollman and Waites 2009; Namaste 2015), which clearly underpins trans feminist work (Namaste 1996, 2015; Serano 2013), is the aim to transform misogynistic gender norms that oppress women. This is certainly possible because, like any social structure, gender systems are culturally contextual and change over time. Yet I argue that this laudable aim is undermined by the extant philosophical underpinnings upon which much contemporary feminist, and, by extension, gender studies, queer and trans theory, is based. In particular, the post-structuralist inclination towards voluntarism and methodological individualism has inhibited the adequate theoretical development of two key aspects of the human experience of gender: first, embodiment (Gunnarsson 2013, 2014) and second, the relation between structure and agency (Martinez Dy et al. 2014). To illustrate, Risman and Davis (2013, p. 740) observe that West and Zimmerman (1987) and Butler (1990) share a similar 'focus on [the] creation of gender by the activity of the actor', but that they 'differ on the ontological reality of the possibility of a self, outside the discursive realm'. Influenced by Nietzsche and Foucault, Butler asserts that there is no 'doer behind the deed' (1990, p. 33). This eschewing of the notion of a relatively autonomous agential subject with its own causal powers (Gunnarsson 2014, p. 30) reflects an unresolved tension in Foucault's work between determinist and voluntarist tendencies (McNay 1999, p. 97). Moreover, not only does the Butlerian conception of gender absent the human agent, but – as Lena Gunnarsson notes – its prioritisation of the discursive also fails to recognise 'any structure or directionality inherent in biology and matter' (2014, p. 41). It is precisely in this space, where agential absence and under-theorised structure meet, that we may find a (critical) realist conceptualisation of sex and gender most fruitful.

Throughout this chapter, I will use the following three umbrella terms: queer, trans and gender non-conforming (GNC) to refer to related but distinct populations who reject normative assumptions regarding gender and/or sexual orientation. I define these terms below. I echo previous work that considers sexual orientation, sexuality, gender identity, and structural discrimination on these bases inextricably bound together (Schilt and Westbrook 2009); as such, while my discussion focuses primarily on issues of gender identity, I make conceptual links to issues of sexual orientation. I also use the word and prefix cis, used by both activists and feminist scholars to refer to people who do not identify as trans (Bettcher 2007; McKinnon 2014; Namaste 1996; Serano 2013); though it is a contested term, I use it purposefully, in order to 'shift the object of analysis from the margins to the centre' (Schilt and Westbrook 2009, p. 441). I do not suggest that cis people are in any way necessarily more comfortable with their biological sex or their gender identity then are trans people, only that they do not identify as trans. Following Katrina Roen's (2001) admonishment of attempts to theorise about transgender issues across cultures, I also note my discussions are based specifically in the Anglo-American context.[1]

A formerly derogatory term, being 'queer' was once denigrated. In the 1990s, the term was reclaimed such that today, 'queer people' is a culturally acceptable way to refer to diverse groups of non-heterosexual people (Rand 2014). Its use suggests an implicit critique of heteronormativity and a foregrounding of alternative and ambiguous sexualities (Driskill et al. 2011), including lesbians, gays, bisexuals, asexuals and pansexuals. Because gender identity is distinct from sexual orientation, trans and GNC people may or may not be queer; nevertheless, I highlight an alignment between queer and trans/GNC political stances as well as a shared history (such as in the 1969 Stonewall Riots that launched the modern gay liberation movement). My use of the terms 'trans' and 'transgender' describes people whose 'internally felt sense of core gender identity does not correspond to their assigned sex at birth or in which they were raised' (MacDonald 1998, p. 5), while 'GNC' refers to people who 'do not follow other people's ideas or stereotypes about how they should look or act based on the sex they were assigned at birth' (SRLP 2017). Included in the GNC category are people who identify as, for example, non-binary, agender, genderfluid, and genderqueer. These usages are not intended to suggest that gender is constrained to individual identity or expression, but refers instead to how structural gender norms are interpreted at the individual level. Finally, biologically intersex people tend to be included in discussions of gender nonconformity, although not always to their agreement. Although estimates of their numbers differ greatly, an accepted figure is somewhere between one third of a per cent to 1 per cent of live births (Ainsworth 2015; Elder-Vass 2012, p. 132; Hull 2006). Together, these populations are often referred to by the acronym LGBT(Q) or, in longer form, LGBTQQIAAP (Schulman 2013). There are, of course, critiques of the ever-growing umbrella acronym, in particular from people who desire greater distinction between issues of sexual orientation and gender identity. While the size of these populations is difficult to measure, a recent study suggests that LGBT people in the US comprise 4 per cent of the population, or 9 million people (Gates 2011).

For much of the mainstream public, the sex-gender distinction and debates over its usefulness (Edwards 1989; Gatens 1983; Oakley 1972; Walsh 2004) are not a significant matter of concern; Moira Gatens notes, for instance, that in the public imagination 'sex' still refers primarily to sexual intercourse while 'gender' is almost a synonym for women, 'as if men don't have a gender'

(Walsh 2004). Yet, the population of people who identify as queer, trans or GNC is growing, both in size and social recognition. In contrast, the social acceptance of these populations appears to be systemically inhibited and canonical understandings of gender are still primarily binaristic and heteronormative in nature (Schilt and Westbrook 2009). Some small changes have occurred; for example, the shift in mainstream usage from the term 'sex' on institutional forms and documents and the like to 'gender'. However, this change is by no means universal. The available options are still usually limited to male or female. While this step is in itself not indicative of any social progress towards inclusivity, however, it illustrates what I perceive as a problematic social conflation between sex – a biological reality – and gender, which today functions at the individual level as a kind of discursive category, into which one can opt-in or out. In this regard, activism in support of trans and GNC people has had some notable effects: for example, in 2017, the US States of Oregon and California as well as Canada have added a gender-neutral option to some legal documents, such as health cards, driving licenses, and birth certificates (BBC 2017; Caron 2017; Sylvester 2017).

Rethinking and reconfiguring (hetero) normative understandings of sex and gender is clearly of critical importance both for queer, trans, and GNC communities and those who support them. At the same time, Butler's assertion that 'queer politics is regularly figured by the orthodoxy as the cultural extreme of politicization' (1997, p. 38) is equally as relevant as ever. The decades-long fight for gay marriage has slowly been won in some countries and continues to be hotly debated worldwide, even within nations themselves (Ball 2015; PRC 2017). Currently, across the US, widespread controversy over so-called 'bathroom bills' that limit access to public toilets for transgender individuals (Kralik 2017) have been a synecdochical example of the way in which trans politics and, by association, trans people are continually rejected by the mainstream. While some of the actors in the 'bathroom debate' were doubtlessly driven by conservative ideas on sexuality and gender, however, there was another, radical feminist stream of criticism concerning the shift from sex-based rights to gender-based rights as well. The organisers of the Michigan Women's Festival, for instance, came under attack for what were perceived as their transphobic policies, and the festival was eventually forced to shut its doors (Karlan 2014; Ring 2015). The widening demands for inclusivity for, in particular, trans and GNC people, has therefore effectively begun to redraw conceptual boundaries as to who deserves legally protected separate spaces, and why.

Yet, a significant indicator of the persistent structural social and cultural inertia around queer, trans and GNC acceptance is the overwhelming amount of institutional and interpersonal violence they face. In the US, queer people are more likely to be the targets of hate crime than any other minority group (Park and Mykhyalyshyn 2016), while 40 per cent of homeless youth served by agencies identify as LGBT (Durso and Gates 2012). Moreover, the number of transphobic hate crimes reported is on the rise in the UK (Yeung 2016). While this rise in reported crimes does not necessarily imply a rise in committed crimes, the high rates of violence against these marginalised populations is deeply troubling. Intersectional issues, of course, apply, with a high incidence of transmisogyny and transmisogynoir (Durham et al. 2013) meaning that trans women and femmes[2] of colour, especially black trans women from poor and working class backgrounds, are the least protected and comprise most trans murder victims (Adams 2017). While a detailed analysis of the ways race, class, labour, and gender interact in these phenomena is necessary to fully understand its dimensions (Namaste 2015, p. 20). Butler's argument that living outside of established gender norms makes it impossible to exist in a 'socially meaningful sense' (1986, p. 41) seems relevant here: social meaning regarding gender appears to remain bound to extant categories, with non-conformists disciplined for their boundary crossing (Schilt and Westbrook 2009). The daily exclusion and violence enacted upon trans bodies (Kidd and Witten 2008) speaks to these conclusions. Although trans people continually reject victimhood and ingeniously find individual and collective ways to live meaningful lives, their continued structural marginalisation is undeniable (Mock 2014; Namaste 2015).

At the same time, the persistent gender binary that privileges men over women, and the masculine over the feminine, has countless negative implications for all people but especially women and femmes. Misogynist violence against girls and women plagues societies around the globe (Garcia-Moreno et al. 2005); as such, it presents an equally important set of challenges driving the feminist project forward. As I believe that these concerns are also at the root of the social inertia around trans issues, following the lead of trans feminist theorists and thinkers (Namaste 2015; Serano 2013) this chapter will outline what I perceive as a space for alliances between movements for trans liberation and feminist agendas (Heyes 2003). While I acknowledge feminist currents that delimit womanhood to biologically female adult bodies, in this chapter I offer a realist view that understands womanhood as an abstraction, distinct from femaleness, such that trans womanhood is a valid gendered subjectivity. In addition, while I take care not to reify trans identity, as transness is not a monolith and all lived experiences will necessarily be intersectional, I note that trans women – particularly those who are poor and/or of colour – are disproportionately socially marginalised and vulnerable to violence. As such, I believe a primary target for both the feminist project and the trans liberation movement should be the elimination of misogyny, as a result of which women and femmes are disproportionately subjected to systemic and interpersonal violence (Heyes 2003; Namaste 2015) on account of their sex and/or gender expression. As a cis, queer, feminist woman, I am thus responding to what Cressida Heyes (2003) calls a responsibility for non-trans feminists to consider trans issues in light of what has historically been a relationship of exclusion (Serano 2013).

This pursuit is, naturally, not without obstacles. In addition to the barriers posed by patriarchal and masculinist structural biases in scholarship and society, persistent and often vitriolic tensions between trans and (radical) feminist standpoints have been well documented (Heyes 2003; MacDonald 1998). For the most part, however, these issues are outside the scope of this piece.

Nonetheless, I believe that bringing critical realist tools, complemented by aspects of James Gibson's theory on affordances (Gibson 1977; Heft 1989), to bear on these discussions can help to illuminate points of alignment between trans and mainstream feminist theory. Though space constraints prevent me from elaborating here, I adopt an intersectional perspective, emphasising that we should carefully attend to multiple dimensions of social structures in order to see privilege as well as oppression, and account for those who may be multiply marginalised or excluded from our analyses (Martinez Dy et al. 2014). I have combined these seemingly diverse approaches to assist us in the much-needed development of theory around gender that more accurately reflects the contemporary social world.

Queering (critical) realist feminist gender theory

A small but significant body of work exists on critical realism, gender and feminism (Gunnarsson et al. 2016), but little work has been done to date to develop queer perspectives based on realism rather than post-structuralism (Griffiths 2016). Recent work has attempted to find points of alignment between critical realist social ontology and intersectionality theory (Gunnarsson 2017, ch. 8 this volume; Martinez Dy et al. 2014), feminist standpoint theory (Mussell 2016), and new materialist perspectives such as those based on Karen Barad's (2003, 2007) agential realism (Gunnarsson 2013; Mussell 2016). This work has shown that a unique set of tools – including its depth ontology, its emergentist/stratified account of being, its transfactual understanding of causality, and more – distinguish critical realism from other contemporary realist perspectives. As I will argue, these tools suit it to the particular intellectual project that this chapter undertakes.

I will take a moment here to define and illustrate the CR concepts that are relevant to my argument by building upon previous realist work on sex and gender more generally. The first of these concepts is 'depth ontology'. Critical realism posits that reality is helpfully conceived of in terms of three concentric spheres, the *real* or the *deep*, the *actual*, and the *empirical*. The deep sphere is all-encompassing, and contains all causal powers, mechanisms and entities in the social and natural worlds, including those that are unexercised. The actual, in contrast, contains the sub-category of causal powers/mechanisms that have been triggered and brought into being as events. The empirical, finally, refers to those events that are observed or observable in experience. This multi-dimensional ontology contrasts with other philosophies of science – like positivist forms of empiricism – that posit a flat ontology (Bhaskar 2008). In addition to this, however, it also facilitates a second CR concept, transfactuality, or the function of causal powers independent from empirical regularities (Bhaskar 2008, p. 14). In other words, while a power may not actualise or have empirical effects, this does not negate its existence. Finally, CR's emphasis on the stratification of being suggests that reality consists of interlinked but irreducible levels; specifically, its theorisation of emergence posits that lower levels of reality provide the ontological conditions that are required for higher order levels to exist. Indeed, these higher order levels are conceived of as being both causally/taxonomically irreducible to lower levels and as characterised by qualitative increases in complexity (Danermark et al. 2002).

From this realist standpoint, sex should be understood as ontologically prior to gender, as social/cultural systems are emergent from natural systems (Gunnarsson 2013; New 2005). Notably, the social categories that appear within the system, such as woman or man, and are defined by hegemonic sets of characteristics, beliefs and behaviours grouped under labels like feminine and masculine (Lorber 1994). As such, they are both properties of the individual agent as well as of the social structure (Else-Quest and Hyde 2016).

Intersectional feminism points out that other categories, of which two of the most significant are race/ethnicity and class, can shape the structural manifestations as well as individual expressions of gender systems (Martinez Dy et al. 2014). As social systems, these interlocked structures enable the reproduction (or transformation) of co-constituted hierarchical social relations of power and subjugation (Anthias 2013; Archer 1995; Davis 1981), such as patriarchal oppression, white supremacy and capitalist exploitation. At the individual level, influenced by reflexive agential choices, this process of reproduction or transformation may be more fluid and dynamic, while at the structural level, it is relatively durable, with structures tending to change slowly over time (Archer 1995). This perspective is particularly useful for theory-building regarding not only feminist, but also queer/trans/GNC issues (Namaste 2015; Overall 2009), as it accounts for the existence of a multiplicity of generative mechanisms at all levels of analysis, influencing human tendencies to identify with either hegemonic feminine or masculine gender expressions, which vary from age to age, society to society, and context to context. It also helps to explain the persistent social inertia to the shifting of gender systems, reading it not as an innocent resistance to change, but instead a question of power relationships and a defence of established social hierarchies.

Combining a stratified ontology featuring extreme openness and complexity in higher order levels (New 2005) with the transfactuality of mechanisms means that both heterosexual attraction and the psycho-social alignment of sex with the expected binary gender expression should be understood as tendencies, not invariant empirical regularities, though they may have some biological basis and are thus relatively common. This emergentist view is identified by David Griffiths as a theoretical opening with the potential to 'recognis[e] the material reality of biological sex, but [also] do some of the queer work which is required in order to destabilise the supposedly strict and stable relations between sex, gender and sexuality' (2016, p. 523). Such a dual-pronged approach can usefully contribute to reconciling realist and post-structuralist contributions to understandings of individual gender expression; a gendered subject is thus both 'a changing and multi-dimensional product of social and discursive processes' as well as a real entity 'irreducible to the process of its production' (Gunnarsson 2014, p. 31). This both/and, as opposed to either/or, thinking is characteristic of critical realism's dialectic turn, which has been employed effectively by Gunnarsson in this context (2013) as well as in relation to intersectionality (2017).

In relation to sex and gender, then, critical realism offers an extraordinarily useful toolkit (Martinez Dy et al. 2014; Rouse and Kitching 2016). In general, a critical (as opposed to naive or empirical) realist perspective upholds the sex/gender and man/woman distinctions not as empirical referents, but primarily as abstract analytical categories (Gunnarsson 2011, ch. 4 this volume). The sex categories of male and female are not seen as socially constructed, but instead are what Dave Elder-Vass (2012) terms *approximate cluster kinds*, that have some natural basis and, significantly, the potential for causal efficacy. Though contentious for feminist theory, which is understandably wary of essentialism, this argument is non-typical in that its reliance on CR conceptions of tendencies and transfactuality results in definitions of femaleness and maleness that are extremely broad and inclusive. He states: 'one may be a member of a particular sex by virtue of possessing a complex of interrelated properties that depend on a set of micro-structural features *that tend to be found together ... but are not always found together*' (2012, p. 135, emphasis mine). Using this definition, arguments that object to delineations of femaleness based upon the dominant presence of hormones like oestrogen and progesterone, female reproductive systems, menstruation or secondary sex characteristics by putting forward counter-examples of females with higher than normal levels of testosterone, who have had uteri or breasts removed, or who do not menstruate, fall short. In other words, the observation of exceptions to structures and kinds does not provide evidence that there are no structures or kinds (Hull 2006, p. 109).

Neither is this cluster kind theory contradicted by the existence of intersex people or emerging work on sex as a spectrum (Ainsworth 2015). For, as Elder-Vass explains, although intersex people have existed throughout history 'there seem to be mechanisms in place that make this unusual' (Elder-Vass 2012, p. 135). Carrie Hull similarly argues that intersex people demonstrate the variability of biological kinds; assuming transfactuality, they do not invalidate the existence of deep causal structures tending to produce males and females (2006, p. 110). Furthermore, this viewpoint is consistent with the claims of trans politics that it is indeed ontologically, not simply discursively, possible to alter one's sex[3], at least to a certain extent. As Elder-Vass notes:

> when the micro-structural feature of a particular object that makes it a member of a particular kind changes so far that it leaves the micro-structural range of the kind concerned ...[it] will cease to be a member of that kind. *Individuals may therefore be members of quite different kinds at different times in their life cycle.*
>
> (2012, p. 130, emphasis mine)

This aim is accomplished by trans people to varying degrees, depending on a combination of their desires and resources. However, at the level of biology, it is thus far not possible for one to completely transform from male to female or vice versa – any gender transition must therefore be understood as an approximation, not a full transformation. Thus, a CR (trans)feminist argument for the shifting of gender norms might read as follows: the natural human tendency towards sexual dimorphism produces approximate cluster kinds of male and female that are given meaning and assigned value in human societies. This meaning and value is stabilized in culturally contextual gender systems and maintained through discourses that are grounded in but irreducible to (and hence not determined by) biology. Hegemonic conceptions of gender are grounded in biology, not individually, but structurally and systemically. A central product of current systems is (trans)misogynist gender-based oppression; therefore, this is an obvious site for the possibility of change, offering space for alignment and solidarity between feminist politics and the trans liberation movement.

Yet, as we see in the political struggles over gay marriage and bathroom bills, gender systems are stubbornly resistant to change; this structural inertia is deserving of theoretical attention. Lois McNay (1999) draws upon Bourdieusian concepts of habitus and the field to theorise issues of embodiment and, in this way, provides some realist conceptual ballast for the idea that 'laissez-faire' (Heyes 2003, p. 1113) accounts of gender result from post-structuralist assumptions of voluntarism. Importantly, she highlights how such assumptions are linked to the consumerist ideology of neoliberalism, in which individuals are presumed predominantly agentic, and concepts of social structure are collapsed into notions of choice and identity (Martinez Dy et al. 2014, ch. 6 this volume; Yuval-Davis 2006). McNay argues that 'overemphasis on the emancipatory expressive possibilities thrown up in late capitalism' gives the impression that 'identity, particularly sexual identity, is fully amenable to a process of self-stylization' that fails to consider 'the embeddedness of sexuality in bodily predisposition' (1999, pp. 97–98). It is this grounding in the body, and the 'relatively involuntary, pre-reflexive and entrenched elements in identity' (1999, p. 98) it precipitates, alongside a view of love and sexuality as relational, that has reinvigorated the realist feminist project (Gunnarsson 2011, 2013, 2014). I argue that it also holds explanatory power for theorising trans politics and social and cultural resistance to them; it is my belief that, by theorising about reality more accurately, we can be more authentically inclusive of trans and GNC people. Although considering the structural embodiment of the habitus and the social conditioning of the field may prove a useful future area of development for realist feminists seeking to shift dominant norms around gender, this chapter instead uses the notion of affordances for theorising embodiment and social relationality. Nonetheless, Bourdieusian and critical realist frames are often complementary[4]; for example, both approaches are temporally grounded and open-ended; McNay deems these conceptual pillars necessary 'if change to dominant norms is to be conceived in terms other than total rupture' (1999, p. 102). It is this potential for change in dominant norms over time to which we now turn.

Gender as an affordance system

Affordance theory was first introduced by James Gibson (1977, 1986) in the field of ecological psychology as a way to conceptualise the relationships of animals to their environment. Defined as 'a combination of physical properties of the environment that is uniquely suited to a given animal' (Gibson 1977, p. 79), it highlights the functional meanings of physical features in the environment (Heft 1989) through which animals interact with their surroundings. As action potentials, affordances are merely potentialities, and as such, the actions they enable must be triggered by an intentional actor (Heft 1989; Pozzi et al. 2014); identifying potential actions as real is in keeping with the critical realist depth ontology that posits causal powers, even if unactualised, as part of the domain of the real (Bhaskar 2008). Affordances are bridges between objects and their perceivers, and thus have both objective and subjective qualities: objective in that they are precipitated by some factual property of the object, and subjective in that a perceiver is needed to provide the frame of reference through which the affordance comes into being (Heft 1989; Pozzi et al. 2014). Gibson argues that the concept cuts across the subjective–objective dichotomy (1977, pp. 69–70). The objective aspects of affordances mean that they should be generally available to similar actors: for example, shoes tend to afford humans foot protection while walking or running; tables tend to afford the possibility of setting things down, and doors afford movement from one defined space to another. However, the subjective aspects of affordances mean that their action possibilities will vary with reference to an individual's unique characteristics – as shoes do not fit all feet, no one pair can provide every individual the same quality of affordance, and Alice's experiences in Wonderland illustrate the problems arising from being too large or too small for a particular table or door.

It is my argument that affordance theory can be used to theorise trans experiences of oppression as well as aspects of the structural conditions that foment it, by treating the body as an object that enables or disables particular affordances. In similar ways, affordance theory has been widely deployed in the Information Systems and innovation literatures (Faulkner and Runde 2009; Orlikowski and Scott 2008; Pozzi et al. 2014) to explore how technological artefacts may or may not enable particular action possibilities. Although the theory of affordances is inextricably linked to the capacities and capabilities of the human body (Heft 1989), it is unusual to point to the human body itself as an object that offers affordances to the subject occupying it. Yet, I suggest that this way of thinking offers a means to address aspects of existing feminist theory that limit its usefulness for understanding trans/GNC issues, as discussed above: first, underdeveloped notions of embodiment, and second, unclear relationality between structure and agency. The theory of affordances aligns with a realist perspective in that both offer accounts of meaning that can exist prior to the development of language, symbolisation and categorisation (Costall and Richards 2013, p. 86; Hull 2006). I suggest developing an understanding of the affordances of bodies within gendered social systems – as possibilities for action – may help steer a path between the Scylla of biological or structural determinism and the Charybdis of voluntaristic accounts of sex and gender that fail to consider their emergence from, and embeddedness in, relationships of natural necessity. Such an understanding may also be used to outline potential ways forward towards a queer, trans, and GNC-positive evolution of gender norms.

Faulkner and Runde (2009) identify two key components to affordances: first, the relevance of the physical form and its ontological capacities, and second, the social creation of meaning (2009, p. 443); taking a realist perspective, I will explore these components in turn.

Embodiment

An application of affordance theory to notions of gender begins with the material affordances of the human body. First, the physical form: the causal powers of the living human body arise from its form and the accompanying generative mechanisms, or 'processes in which the parts of the entity interact to produce its powers' (Elder-Vass 2012, p. 17). Basic human causal powers – for example, breathing air, moving, swallowing, interacting with the world via the senses – arise from the chemical, cellular, and physiological mechanisms of the body, and can be enacted from birth. These lower-order powers offer us a biological system of affordances – the action potentials of living on land, taking shelter from inclement weather, nourishing ourselves, and experiencing our surroundings, respectively. However, a higher-order causal power, the ability to speak, exists in potentia and is only realised through continuous contact with other humans (Hull 2006, p. 119); the trained vocal cords and larynx offer us the affordance of verbal communication. Higher-order still is the ability to reproduce, another power that requires contact with other humans to be realised: specifically, contact with the gametes of the opposite sex, offering humans with male reproductive systems the biological affordance of fertilisation, and humans with female reproductive systems the biological affordance of conception, pregnancy, and birth. We share this sexual dimorphism with many other creatures, our evolution most closely resembling that of other complex animals with large neocortexes (Hull 2006). It has causal efficacy, and is not limited to the cultural or discursive realms (Elder-Vass 2012; Hull 2006; New 2005). The biological affordances of sexed bodies, combined with evolutionary processes, produce particular higher order (psychological, social) affordances within gendered systems. As such, they are also culturally and geo-historically specific.

One of the key social affordances humans are offered by our dimorphic bodies is genderability, defined as the action possibility of attaching psychological and social meaning to sexual cluster kind characteristics.[5] This is reflected in Butler's observation that 'Gender seems less a function of anatomy than one of its possible uses' (1986, p. 46). Genderability does not work alone: Caroline New points out that sexual difference is but one of many mechanisms that produce the variety of gender orders that exist and have existed throughout history (2005). Alongside other visual ascriptive characteristics, for example, race, age, or body size, amongst others, the first gender-related affordance one's body enables is intelligibility within gendered social systems, functioning as a central way in which meaning and value is given to one's physicality: this is why the sexing of an infant at birth is such a fundamental component of human experience (Butler 1990). Placed into these specific gendered systems of affordances and socio-sexual behaviours that are emergent from the biological (Gunnarsson 2014), the body itself is the object, or the vehicle, by which particular gendered action possibilities are enabled.

Furthermore, a person whose body has certain characteristics is afforded a cascade of gendered action potentials over the course of their life, where a series of affordances builds on those that precede them (Michael 2000 as cited by Bloomfield et al. 2010).

For example, if one's bodily features tend to correspond to the female cluster kind, the social affordances of being read as a woman for this subject should allow them to enter a public toilet designated for women without expectation of rejection, resistance or violence on the basis of gender incongruence. The affordance of using a public toilet then affords the subsequent action possibility of inhabiting public spaces for more than a few hours at a time without fear, due to the regularity of the physical need to relieve oneself. This affordance would then enable the subject to, for example, go to school, or work with others without hindrance due to the need for a safe toilet facility (Cox 2017).[6] This privilege is, of course, relational; while being 'read' (perceived by another) as a woman is not a privilege in the normative gender binary that privileges men over women, it is a privilege in relation to trans women, who are at risk for violence *because* they wish to be read as women but instead are perceived as errant men. Similarly, when trans men are read as women in men's clothing, they may be subjected to violence for being errant women, while GNC people are subjected to violence for not conforming to the norms associated with their assigned sex. In both cases, the cascades of physical affordances of the body are policed through violence. Using affordances in this manner we can thus theoretically conceptualise key aspects of what trans theorists refer to as cisgender privilege (Serano 2014), or the privilege experienced by people whose individual gender expression appears to correspond to the sex they were assigned at birth. The people have access to similar cascades of affordances to those here described, producing effects at every level of analysis. Such privilege is both relational and transfactually situational, as it may not operate in every situation. Trans people who are able to 'pass' for the gender identity to which they transitioned may even experience cis privilege until a particular marker or tell, say, a voice in a higher or lower register than expected, 'outs' them.

In the original formulation of affordance theory, it is simply the physical characteristics of the object that determine its particular affordances, not the perceiver's mental processes (Gibson 1977; Heft 1989, p. 25) that bestow them. A shoe may still be used for foot protection, or a table for the setting down of items, whether or not the perceiver realises this. However, these objects lack perception of themselves, whereas a living human does not; thus, in our application, the perceiver's mental processes of discernment and selection are crucial. In keeping with the theory, a subject's perception of their own body does not *bestow* affordances per se, but it is nevertheless central to evaluating the attractiveness of various action possibilities, and the emotional responses that would arise through their pursuit. So, in this context, consideration of the subject's socially conditioned, yet reflexive, evaluation of action possibilities (Elder-Vass 2007)[7], and the inner life from which they emerge (Hull 2006, p. 121), is justified. For example, a body with characteristics typical of the male cluster kind is afforded by gender systems the action possibility of wearing boy's or men's clothing, maintaining short hair and otherwise producing masculine gender signals, yet these signals may not feel comfortable or appropriate to the embodied subject, as Janet Mock describes in her memoir of her childhood and adolescence (2014).

Structure and agency: natural, canonical and designed affordances

It may be countered that the same person, in the body with characteristics typical of the male cluster kind, is still technically afforded the action possibility of wearing clothing designated for girls or women, as Janet Mock describes doing in her teenage years (2014). Yet strict gender norms foreclose the possibility of some affordances that are technically available at the physiological level (Janet could potentially wear any skirt that fit her body), but at the social level, in some situations, are made unavailable (her high school principal would send her home if she wore skirts, telling her they were inappropriate for boys, causing her to miss school and be further punished for it). Thus, a natural affordance of the body, to wear any clothing that physically covers it, may be superseded by what affordance theorists would understand to be 'canonical affordances', or the socially understood and accepted action possibilities for a thing, due to gendered expectations. Similarly, a natural affordance of the body is for socio-sexual interest and pleasure (Gunnarsson 2014) with other people, whether their bodies exhibit characteristics of the same cluster kind, or not (Hull 2006). However, amongst some individuals and societies, this natural affordance is limited by the canonical acceptance as 'valid' only that socio-sexual interest in those people whose bodies are of the opposite cluster kind. This is consistent with Harry Heft's observation that the affordances of the environment, in concert with the body, 'constrain the range of intentional acts that can be expressed' (1989, p. 12). Nonetheless, any object with a canonical affordance still affords other uses and meanings (Costall and Richards 2013, p. 88). These are encapsulated in the term 'designed affordances', or those known to the developer (van Osch and Mendelson 2011) and shared through social processes of meaning-making. For instance, although it is generally accepted that shoes are for wearing, the Arab insult of showing the bottom of a shoe to a disliked person (Gammell 2008) might be read as a designed affordance.

Canonical affordances of gender can and are frequently subverted, and new affordances designed, though this must be done in the context of a durable gender system that, like other social structures, changes slowly, over time (Archer 1995). Structures predate agency, and people reflexively decide to reproduce or transform them through their constellation of concerns and their internal conversations, which enable them to decide upon and pursue particular courses of action (Archer 2007; Elder-Vass 2007). To this end, queer, trans and GNC individuals frequently decide to employ gendering technologies (including, but not limited to, clothing, makeup, hairstyles, hormones, and surgery) to design affordances for their bodies that enable them to move through and/or destabilise hostile gender systems. This is not to say that this process is unproblematic – while individuals may wish to prioritise safety or family continuity through cisgender conformity, they may at the same time be unable or unwilling to do so. Such difficult experiences and the emotional trauma they foment are evidenced by exceptionally high rates of suicide attempts and suicidal ideation amongst trans and GNC people (Haas et al. 2014).

There are now numerous compelling accounts of how to decouple one's biological sex from individual gender expression, thus illustrating how designed affordances of the body can result in more positive outcomes for people who are marginalised by the gender system. Nonetheless, an expectation that trans liberation will be accomplished through individuals essentially designing their own personal genders through technologies, medical and otherwise, is problematically based on post-structuralist and constructivist approaches that presume atomism, ignore relationality and reject notions of structures and kinds, while conceiving of individuals as the 'building blocks of existence' (Hull 2006, p. 119). As mentioned, access to medicalised transitioning technologies, not to mention individual perception of this action possibility, varies greatly; thus, while there is great value in making these technologies, and trans-sensitive medical care in general, more widely available, a push for the trans-positive development of canonical affordances is perhaps even more urgent. Drawing inspiration from the social model of disability (Burchardt 2004), canonical affordances of bodies could be made more gender-neutral. This could help to shift the responsibility away from trans individuals who are currently compelled to alter themselves to fit better into the world towards the acknowledgment of a social responsibility to make our systems more amenable to trans people. Notably, this echoes an early radical feminist aim, which was to eradicate the cultural significance of the sex distinction itself (Firestone 1979).

Mainstream understandings of sex and gender remain embedded in the binary, due to the real causal powers emerging from human dimorphic sexual difference and relationship of natural necessity between female and male cluster kinds (Elder-Vass 2012; Gunnarsson 2014; Hull 2006). Such understandings are not emergent from individual bodies or agents but pre-exist them as part of social structures which shape the internal conversations of agents (Archer 1995,

2007): the action possibilities for a body are thus mediated through the distorting mirror of social structure. Queer, trans and GNC politics seek to disrupt this structure for its constraining and oppressive tendencies, not unlike the feminist project that seeks to counteract the subordination of women within the same structure (queer and trans feminist perspectives, of course, align the two). However, for this to be accomplished, we must counter laissez-faire accounts of gender as something that is determined by atomistic notions of human nature and resist methodological individualism by drawing on the concept of emergence. Further, we should recognise the embeddedness of sex and sexuality in bodies that are malleable only to a certain extent, as well as the structural relationality and relationship of natural necessity between the sexes, which is arguably even less malleable (Heyes 2003; Hull 2006; McNay 1999; New 2005). While there is ideological value in imagining a world in which 'gender is over',[8] Hull persuasively argues that the elaborate nature of the human sexual form conveys a felt sense prior to language, a meaning structured in nature precisely to be understood by other humans (2006, p. 128), and as such, is unlikely to be completely abolished.

Affordance theory, due to its emphasis on relationality, complements a realist perspective in that it reminds us of not only our own relationships to our bodies and the action possibilities provided there, but also our role as agents in our environment (Heft 1989, pp. 3–4). Trans people's accounts have clearly identified both of these as constraining or enabling forces (Cox 2017; Mock 2014; Serano 2013). It is often through other's responses to our self-presentation that structural enablement and constraint is enacted. Gender, along with race, age, ability, body size, and more, contributes to the way the body is 'read' by an observer who decides, often pre-reflexively or involuntarily (McNay 1999) how to treat the other – with sexual interest, friendliness, caution, suspicion, fear, competition, or something else altogether. Ann Costall and Alan Richards suggest that affordances are not confined to actors and objects in isolation, but depend on a constellation that includes events (2013, p. 86); external others must be accounted for in any such constellation. This points to the role of social influences, such as widespread education and positive media representation, in normalising and encouraging acceptance of queer, trans and GNC people.

The value of affordance theory for critical realist feminism

Affordance theory provides a number of conceptual contributions to a critical realist feminist perspective on gender. First, an affordance-based theory allows us to more deeply understand the manifestations of gender at multiple levels of analysis, specifically: the biological/physiological, the psychological, and the social. At the biological level, gender structures the emergent properties of dimorphic sexed bodies via social processes, which carry with them particular physiological affordances in a non-deterministic way (Gunnarsson 2013; Hull 2006; New 2005). Gender is one of many social influences on our physiology, most noticeably upon the neural networks in our plasticine brains (Fine 2010, 2017), and may lead us to seek new psychological and social affordances through the alteration of our physical bodies (Heyes 2009). At the psychological level, gender may usefully be conceived of as a system of affordances (Gibson 1977; Heft 1989), indicating the range of natural, canonical, or designed action possibilities related to the enactment of masculinity or femininity for embodied subjects, as well as the appeal of some over others. At the interpersonal level, it is communicated through a set of signifiers (such as clothes, hair, makeup, vocal register, body carriage and other aspects of self-expression) combined with processes of interpretation that make bodies intelligible to social others, and as such engender particular social affordances. Lastly, at the structural level, gender can be conceptualised as an overarching social stratification structure with multilevel consequences, on par with politics and economics (Risman 2004).

Second, notions of affordance enable an alternative theory of gender that is less reliant upon individual issues of identification, and more aware of available action possibilities. This attention to the affordances offered to different kinds of bodies within social structures can contribute to de-pathologising individuals who conform to, defy, or disrupt gender norms by illustrating the constraints and enablements shaping their possibilities for action, and eventually, paving the way for more structural solutions. Thus, affordance theory holds particular value for the development of a queer and trans feminist realism. It offers a means by which to challenge hetero – and cis-normativity within theory by more accurately reflecting the perspectives of queer and trans people and theorising cis privilege, which, like most privilege, is invisible to those who possess it. Using the language of affordances, we can argue that, generally speaking, trans people's bodies do not afford them the same gendered action possibilities as cis people. Such an analysis explains the motivation of many trans people to transition, no matter the physical, psychological, social or monetary cost. If trans people are unable to access the same simple cascade of affordances as cis people, this justifies the demand for the availability of, for example, gender-neutral toilets, based upon notions of equal treatment and non-discrimination. Furthermore, the notions of natural, canonical and designed affordances helps lend explanatory power to theories on the social inertia around gender norms through illustrating how canonical affordances are contextual and – at least theoretically – open to transformation, yet with a realist acknowledgement of the natural structural relations in which they are embedded.

Third, an affordance-based theory of gender can be used to extend the contributions of a materialist feminist perspective (Gunnarsson 2013), for example by theorising phenomena related to trans and femme labour and relations to capital, which Namaste (2015, p. 21) highlights as a glaring omission in feminist theory. Such an investigation might explore how, due to structural discrimination, the labour affordances for people with trans bodies, especially those of colour and with few resources to medically transition, are dramatically narrowed, leaving sex work as often the most lucrative, if not the only, form of labour available to them (Mock 2014), disproportionately exposing them to violence and disease (Namaste 2015). This could then justify increasing access to trans-positive medical procedures and making the provision of trans-sensitive health care mandatory and widely available, which may expand the portfolio of available labour affordances, not to mention improve mental health outcomes (Durwood et al. 2017). Finally, affordance theory offers new insights into the gendered mechanisms, constraints and enablements acting at all levels of reality and the relationships between them, thereby advancing our efforts to develop explanations of both variability and regularity, such that more equal and inclusive societies can be encouraged (Hull 2006; New 2005).

Future research

There is significant scope for future realist gender research using affordance-based conceptualisations. The first and most obvious for contemporary feminism is using the notion of affordances to develop an intersectional perspective in which gender is but one dimension of intersecting social hierarchies that are causally efficacious in producing nuanced and complex experiences of power, privilege and oppression. Affordance theory provides a useful set of conceptual tools, which, combined with critical realist concepts, can be used to theorise – in an intersectional way – how privilege and oppression may be co-constituted on the subject level, an area that has been identified by intersectionality scholars as underdeveloped (Nash 2008, p. 11). For example, a subject may be privileged with access to some affordances while denied access to others; the shared geohistorical and contextual awareness posited by intersectionality, affordance theory and realist feminism means that these affordances are understood not as static but changeable over space and time. There is also room for deeper exploration of the subject perception of affordances, and how this may factor into reflexive processes of decision-making, thus enabling a fuller conceptualisation of the social conditioning and internal conversations that are enacted in agency (Elder-Vass 2007). We may apply insights from affordance theory to better understand the action possibilities open to people experiencing particular structural conditions, and thus better theorise and empirically investigate the murky area at the point where structure and agency meets: how structural conditions manifest in everyday life (Archer 2007).

Conclusions

Feminist, gender and trans theory are facing a methodological quagmire, as contemporary assumptions of atomism and voluntarism stemming from the post-structuralist legacy clash with social power structures that stubbornly resist individual expressions of choice and agency in relation to sexuality and gender. This chapter has drawn upon the critical realist theoretical toolkit to explain some of the persistent structural and cultural inertia inhibiting the transformation of gender norms, and argued for an affordance-based theory of gender that explicitly addresses extant theoretical gaps around embodiment, structure and agency. In so doing, it offers a novel theoretical framework in which canonical affordances not based in relationships of natural necessity can be identified, critiqued, and intentionally redesigned, moving us towards a world in which gender, if not 'over', simply matters less, so that a fairer and more just society can emerge.

Notes

1 A predominantly Western, individualistic perspective, with its clear distinction between sexuality and gender, and specific labelling of categories, may be rejected by people from non-Western or indigenous cultures that may possess alternative, often more relational, concepts of gender, sexuality, and social identity (Roen 2001).
2 People identifying with traditional femininity.
3 Similar arguments that have recently been made for the viability of trans-racial individuals, I contend, do not hold, for the notion of the human species being divided into various racial kinds has long been scientifically disproven (New 2005; Omi and Winant 1994). This position and the historical context it emphasises is discussed thoroughly by Cressida Heyes (2003, pp. 1102–1103; 2009). However, this remains a highly divisive subject for feminist philosophy, evident in a recent controversy within the discipline regarding an article published in the feminist theory journal Hypatia (Schuessler 2017).
4 Elder-Vass (2007) draws together the Bourdieusian focus on habitus and the role of social conditioning with Margaret Archer's work on reflexive deliberation, arguing that they can be reconciled in a single emergentist theory of human action; this may be another productive area for future theoretical development regarding how gender structures are enacted by individuals.
5 I attach no moral judgment to this possibility but note that the similar conditions that produced racialisability have historically been used to cause the pain and suffering of countless racialised groups and individuals.
6 I note here that Laverne Cox, Julia Serano and Janet Mock are activist authors and not academic philosophers. This is not to discredit them, but simply to point out their writings are motivated neither by academic nor explicitly philosophical aims.
7 Elder-Vass (2007) draws together the Bourdieusian focus on habitus and the role of social conditioning with Margaret Archer's work on reflexive deliberation, arguing that they can be reconciled in a single emergentist theory of human action; this may be a productive area for future theoretical development regarding how gender structures are enacted by individuals.
8 A slogan from a contemporary gender abolition project: http://genderisover.com/.

References

Adams, N. 2017. "GLAAD Calls for Increased and Accurate Media Coverage of Transgender Murders." *GLAAD*. Available at: www.glaad.org/blog/glaad-calls-increased-and-accurate-media-coverage-transgender-murders.

Ainsworth, C. 2015. "Sex Redefined." *Nature*, 518. Available at: www.nature.com/news/sex-redefined-1.16943.

Anthias, F. 2013. "Hierarchies of Social Location, Class and Intersectionality: towards a Translocational Frame." *International Sociology* 28(1): 121–138.

Archer, M. 1995. *Realist Social Theory: the Morphogenetic Approach*. Cambridge: Cambridge University Press.

———. 2007. *Making our Way Through the World*. Cambridge: Cambridge University Press.

Ball, M. 2015. "How Gay Marriage Became a Constitutional Right." *The Atlantic*. Available at: www.theatlantic.com/politics/archive/2015/07/gay-marriage-supreme-court-politics-activism/397052/.

Barad, K. 2003. "Posthumanist Performativity: toward an Understanding of How Matter Comes to Matter." *Signs: Journal of Women in Culture and Society* 28(3): 801–831.

———. 2007. *Meeting the Universe Halfway: Quantum Physics and the Entanglement of Matter and Meaning*. Durham: Duke University Press.

BBC. 2017. "Canadian Baby 'First without Gender Designation' on Health Card." *BBC News*. Available at: www.bbc.co.uk/news/world-us-canada-40480386.

Bettcher, T.M. 2007. "Evil Deceivers and Make-Believers: on Transphobic Violence and the Politics of Illusion." *Hypatia* 22(3): 43–65.

Bhaskar, R. 2008. *A Realist Theory of Science*. 2nd edition. London: Verso.

Bloomfield, B., Y. Latham and T. Vurdubakis. 2010. "When Is an Affordance? Bodies, Technologies and Action Possibilities." *Sociology* 44(3): 415–433.

Bornstein, K. 1995. *Gender Outlaw: on Men, Women, and the Rest of Us*. New York: Vintage.

Burchardt, T. 2004. "Capabilities and Disability: the Capabilities Framework and the Social Model of Disability." *Disability & Society* 19(7): 735–751.

Butler, J. 1986. "Sex and Gender in Simone De Beauvoir's Second Sex." *Yale French Studies* 72: 35–49.

———. 1990. *Gender Trouble: Feminism and the Subversion of Identity*. New York, NY: Routledge.

———. 1993. *Bodies that Matter*. New York and London: Routledge.

———. 1997. "Merely Cultural." *Social Text* 52–53: 33–44.

Caron, C. 2017. "Californians Will Soon Have Nonbinary as a Gender Option on Birth Certificates." *New York Times*. Available at: www.nytimes.com/2017/10/19/us/birth-certificate-nonbinary-gender-california.html.

Costall, A. and A. Richards. 2013. "Canonical Affordances: The Psychology of Everyday Things," in P. Graves-Brown, R. Harrison and A. Piccini (eds.) *The Oxford Handbook of the Archaeology of the Contemporary World*. pp. 82–93. Oxford: Oxford University Press.

Cox, L. 2017. "Laverne Cox: bathroom Bills 'Criminalize Trans People' And No One Is Talking About It." *Media Matters*. Available at: www.mediamatters.org/video/2017/02/14/laverne-cox-bathroom-bills-criminalize-trans-people-and-no-one-talking-about-it/215336.

Danermark, B., M. Ekstrom, L. Ekstrom and J. Karlsson. 2002. *Explaining Society: Critical Realism in the Social Sciences*. London and New York: Routledge.

Davis, A. 1981. *Women, Race and Class*. New York: Random House.

de Beauvoir, S. 1989. *The Second Sex*. New York: Vintage Books.

Driskill, Q.-L., C. Finley, B. J. Gilley and S. L. Morgensen (eds.) 2011. *Queer Indigenous Studies: Critical Interventions in Theory, Politics and Literature*. Tuscon: University of Arizona Press.

Durham, A., B. C. Cooper and S. M. Morris. 2013. "The Stage Hip-Hop Feminism Built: a New Directions Essay." *Signs: Journal of Women in Culture and Society* 38(3): 721–737.

Durso, L. E. and G. J. Gates. 2012. *Serving our Youth: findings from a National Survey of Services Providers Working with LGBT Youth Who are Homeless or At Risk of Becoming Homeless*. Los Angeles.

Durwood, L., K. A. McLaughlin and K. R. Olson. 2017. "Mental Health and Self-Worth in Socially Transitioned Transgender Youth." *Journal of the American Academy of Child and Adolescent Psychiatry* 56(2): 116–123.

Edwards, A. 1989. "The Sex/gender Distinction: has It Outlived Its Usefulness?." *Australian Feminist Studies* 4(10): 1–12.

Elder-Vass, D. 2007. "Reconciling Archer and Bourdieu in an Emergentist Theory of Action." *Sociological Theory* 25(4): 325–346.

———. 2012. *The Reality of Social Construction*. Cambridge: Cambridge University Press.

Else-Quest, N.M. and J. S. Hyde. 2016. "Intersectionality in Quantitative Psychological Research: II. Methods and Techniques." *Psychology of Women Quarterly* 40(3): 319–336.

Faulkner, J. and P. Runde. 2009. "On the Identity of Technological Objects and Users Innovation in Functions." *Academy of Management Review* 34(3): 442–462.

Fine, C. 2010. *Delusions of Gender: How Our Minds, Society, and Neurosexism Create Difference*. New York: W.W. Norton & Company.

Fine, C. 2017. *Testosterone Rex: Unmaking the Myths of Our Gendered Minds*. London: Icon Books.

Firestone, S. 1979. *The Dialectic of Sex: the Case for Feminist Revolution*. London: The Women's Press.

Gammell, C. 2008. "Arab Culture: the Insult of the Shoe." *The Telegraph*. Available at: www.telegraph.co.uk/news/worldnews/middleeast/iraq/3776970/Arab-culture-the-insult-of-the-shoe.html.

Garcia-Moreno, C., L. Heise, H. A. Jansen, M. Ellsberg and C. Watts. 2005. "Violence Against Women." *Science* 310(5752): 1282–1283.

Gatens, M. 1983. "A Critique of the Sex/gender Distinction," in J. Allen and P. Patton (eds.) *Beyond Marxism? Interventions after Marx*. pp. 143–160. Leichhardt, NSW: Intervention Publications.

Gates, G. J. 2011. "How Many People Are Lesbian, Gay, Bisexual, and Transgender?" *The Williams Institute*.

Gibson, J.J. 1977. "The Theory of Affordances," in R. Shaw and J. D. Bransford (eds.) *Perceiving, Acting and Knowing: Toward an Ecological Psychology*. pp. 127–143. Hillsdale, NJ: John Wiley & Sons Inc.

———. 1986. *The Ecological Approach to Visual Perception*. Hillsdale: Lawrence Erlbaum Associates.

Griffiths, D.A. 2016. "Queer Genes: Realism, Sexuality and Science." *Journal of Critical Realism* 15(5): 511–529.

Gunnarsson, L. 2011. "A Defence of the Category 'Women'." *Feminist Theory* 12(1): 23–37.

———. 2013. "The Naturalistic Turn in Feminist Theory: a Marxist-realist Contribution." *Feminist Theory* 14(1): 3–19.

———. 2014. *The Contradictions of Love*. London and New York: Routledge.

———. 2017. "Why We Keep Separating the 'Inseparable': Dialecticizing Intersectionality." *European Journal of Women's Studies* 24(3): 114–127.

———, A. Martinez Dy and M. van Ingen. 2016. "Critical Realism, Gender and Feminism: exchanges, Challenges, Synergies." *Journal of Critical Realism* 15(5): 433–439.

Haas, A.P., P. L. Rodgers and J. L. Herman. 2014. "Suicide Attempts among Transgender and Gender Non-Conforming Adults: findings of the National Transgender Discriminatory Survey." in *American Foundation for Suicide Prevention.*

Heft, H. 1989. "Affordances and the Body - an Intentional Analysis of Gibson Ecological Approach to Visual-Perception." *Journal for the Theory of Social Behaviour* 19 (1): 1–30.

Heyes, C.J. 2003. "Feminist Solidarity after Queer Theory: the Case of Transgender." *Signs: Journal of Women in Culture and Society* 28(4): 1093–1120.

———. 2009. "Changing Race, Changing Sex: the Ethics of Self-Transformation," in L. J. Shrage (ed.) *"You've Changed": sex Reassignment and Personal Identity.* pp. 135–154. New York: Oxford University Press.

Honeychurch, K.G. 1996. "Researching Dissident Subjectivities: queering the Grounds of Theory and Practice." *Harvard Educational Review* 66(2): 339–356.

Hull, C. 2006. *The Ontology of Sex: A Critical Inquiry into the Deconstruction and Reconstruction of Categories.* New York: Routledge.

Karlan, S. 2014. "Michigan Womyn's Music Festival Releases Statement Concerning Trans Women." *Buzzfeed.* Available at: www.buzzfeed.com/skarlan/michigan-womyns-music-festival-releases-statement-concerning?utm_term=.xs4vdQjm8#.to0YyLW2D.

Kidd, J.D. and T. M. Witten. 2008. "Transgender and Trans Sexual Identities: the Next Strange Fruit-Hate Crimes, Violence and Genocide against the Global Trans-Communities." *Journal of Hate Studies* 6(1): 31–63.

Kollman, K. and M. Waites. 2009. "The Global Politics of Lesbian, Gay, Bisexual and Transgender Human Rights: an Introduction." *Contemporary Politics* 15(1): 1–17.

Kralik, J. 2017. "Bathroom Bill Legislative Tracking." *National Conference of State Legislators.* Available at: www.ncsl.org/research/education/-bathroom-bill-legislative-tracking635951130.aspx.

Lorber, J. 1994. *Paradoxes of Gender.* New Haven, CT: Yale University Press.

MacDonald, E. 1998. "Critical Identities: rethinking Feminism through Transgender Politics." *Atlantis: Critical Studies in Gender, Culture & Social Justice* 23(1): 3–12.

Martinez Dy, A., L. Martin and S. Marlow. 2014. "Developing a Critical Realist Positional Approach to Intersectionality." *Journal of Critical Realism* 13(5): 447–466.

McKinnon, R. 2014. "Stereotype Threat and Attributional Ambiguity for Trans Women." *Hypatia* 29(4): 857–872.

McNay, L. 1999. "Gender, Habitus and the Field." *Theory, Culture & Society* 16(1): 95–117.

Mock, J. 2014. *Redefining Realness: my Path to Womanhood, Identity, Love & So Much More.* New York: Atria.

Mussell, H. 2016. "The Truth of the Matter." *Hypatia* 31(3): 537–553.

Namaste, K. 1996. "Tragic Queer: theory's Erasure of Transgender Subjectivity," in B. Beemyn and M. Eliason (eds.) *Queer Studies: a Lesbian, Gay, Bisexual and Transgender Anthology.* pp. 183–203. New York and London: New York University.

Namaste, V. 2015. "Undoing Theory: the 'Transgender Question' and the Epistemic Violence of Anglo-American Feminist Theory." *Hypatia* 24(3): 11–32.

Nash, J.C. 2008. "Re-thinking Intersectionality." *Feminist Review* 89(1): 1–15.

New, C. 2005. "Sex and Gender: a Critical Realist Approach." *New Formations* 56: 54–70.

Oakley, A. 1972. *Sex, Gender and Society.* Ashgate Publishing, Ltd.

Omi, M. and H. Winant. 1994. *Racial Formation in the United States: from the 1960s to the 1990s.* New York: Routledge.

Orlikowski, W.J. and S. V. Scott. 2008. "Challenging the Separation of Technology, Work and Organization." *The Academy of Management Annals* 2(1): 433–474.

Overall, C. 2009. "Sex/Gender Transitions and Life-Changing Aspirations," in L. Schrage (ed.) *'You've Changed': sex Reassignment and Personal Identity.* pp. 11–27. New York: Oxford University Press.

Park, H. and I. Mykhyalyshyn. 2016. "L.G.B.T. People are More Likely to Be Targets of Hate Crimes than Any Other Minority Group." *New York Times.* Available at: www.nytimes.com/interactive/2016/06/16/us/hate-crimes-against-lgbt.html?mcubz=3.

Pozzi, G., F. Pigni and C. Vitari. 2014. "Affordance Theory in the IS Discipline: a Review and Synthesis of the Literature." *Twentieth Americas Conference on Information Systems, Savannah.* 13: 1–12.

PRC. 2017. "Gay Marriage around the World." *Pew Research Center, Religion and Public Life.* Available at: www.pewforum.org/2017/08/08/gay-marriage-around-the-world-2013/.

Rand, E. 2014. *Reclaiming Queer: activist and Academic Resistance.* Tuscaloosa: University of Alabama Press.

Ring, T. 2015. "This Year's Michigan Womyn's Music Festival Will Be the Last." *The Advocate.* Available at: www.advocate.com/michfest/2015/04/21/years-michigan-womyns-music-festival-will-be-last.

Risman, B.J. 2004. "Gender as a Social Structure: theory Wrestling with Activism." *Gender and Society* 18(4): 429–450.

———. and G. Davis. 2013. "From Sex Roles to Gender Structure." *Current Sociology* 61 (5–6): 733–755.

Roen, K. 2001. "Transgender Theory and Embodiment: the Risk of Racial Marginalisation." *Journal of Gender Studies* 10(3): 253–263.

Rouse, J. and J. Kitching. 2016. "Entrepreneurial Practice in Pregnancy: a Framework and Research Agenda." *Academy of Management Proceedings* 1.

Schilt, K. and L. Westbrook. 2009. "Doing Gender, Doing Heteronormativity: 'gender Normals', Transgender People, and the Social Maintenance of Heterosexuality." *Gender and Society* 23(4): 440–464.

Schuessler, J. 2017. "A Defense of 'Transracial' Identity Roils Philosophy World." *New York Times.* Available at: www.nytimes.com/2017/05/19/arts/a-defense-of-trans racial-identity-roils-philosophy-world.html.

Schulman, M. 2013. "Generation LGBTQIA." *The New York Times.* Available at: www.nytimes.com/2013/01/10/fashion/generation-lgbtqia.html?mcubz=3%0A.

Serano, J. 2013. *Excluded.* Berkeley: Seal Press.

———. 2014. "Julia Serano's Compendium on Cisgender, Cissexual, Cissexism, Cisgenderism, Cis Privilege, and the Cis/trans Distinction." *Whipping Girl.* Available at: http://juliaserano.blogspot.co.uk/2014/12/julia-seranos-compendium-on-cisgender.html.

Sparkes, M. 2014. "Facebook Sex Changes: which One of 50 Genders are You?" *Telegraph.* Available at: www.telegraph.co.uk/technology/facebook/10637968/Facebook-sex-changes-which-one-of-50-genders-are-you.html%0A.

SRLP. 2017. "Fact Sheet: transgender & Gender Nonconforming Youth In School." *Sylvia Rivera Law Project*. Available at: https://srlp.org/resources/fact-sheet-transgender-gender-nonconforming-youth-school/.

Sylvester, T. 2017. "Male, Female or X? Oregon Adds Third Option to Driver's Licenses." *Reuters*. Available at: http://uk.reuters.com/article/us-oregon-lgbt-license-idUKKBN196300.

van Osch, W. and O. Mendelson. 2011. "A Typology of Affordances: untangling Sociomaterial Interactions through Video Analysis," in *Thirty Second International Conference on Information Systems*, pp. 1–18. Shanghai: ICIS.

Walsh, M. 2004. "Twenty Years since 'A Critique of the Sex/gender Distinction': a Conversation with Moira Gatens." *Australian Feminist Studies* 19(44): 213–224.

West, C. and D. Zimmerman. 1987. "Doing Gender." *Gender and Society* 1(2): 125–151.

Yeung, P. 2016. "Transphobic Hate Crimes in 'Sickening': 170% Rise as Low Prosecution Rates Create 'Lack of Trust' in Police." *The Telegraph*. Available at: www.independent.co.uk/news/uk/home-news/transphobic-hate-crime-statistics-violence-transgender-uk-police-a7159026.html.

Yuval-Davis, N. 2006. "Intersectionality and Feminist Politics." *European Journal of Women's Studies* 13(3): 193–209.

Part II

Critical realism and intersectionality

If the first section served to examine those features of critical realist philosophy that are of most general relevance to feminism and gender studies, its second section – consisting of three chapters – uses the tools developed therein to critically engage with the topic of intersectionality. In particular, while intersectionality has commonly been lauded as a feminist success story, these chapters suggest the need for a more nuanced appraisal of its (otherwise very real) achievements. Angela Martinez Dy, Lee Martin, and Susan Marlow's chapter, for instance, notes the existence of numerous 'disparate approaches and methodological rifts' (p. 144) in the literature on this topic, while Sue Clegg's chapter adds that the ambiguities that characterise intersectional analysis are a weakness rather than a strength. Importantly, such statements should not be mistaken for an opposition to intersectional theory/praxis as such. Despite Gunnarsson's earlier claim that paying attention to people's multiple positions is perhaps 'a rather unspectacular undertaking' (p. 100), the three chapters that follow (1) trace the philosophical, historical, and geographical roots of influential theorisations of intersectionality, and (2) aim to move beyond the rifts, ambiguities and elisions that characterise them. As such, these chapters do not just (historically and geographically) situate and critique prominent approaches to intersectionality, they also advance a new approach to its theorisation and practical application that is rooted in critical realist philosophy.

Martinez Dy, Martin, and Marlow's chapter begins, however, by arguing – in specifically *negatory* fashion – that 'the scope and explanatory power of intersectionality theory is limited by implicit philosophical assumptions stemming from [its] roots in [the] positivist and hermeneutic traditions' (p. 159). They then proceed – in *affirmatory* fashion – by arguing that critical realist philosophy provides 'the conceptual tools necessary to augment intersectionality theory and rectify some of its problematic limitations' (ibid.). Of particular importance in this regard are the *epistemic fallacy* (as discussed in the first section introduction on p. 10 and New on p. 92), *ontological depth* (as discussed by New on pp. 83–88, Clegg on pp. 167–168, Parr on p. 264 and van Ingen on pp. 244–251), and *transfactual causality* (the idea that causal powers may operate 'independently of any particular sequence or pattern of events' (Bhaskar 2008 [1975], p. 3)).

These concepts are central to the new ontology that critical realist philosophy proposes. As Martinez Dy, Martin, and Marlow show, however, this new ontology also holds significant promise when it comes to (re)theorising key feminist and gender studies terms like 'privilege'. In line with intersectional theorising more generally they begin by stressing that privilege is commonly 'normalized and made to seem natural' and, as a result, 'tends to go unacknowledged and unrecognized, particularly by those whom it benefits' (p. 152). Hence 'it is entirely possible and likely quite common that someone could believe [that] they are not privileged on the basis of their normative race, dominant gender, or higher social class, and for this belief to be incorrect' (ibid.). Such claims are common in the wider intersectionality literature. As Martinez Dy, Martin and Marlow note, however, the intelligibility of such statements is, in fact, dependent on an understanding of reality as possessing depth (and hence on a critique of the epistemic fallacy), a transfactual understanding of causality, and a distinction between open and closed systems.

For instance, if it is possible for people (privileged or otherwise) to be incorrect about, or at least have only a partial understanding of, the sociocultural context which they inhabit, this suggests that it is necessary to maintain a distinction between, on the one hand, people's corrigible experience and understanding of what is happening and, on the other, what is actually occurring; or, to put this in the depth-ontological terms that critical realists favour, what is required – in addition to the idea that competing explanatory claims are indeed subject to *judgmentally rational* evaluations – is a distinction between the *empirical* and the *actual* realms. Moreover, the critical realist distinction between the realms of the *actual* and the *real* is arguably at the heart of existing forms of intersectional theorising as well. Specifically, the depth-ontological claim that *actual* (and *empirical*) events occur when and where *real* causal powers/mechanisms are triggered, combined with the claim that these powers/mechanisms operate very largely outside closed systemic settings, sheds light on the persistent variation that characterises (gendered/classed/racialised, etc.) events. As Martinez Dy, Martin and Marlow highlight, it is common for *particular* women (of colour) to advance within an organisational hierarchy (e.g. a corporation) while more *general* patterns of discriminatory hiring and/or promotion remain firmly in place. The existence of such exceptions has always posed a significant – and arguably insurmountable – challenge for positivist philosophy, which has stubbornly persisted in its efforts to identify (strict or probabilistic) empirical event regularities. From a critical realist perspective that stresses both the prevalence of open systems and the need to maintain a distinction between *real* causal powers/mechanisms and *actual/empirical* events, however, such exceptions do not pose an explanatory challenge. Rather, from this perspective it is fully anticipated that a power/mechanism will be counteracted, whether partially or wholly, by other powers/mechanisms, and that – despite the existence of e.g. a strong actual/empirical trend towards discriminatory outcomes – exceptions to this trend will occur. This is, after all, perfectly in line with its abovementioned notion of transfactual causality.

A similarly promising avenue for a critical realist contribution to intersectional theorising is discussed both in Clegg's chapter and Martinez Dy, Martin and Marlow's chapter. Specifically, both of these contributions – along with a significant number of the other contributions to this reader – repeatedly draw our attention to the ways in which the proponents of critical realist philosophy have theorised agency, structure, and their (dialectical) interaction.

As Clegg notes with regard to the first of these topics, critical realist philosophy – in contrast with especially the unidirectional textualism of much post-structuralist work and the nomotheticism of positivist philosophy – provides useful resources for theorising agency (see also van Ingen on pp. 232–234). In developing this claim, Clegg draws especially on the social-theoretical defence and elaboration of critical realist philosophy that is advanced by Margaret Archer (1995, 1996, 2000, 2003, 2007). She highlights, for instance, that Archer's work 'breaks with the disembodied subject of "modernity's man"' – as epitomised particularly by the tenets of rational choice theory – and develops an alternative theorisation of human beings that conceives of them both as irreducibly agential and as 'fundamentally evaluative in their relations with reality' (p. 172).[1] More specifically, Archer's work develops an analytical framework that is rooted in the idea that human beings form complex evaluative and behavioural commitments by engaging in what she terms an 'internal conversation'. The adoption of such an approach, Clegg stresses, is crucial for understanding the emergence of social movements like feminism and – furthermore – it is of the utmost importance if feminist and gender studies authors are to 'sustain the normative intent of intersectional analysis and the political projects that underpin it' (p. 164).

If intersectional analysis and politics are to be provided with a robust philosophical basis, however, much more is clearly needed than any account of agency, however sophisticated, is capable of providing; specifically, it is vital that an equally robust understanding of both sociocultural structures and their mode of interaction with human agents is also supplied.

It is worth highlighting, therefore, that previous chapters have already made significant headway in this regard. Caroline New's chapter, for instance, noted that 'gender regimes condition the embodied agents positioned within them, who, collectively and severally, reproduce, modify and over time transform' them (p. 80). Tony Lawson's chapter further expanded such broad theoretical statements by making a number of distinct but interconnected arguments; first, it argued that 'the social world is a highly internally related, intrinsically dynamic process, and [...] is dependent upon, if irreducible to, transformative human agency' (p. 24); second, it claimed that 'human subjectivities, human experiences, and social structure cannot be reduced one to another' (p. 36); and finally, it suggested that, 'because social structure both depends upon human agency and in turn conditions it, a switch of emphasis in social analysis is necessitated, away from [...] *creation* and *determination*, to [...] *reproduction* and *transformation*' (p. 21, emphasis added).

Such claims provide clear echoes of the relational and emergentist understanding of social structures that was developed by Roy Bhaskar in *The Possibility of Naturalism* (1998 [1979]), especially his 'Transformational Model of Social Activities' (TMSA). Importantly, this model provides numerous resources for the purpose of grounding intersectional theory and praxis at a philosophical level. For instance, as Bhaskar noted (in a different intellectual context), one significant advantage of the TMSA is that it 'allows one to focus on a range of questions, having to do with the distribution of the structural conditions of action, and in particular with differential allocations of: (a) productive resources (of all kinds, including for example cognitive ones) to persons (and groups) and (b) persons (and groups) to functions and roles (for example in the division of labour)' (ibid., p. 45). Or, in Lawson's words, it results in a conception of the social as 'highly segmented in terms of the obligations and prerogatives that are on offer' (p. 22). In conceiving of the social realm as such, importantly, the TMSA also situates 'the possibility of different (and antagonistic) interests, of conflicts within society' (Bhaskar 1998 [1979], p. 45).

The three chapters that follow both reiterate and build on such claims. Martinez Dy, Martin and Marlow, for instance, stress that critical realist philosophy 'rejects both determinism and voluntarism in favour of a dialectical, interactionist and mutually constitutive approach to the explanation of social phenomena' (p. 155). As such, they argue that it provides us with a more robust approach to the structure/agency problematic than do existing approaches to intersectionality. Similarly, Clegg emphasises that 'substantive analyses would be better if [they were] not hobbled by inadequate accounts of structure and agency' (p. 177). Like before, she develops this point by drawing on Archer's work. Clegg claims, for instance, that Archer's ('morphogenetic') approach provides a more robust ground for analysing the cross-cutting oppressions that intersectional theory highlights because it does not conflate experience with structural and cultural conditions and their elaboration. Like Lawson's chapter, then, Clegg's contribution to this volume maintains that '[i]t makes no more sense [...] to reduce structural problems to individual experience than it does to think that experience can be deduced from structure' (p. 167). In contrast, the challenge faced by current approaches to intersectionality is that 'analytical distinctions between structure and agency, and between culture and agency, are elided' (p. 163)

If the first two chapters argue that critical realist accounts of agency, structure, and their interaction can help to move us past the rifts, ambiguities and elisions that characterise current forms of intersectional theorising/politics, however, its third chapter – by Lena Gunnarsson – explicitly aims to deepen such claims by foregrounding dialectics. Gunnarsson begins by noting that '[d]isputes about how to understand intersectional relations often pivot around the tension between separateness and inseparability, where some scholars emphasize the need to separate between different intersectional categories [gender, 'race', class, etc.] while others claim they are inseparable' (p. 180). These disputes, she suggests, have resulted in 'an unnecessary and unproductive polarization' (ibid.) which reproduces 'absolutist and undifferentiated notions of difference as well as unity' (p. 182). Critical realist philosophy, in contrast, takes issue '*both* with accounts that obscure the co-enfoldment of phenomena *and* with claims that phenomena cannot be at all separated if they have intrinsic ties to one another' (ibid.). In accordance with this orientation, Gunnarsson (1) problematises the either/or logic that characterises much of the intersectionality literature, and (2) suggests the need to dialecticise this literature by thinking of intersectional categories as well as different ontological levels as both distinct and unified. Such claims are rooted in the emergentist ontology that critical realist philosophy favours; in particular, they are rooted in its emergentist notion of ontological unity-in-difference, which provides a challenge to 'the most basic and problematic of all dualisms, that between separateness and inseparability itself' (p. 182). As a result, an approach to intersectional theory and praxis that is rooted in critical realism simultaneously negates *and* provides a synthesis of Leslie McCall's (2005) well-known 'anticategorical' and 'intercategorical' analytical frameworks.

On the whole, the picture of critical realist feminism and gender studies that emerges is – once again – a preservative and heterodox one. Whereas the first section of this reader highlighted that critical realist philosophy provides *both* natural scientific *and* human/social scientific approaches with a 'seat at the table', however, this second section places centre-stage the fact that it brings together structure *and* agency, separability *and* inseparability, etc. More specifically, the three chapters that follow show that an approach to feminism and gender studies which is rooted in critical realism is able to provide the literature on intersectionality with (1) a more robust account of agency, structure, and their interaction than has been available to it thus far, and (2) a dialectical alternative to the choice that is supposedly to be made between ontological unity and ontological difference, the adoption of an anticategorical approach and the adoption of an intercategorical approach, etc. The final section of this reader will conclude by showing that this negation of the choice between purportedly incompatible, opposing pairs – along with the affirmation of a synthetic alternative which accompanies it – also provides feminist and gender studies authors with both a sound philosophical basis for empirical research and clear guidelines on how to navigate the treacherous terrain of (discussions about) methodology and methods.

Note

1 A similar approach is developed in the (critical realist) work of Andrew Sayer (2011).

References

Archer, M. S. 1995. *Realist Social Theory: The Morphogenetic Approach*. Cambridge: Cambridge University Press.

———. 1996. *Culture and Agency: The Place of Culture in Social Theory*, revised edition. Cambridge: Cambridge University Press.

———. 2000. *Being Human: The Problem of Agency.* Cambridge: Cambridge University Press.

———. 2003. *Structure, Agency and the Internal Conversation.* Cambridge: Cambridge University Press.

———. 2007. *Making Out Way through the World: Human Reflexivity and Social Mobility.* Cambridge: Cambridge University Press.

Bhaskar, R. 2008 [1975]. *A Realist Theory of Science.* London; New York: Verso.

———. 1998 [1979]. *The Possibility of Naturalism: A Philosophical Critique of the Contemporary Human Sciences*, 3rd edition. London: Routledge.

McCall, L. 2005. "The Complexity of Intersectionality." *Signs: Journal of Women in Culture and Society* 30(3): 1771–1800.

Sayer, A. 2011. *Why Things Matter to People: Social Science, Values and Ethical Life.* Cambridge: Cambridge University Press.

6 Developing a critical realist positional approach to intersectionality[1]

Angela Martinez Dy, Lee Martin, and Susan Marlow

Introduction

Intersectionality has emerged over the past thirty years as an interdisciplinary approach to analysing the concurrent impacts of social structures, with a focus on theorising how belonging to multiple exclusionary social categories can influence political access and equality (Hancock 2007). It conceptualises the interaction of categories of difference such as gender, race and class at many levels, including individual experience, social practices, institutions and ideologies, and frames the outcomes of these interactions in terms of the distribution and allocation of power (Davis 2008, pp. 67–68; Hurtado 1989). As a form of social critique originally rooted in black feminism (Dhamoon 2011; e.g. Combahee River Collective 1977; Crenshaw 1989; Davis 1981; Hill Collins 1990; hooks 1981), intersectionality is described by Jennifer Nash as 'outsider knowledge' that has 'transversed disciplinary borders and gained institutional legitimacy' (2011, pp. 446–47; see also Oleksy 2011). Eventually adopted into mainstream feminist discourse, intersectionality is now acknowledged as a significant contribution to feminist scholarship.

However, the scholarly discourse underpinning intersectionality encompasses a range of philosophical, methodological and practical positions that differ greatly in their approaches to analysing the varying impacts of categories (Davis 2008), and indeed, in their stances on whether this is even possible. Although it is generally accepted that understanding intersectionality helps make visible the influences of multiple categories of oppression, when researchers have attempted to tease out the related forces involved, their approaches have been problematised and their methods critiqued. The inconsistency amongst approaches combined with lack of ontological discussion has led some to suggest that the widespread uptake of intersectionality in feminist theory may be obscuring relevant debates within the field, such as those between liberal, post-structuralist, and black standpoint perspectives (Carbin and Edenheim 2013). Additionally, due to its original aim of analysing the impacts of intersecting forces of oppression, both theory and research have tended to pay less attention to questions of agency and privilege (Nash 2008). Together, these issues have precipitated something of a methodological crisis for intersectionality.

One conceptual approach that has been heavily problematised is the idea that the intersections of certain categories affect identities in a fixed or static way. In response, a more fluid notion of social positionality has been put forward. Positionality builds upon the importance intersectionality places on multiple identities, but concentrates instead on broader social locations and processes that are context-, meaning-, and time-specific, explicitly located within social hierarchies, and tied to both material and cultural resource distribution (Anthias 2001a, 2001b, 2002, 2006, 2008). The move towards positionality is clearly articulated by Floya Anthias, for whom intersectionality is a social process of practices and arrangements giving rise to particular forms of positionality, which tend to involve shifts and contradictions (2008). She suggests that from a temporal view, positionality encompasses both the present outcome of intersectionality – i.e. the being – as well as the process of development that is continually occurring, or the becoming. Like intersectionality, positionality is held to have present effects, yet also be dynamic and subject to changing social and individual circumstances. But in its acknowledgement of potential contradictions, positionality is arguably better equipped than its precursor to articulate discussions of agency and privilege as well as oppression and disadvantage.

There is now a rich history informing intersectionality and positionality theorising and research, yet the literature rarely calls into question the underlying assumptions that have led to such disparate approaches and methodological rifts. Whilst there have been significant contributions made in identifying and categorising intersectional approaches (McCall 2005; Mehrotra 2010), the various philosophical underpinnings of these approaches are not often clearly elucidated, nor are the effects of their foundations subject to critique (Carbin and Edenheim 2013). Thus this article will draw upon the philosophy of critical realism to explore some of the philosophical roots of intersectionality theory and argue that key ontological and epistemological assumptions across the various approaches have led intersectionality into its present crisis of method. We suggest that a number of current limitations can be overcome if critical realism is used to inform theory development. To make this argument, the article is structured as follows. First, contemporary reviews and critiques of intersectionality are examined. Second, the theoretical limitations identified are mapped to implicit roots in positivist and hermeneutic philosophical traditions and the methodological problems engendered by such assumptions articulated. Finally, we propose an outline of a critical realist approach to intersectionality that addresses how these problems can be reconciled, and in so doing, offer an alternative philosophical foundation for future intersectional research.

Intersectional complexity and the limitations of current approaches

Because of ambiguity in basic definitions and the complexity of the subjectivities with which it grapples, there is a notable lack of consensus about key elements of intersectionality theory. A case in point concerns inconsistency in conceptualisation: depending on the author or context, intersectionality has been considered a theory, a paradigm, a framework, a method, a perspective, or a lens (Mehrotra 2010). Such vagueness and ambiguity has been both heralded for its flexibility and usefulness (Davis 2008, p. 76) as well as identified as a central tension within the literature (Nash 2008). There is also a conspicuous dearth of explicit ontological and epistemological discussions within the field (Carbin and Edenheim 2013). Combined, these issues have meant there is currently a limited range of methodological tools with which to research intersectionality, leading to the conclusion that intersectionality is methodologically under-theorised (Bowleg 2008; McCall 2005).

One exception is found in Leslie McCall's work. Defining methodology as encompassing the philosophy and methods that underpin the research process and production of knowledge, she identifies three distinct methodological strands within intersectional research: anti-categorical complexity, intra-categorical complexity, and inter-categorical complexity (2005). Anti-categorical approaches attempt to deconstruct and reject analytical categories, starting from the assumption that categories, including race and gender, are too simplistic to capture the complexity of lived experience (Nash 2008; c.f. McCall 2005). Intra-categorical approaches, representative of the original approach of intersectionality, attempt to focus on social groups at neglected points of intersection. Inter-categorical approaches, described as the 'strategic use' of categories, 'begins with the observation that there are relationships of inequality among already constituted social groups, as imperfect and ever changing as they are, and takes those relationships as the centre of the analysis' (ibid., pp. 1784–85). McCall notes that not all research on intersectionality can be categorised into one of the three types of approaches, that some will cross categorical boundaries, that there may not be homogeneity within the categories, and that she may have misunderstood or misclassified some pieces of research (ibid., p. 1774). However, the methodological strands she describes provide a useful framework for analysing extant intersectional methodology, particularly because the framework presented does not reflect upon the ontological and epistemological underpinnings of intersectional research. It will be later argued that the current limitations of intersectional theory correspond to problematic ontological and epistemological assumptions underpinning the various types of approaches outlined by McCall.

Positivism in intersectionality theory

Positivism is a philosophy of science that underpins much of the natural sciences. There are many forms of positivist thought, but some of the most influential forms were developed from the work of Comte and Hume. For Hume, causality was synonymous with regularity between events, i.e. if event x and event y are regularly conjoined, it is presumed that one causes the other. His philosophy of science, therefore, emphasises the importance of empirical observation for uncovering such causal laws, and that knowledge claims about the natural world should be limited to such uncovered events. Roy Bhaskar recognised that this set of ideas and the principles of the related philosophy of empiricism contained the implicit ontological assumption that reality is limited to that which is observable and measurable. He termed this the epistemic fallacy: what we consider real is limited to what we can know (1998 [1979]).

Feminist theory has also critiqued dominant philosophical frameworks; in particular, for their privileging of men and lack of grounding in women's experiences (Harding 1986). It has challenged the forms of positivism described above for their insistence on the primacy of masculinist empirical observation for the construction of knowledge (McCall 2005). Multiple feminist interdisciplinary methodological approaches have thus been developed, including feminist empiricism, standpoint theory and postmodern perspectives, some of which have themselves been critiqued for similar exclusionary limitations (Harding 1986, 1991; Letherby 2003; New 1998). Intersectionality as a diverse and pluralist paradigm has drawn and built upon all of these, with particular grounding in structuralist standpoint feminism (Carbin and Edenheim 2013). And whilst its philosophical underpinnings have not tended to be at the forefront of the conversation, McCall notes that those in anticategorical and intra-categorical camps tend to associate advanced quantitative techniques, large data sets, and surveys with the negative legacies of positivism (2005, p. 1791). However, whilst intersectionality has clearly been influenced by both feminist standpoint theory and postmodern perspectives, it will be argued that the positivist and feminist empiricist traditions have had a larger impact upon intersectional theory building than has been previously acknowledged.

Some of the inter- and intra-categorical intersectional approaches identified by McCall seem to contain implicit positivist assumptions as they attempt to theorise the nature and kind of causes at work in structures of domination, as well as to articulate the historically specific conditions under which they exist. The concern with identifying such causes means that some of this research has treated categories such as race and class as discrete and separable. Subsequently, race, class and gender have been portrayed and analysed as fixed categories with discrete, consistent and measurable effects (Mehrotra 2010; Nash 2011) when they are in fact 'shifting, slippery, [and] highly contextual' (Nash 2011, p. 461). This is an issue within identity-centred intersectionality scholarship in general, as identity – and by extension, difference and inequality – may be treated as static and possessive attributes of individuals or groups (Anthias 2006 t2008). Gita Mehrotra points to the predominance of mathematical and geometric metaphors invoked to structurally describe intersectionality, including vectors of difference, matrices of oppression, and axes of power (2010, pp. 420–21), along with the problematic additive model, and its cousin, the multiplicative model (Nash 2008, p. 7). These metaphors suggest that gender, race, and class can be considered separately and so, understood and analysed through, for example, additive calculation (Mehrotra 2010, p. 421). The extensive use of mathematical tropes to portray structural conditions is clearly reflective of a positivist legacy and has created a conceptual cul-de-sac that makes it difficult to imagine other ways in which structures might interact.

Additionally, Hume's philosophy of science informed positivist methodologies that suggest hypothesis development and the prediction of the results of empirical investigation are important to knowledge formation. Tendencies towards prediction are arguably at the root of why simplistic quasi-predictive conceptualisations, such as the additive approach, wherein experiences of oppression explained in terms of the sum total of the oppressions of the relevant marginalised categories, became popular. Such conceptualisations, however, have now been roundly critiqued as both unlikely and essentialising (e. g. Bowleg 2008; Hancock 2007; Yuval-Davis 2006). Ironically, it was just this kind of quasi-predictive approach that was specifically challenged in seminal intersectional work, which served to complicate essentialist notions of womanhood espoused by second wave feminism through challenging the assumption that categories such as 'woman' or 'black' affect everyone within their bounds in a similar manner, whilst taking the assumed stability of those boundaries to task. For example, Patricia Hill Collins stressed that common challenges did not necessarily produce common experiences (2000 [1990]). But Nash notes that early theorists' work on the intersections of race and gender in particular, pushed these two constructs to the fore, and away from grappling with other issues of multiple marginality. The legacy of this early work is still present: Nash points out that 'intersectional projects often replicate precisely the approaches that they critique' (2008, p. 6, 2011) by reifying categories or overlooking heterogeneity due to bracketing or ignoring categories with which they are not explicitly concerned.

Black feminist critiques of theory as elitist and exclusionary (e.g. Hill Collins 2000 [1990]) were concordant with other feminist critiques of the androcentric construction of 'knowledge' in the natural sciences, which pointed out that a science created by Western, bourgeois, white heterosexual men can only be subjective (e.g. Haraway 1988; Harding 1986, 1991). Despite these critiques, intersectional scholars have yet to address the epistemic fallacy (Bhaskar 1998 [1979], p. 133; 2008 [1975], p. 13, p. 36) within their epistemologies. In their attempt to contest the idea of theory as neutral, Nash points out that the black feminist scholarship in which intersectionality is grounded intentionally 'collaps[ed] the distinction between theory and experience' (2011, pp. 462–463). Yet, in spite of such justifiable intentions, it still results in problems of being becoming conflated with problems of knowing. Thus, the conflation of experience, theory, and knowledge that feminism critiqued in the scientific tradition can be seen to have been replicated within this category of intersectionality theory, albeit with important differences; the vantage point was now articulated and embodied. It was no longer elite, but instead occupied a subjugated position in the social hierarchy. As such, from the perspective of feminist standpoint theory, it had the potential to precipitate an acute awareness of relationships of power, described by Donna Haraway as 'vision [...] from below' (1988, p. 583). Although there is undeniable value in the demarginalisation of subjugated worldviews, intersectional theories suffer from the epistemic fallacy when they do not separate ontological claims from their epistemological origins. As a result of this philosophical legacy, intersectionality scholarship risks omitting from its theories that which may be unexercised, unactualised, or unobserved; this will be explored in more detail later.

The hermeneutic tradition and intersectional identity

Hermeneutics has its origins in ancient Greek philosophy, although modern hermeneutics is derived from many thinkers, such as Heidegger, Gadamer and Habermas. Whilst there is heterogeneity in these approaches, what links them is a focus on meaning via textual interpretation or sense-making. Phenomenology, the study of the structures of experience, and constructivism, the argument that all knowledge is a social construction, are derived, in some way, from this hermeneutic tradition, whilst post-structuralism can be considered part of its radical intellectual evolution. Like phenomenology, post-structuralism is primarily concerned with how people experience and make sense of the world and warns against research that seeks to uncover underlying truths (Brown and Heggs 2005). What makes it radical is the basic premise that it is fundamentally impossible to accurately represent the world (Carbin and Edenheim 2013). Although differences between authors are acknowledged, for the purpose of this article, these schools of thought will be subsumed under the umbrella of the hermeneutic tradition. Contemporary work on intersectionality is predominantly associated with the anti-categorical approaches identified by McCall, which, taking broadly defined hermeneutic (predominantly constructivist and post-structural) positions, tend to view categories as 'simplifying social fictions' (2005, p. 1773) based upon the idea that social reality is a fluid and co-constitutive phenomenon that cannot be depicted in simplistic, categorical and discrete ways (Mehrotra 2010, p. 421). Within such intersectionality research, these approaches have helped to further complicate notions of categories of belonging, highlighting their political function. However, the retained focus on interpretation, due to what is perceived to be the impossibility of truth claims, carries the risk that such research will be 'drained of causal import' (Bhaskar 1998 [1979], p. 12) as it attends primarily to individual interpretations of reality.

Importantly, neither hermeneuticist nor positivist traditions articulate an ontology that includes a notion of transfactuality, i.e. that causes can exist and endure without our knowledge of them. For Bhaskar, the lack of an articulated ontology concerning causality results in the tacit adoption of an implicit one. Critiquing the hermeneutic tradition for the way it regards the key problems of philosophy arising from the 'conditions, limits and forms' of language (ibid., p. 133), he argues that the consequence of the implicit ontological assumptions within the hermeneutic tradition is that society is entirely conceptual in character, with its central category being that of meaning (ibid., pp. 133–135). Although prominent post-structuralists such as Judith Butler have argued that categories are still relevant and that hegemonic discourses do have significant material consequences (Butler 1990,

1998), the problematic methodological implication of this line of thinking when translating these abstract arguments to research is that structural issues tend to be analysed primarily in terms of individual experiences and related understanding of them, to the detriment of the analysis of unrecognised structural impediments (Yuval-Davis 2006) and their relationship with individual agency (Clegg 2006; see also Carbin and Edenheim 2013).

The tendency of anti-categorical intersectionality theorists to focus ever more closely on the meaning-making processes of the individual reflects the methodological restriction imposed through this tradition. Within anti-categorical discourse, notions of positionality or structural discrimination are often collapsed into the concept of 'identity'. Yuval-Davis defines identities as individual and collective narratives that answer questions of who we are. She notes, however, that in contemporary literature, concepts of identity are often required to perform analytical tasks beyond their abilities (2006). For example, the study of identity at the level of the individual seems ill-suited to providing wider contextual analysis for a given social condition. Although exploring identity can provide insight into how people perceive, make sense of and cope with particular circumstances, it cannot speak decisively about how structural components of those circumstances may be determined by the wider social field. The predominance of inquiries into intersectional identity is herein argued to be a continuation of the hermeneutic focus on the discursive construction of reality as it manifests at the micro level. Concurrently, there is a conspicuous lack of theory on the intersecting structural conditions that engender these realities (Acker 2000, 2006; Yuval-Davis 2006), in which resource inequalities of various kinds produce complex experiences of discrimination and privilege (Anthias 2001b; Nash 2011). This poses significant challenges for intersectional scholars seeking to explain macro-level conditions without contradicting their philosophical tradition.

Table 1 shows the three existing approaches to intersectional methodological complexity (McCall 2005; Mehrotra 2010; Nash 2008). Drawing upon critical realist perspectives (Bhaskar 1998 [1979]; Gunnarsson 2011, ch. 4 this volume), it illustrates how these approaches are implicitly informed by the positivist and/or hermeneutic traditions, and highlights some of the common problematic outcomes that occur as a result.

Whilst many post-structuralist scholars have embraced intersectionality and vice versa, Maria Carbin and Sara Edenheim have critiqued intersectionality's apparent hegemony within current feminist theory, arguing that there is no room in the field of intersectionality for a post-structuralism based on the premise that reality is inherently unknowable, and which does not share the 'dream of a common feminist language' (2013, p. 232). They lend temporal and political context to the debate when they argue that intersectionality's widespread adoption into feminist theory, constructivist intersectionality especially, has come to signal a 'liberal consensus-based project [...] in an increasingly neoliberal and conservative European context' (ibid., p. 245). Intersectionality has also been challenged by feminist new materialists Evelien Geerts and Iris van der Tuin,

Table 1 Extant intersectional approaches to methodological complexity

Approach to complexity	*Inter-categorical (categorical)*	*Intra-categorical*	*Anti-categorical*
Approach to categories	Provisionally adopt	Categories inadequate, but identify complexity	Deconstruct and reject
Predominant philosophical Influence	Post-positivist	Positivist-hermeneutic	Hermeneutic (discursive approach)
Problematic assumptions	Categories fixed, can be analysed discretely	Intersections fixed, experience = theory	Categories fictional and thus, irrelevant
Problematic outcomes	Additive approach, mathematical tropes	Epistemic fallacy	Focus limited to 'identity' or 'discourse'

who critique what they see as its denial of agency and, addressing the gap around intersectional ontology, follow Karen Barad in arguing for an explicit onto-epistemology, or 'entanglement' between being and knowing (2013). Thus, it is both useful and timely to introduce the concepts of critical realism to intersectionality theory. A philosophy of science that accepts the transfactual existence of causal powers emerging from structural categories and positions, and which explains how agency interacts with, reproduces, and changes these structures, offers the opportunity to strengthen intersectionality's philosophical underpinnings and move beyond these restricting debates.

Towards a critical realist intersectionality

Critical realism can help address the limitations of existing intersectionality theory by providing an alternative ontology and epistemology to those that currently predominate. The critical realist philosophy contains a conception of causality that enables an understanding of how the social world can exist independently from our knowledge of it. Bhaskar's philosophy of science arose from asking the question: What must the world be like in order for science, as we understand it, to be possible? Arguing that because it is possible to identify correlations and causation through experimental activity, his conclusion was there must be underlying causal mechanisms enabling such events to be measured. Because these correlations may not endure outside of this experimental activity (as they require scientific work in order to be identified) the causal mechanisms that lead to them must be considered separate from the events they generate. In other words, causes have essential properties that operate continuously, regardless of any immediate effect (2008 [1975]). Bhaskar then proposed that these causal mechanisms underpin events, and that mechanisms can be considered real if they 'have an effect or make a difference' (Fleetwood 2004, p. 29). This logic enabled the conclusion that the social world must be stratified into at least three domains: the empirical, in which events are observed and measured; the actual, in which events occur irrespective of our knowledge of them; and the real or the deep, where causal powers can be exercised (formed but not necessarily acting) or un-exercised (yet to be formed but possible given current conditions) (Mole 2012; cf. Bhaskar 2008 [1975]).

Whilst acknowledging important contributions to knowledge from both positivist and hermeneutic traditions, Bhaskar points out two fundamental oversights. First, both strands of thought predicate a flat and positive ontology, which he terms 'ontological monovalence' (2008 [1993]). Here both philosophies make implicit assumptions that there can be no absence, and no potential, in the world. Positivism assumes only that which can be measured exists; hence, the unobserved cannot be considered part of reality. The hermeneutic tradition implicitly assumes that if something is not registered within the subjective perception or sense-making processes of an individual we can make no claim to knowing it, and by consequence it cannot be considered part of the social world. This again restricts what can be theorised about the unsaid, the unknown, the absent and what may lie in potential. Second, he identified that neither philosophical approach allows for the possibility of transfactuality: the idea that causal powers can exist without being actualised in events or recognised by observers (1998 [1979]; 2008 [1975]. Instead, only causes or mechanisms that are observed, experienced and measured are acknowledged, with no means of accounting for that which may not be actualised or recognised. Thus, according to both traditions, any social cause or mechanism that is either unactualised or unrecognised by actors cannot be assumed to exist. Bhaskar proposes transfactuality as a path through this divide, in which causal mechanisms are considered real and external to individuals, but transcendentally so. Accordingly, they may exist actualised or unactualised, perceived or unperceived. The possibility of knowing their existence is pursued through the development of fallible theories, including that of their potential transfactuality.

This logic provides a means with which to reconcile some key problems facing current intersectionality theory. For example, there is a tendency within intersectionality theory to avoid conceptualising privilege (Nash 2008). This means theory has not clearly articulated ways in which individuals may be subject to oppression by certain mechanisms whilst benefiting from privilege because of others. Nash articulates this need when she comments that 'progressive scholarship requires a nuanced conception of identity that recognises the ways in which positions of dominance and subordination work in complex and intersecting ways to constitute subject experiences of personhood' (ibid., p. 10). This could be addressed by incorporating a notion of transfactuality into intersectionality's conceptualisation of complexity. Transfactuality enables the conceptualisation of causal mechanisms emerging from the level of society that in some cases are unactualised or unrecognised and yet, which are still held to function. For example, it is particularly useful for theorising privilege, since the ways it is normalised and made to seem natural (Maier 1997; McIntosh 1989) mean that it tends to go unacknowledged and unrecognised, particularly by those whom it benefits (Frankenberg 1993; Ahmed 2012). Thus, it is entirely possible and likely quite common that someone could believe they are not privileged on the basis of their normative race, dominant gender, or higher social class, and for this belief to be incorrect. Another way of conceptualising privilege could utilise the critical realist notion of absence (Bhaskar 2008 [1993]); in this case, privilege could mean the absence of additional obstacles to success as a result of belonging to the dominant race, class, or gender. These concepts would be especially useful for enabling intersectionality theory to explain how individuals may be subject to oppression in some ways but privileged in others.

In another example, an institution or organisation may have an implicit culture of sexism and racism in relation to career progression and the allocation of financial rewards, yet these mechanisms may not be perceived by those benefiting from them, and unacknowledged by those perpetuating them. However, the transfactuality of mechanisms of privilege and discrimination means that they operate whether or not they are acknowledged to exist. It also explains why, within the same organisation, individual women and people of colour might advance, but the demographic composition of the management structure remains predominantly white and male. Though the overall tendency of the structure is governed by the dominant mechanisms of sexism and racism, discriminatory mechanisms may not be actualised in all cases, and other mechanisms – say, a corporate call for diversity or an equal opportunities policy – may potentially provide some countervailing forces. Incorporating the concepts of transfactuality and absence in this way can help advance intersectional theory at both the micro- and macro-levels, in order to more accurately theorise the nature of systems of oppression and privilege.

Critical realist feminism in an intersectional framework

Although critical realism has seen only initial deployment within feminist theory in general (e.g. Clegg 2006) and intersectionality theory in particular (e.g. Walby et al. 2012), critical realist feminists such as Lena Gunnarsson and Caroline New have responded to the post-structuralist and anti-categorical approaches that feature prominently in intersectional literature. Gunnarsson notes that as a result of these approaches, the category 'woman' is now assumed to have little positive theoretical validity in feminist literature (2011). This is corroborated by McCall, who observes that anti-categoricalism has led to 'great scepticism about the possibility of using categories in anything but a simplistic way', and highlights the potential value of critical realism to intersectionality theory (2005, p. 1773). Gunnarsson explains that the rejection of the category 'woman' stems from 'deny[ing] categories any analytical validity by virtue of their empirical inseparability' (2011, p. 26); however, she maintains that it is not impossible to distinguish gender analytically from other categories. Indeed, she argues that an intersectional standpoint is premised upon a category called 'gender' being analysed in conjunction with other categories. But for anti-categoricalists, notes Gunnarsson 'the notion that gender is constructed entails that it is a fiction' (ibid., p. 29). In contrast, critical realist feminists maintain that women are a real group, joined by the abstract social category of 'woman' (ibid., p. 32), who, New argues, may have some universal interests despite the reality of heterogeneity (2003). So, although categories like race, ethnicity and gender are understood to be constructions, and as such are not based on embodied reality or any 'essential truth' about a group, this does not negate the fact that they have significant social meaning.

Gunnarsson details a realist understanding of categories such as race/ethnicity, class and gender as neither essential nor analytically inseparable, but instead as abstractions with real social, political, cultural and economic implications within their respective contexts. Categories are seen to have real material and social effects, particularly on what Anthias refers to as the 'set of outcomes relating to life conditions, life chances and solidarity processes' (2001b, p. 367). They serve to enable or constrain opportunities, resources, perception by self and others, and treatment in social settings. However, the usefulness of even abstract categories is still under debate within critical realist feminism; Sylvia Walby et al. argue for a move away from concepts such as 'category' that connote unity, and toward phrases like 'regimes' or 'set of unequal social relations' (2012, p. 230, p. 236). Thus, any critical realist understanding of categories as abstractions 'implies neither essentialism nor homogenisation' (Gunnarsson 2011, p. 24) of the people to whom the categories refer. Instead, it is the social meanings that categories convey, and the structural positions to which they correspond, that lead to such essentialising perceptions, resulting in treatment that reproduces or exacerbates inequalities in social conditions.

Finally, Bhaskar's notion of concrete universality (Bhaskar 2008 [1993]) provides the necessary theoretical links between the category-as-abstraction and heterogeneous individual experiences. He describes abstract universal categories (e.g. woman) as being mediated by intersecting factors (including race, class, age, sexual orientation, ability, etc.) and framed in a particular geopolitical and historical context. This, combined with the irreducible uniqueness of individuals, defines the concept of a concrete universal, in which abstract categorical belonging is held to be located in a particular spatial/temporal context, mediated by social positionality, and concretised in the life experiences of individuals. It enables elaboration upon critical realist feminist perspectives on the validity of the category 'woman' (Gunnarsson 2011; New 2003) whilst at the same time preserving important intersectional critiques of categorical essentialism by articulating the key factors that produce heterogeneity of experience, therefore, broadening the understanding of what a 'universal' category is able to encompass.

Structure and agency in intersectional theory

The lack of a well-defined relationship between structure and agency, as well as between structures themselves, are further hurdles within intersectional theory that a critical realist approach could help to clarify. It may be the case that since the so-called post-structural turn in feminism, implicit influences from the hermeneutic tradition contributed to the current tendency to avoid theorising structure within intersectional theory, although a number of pioneering structuralist scholars (e.g. Anthias and Yuval-Davis 1992; Davis 1981; Hill Collins 2000 [1990]; hooks 1981) have made significant contributions in this area. But with the current predominance of anti-categorical approaches, attention has been much more heavily focused on individual interpretations of social reality. The relationship between structure and agency has therefore, been arguably under-theorised as a result, as has the interaction between agency and the replication of the structures of domination, gaps which are highlighted in contemporary critiques of the literature (McCall 2005; Nash 2008; Yuval-Davis 2006). Thus far, neither positivist nor post-structuralist approaches have conceptualised this relationship between structure and agency in a way that has been widely adopted by intersectionality theory, leaving one of its key aims unfulfilled: Nash observes that due to the lack of a comprehensive theory of agency, intersectionality theory has thus far been unable to 'answer [...] questions about the fit between intersectionality and lived experience of identity' (2008, p. 11).

Conceptualising structure and agency, and the relationship between them, is a widely contested area of social theory (Archer 1995; Bhaskar 1998 [1979]; Bordieu 1977; Butler 1990; Giddens 1979; McNay 2000), replete with vigorous debate that due to limitations of space it is not possible to engage with here. For now, however, we turn to realist sociologist Margaret Archer's conceptions of structure and agency, as they are rooted in critical realism and contain much promise for propelling intersectional theory forward past these intellectual hurdles. In Archer's model, termed the morphogenetic approach, structures are regarded as products of past human agency, influencing actors in the present who can then contribute to either the reproduction or transformation of these pre-existing structures. The influence of structure upon actors is two-pronged. First, structure is held to affect life-chances, endowing them with initial interests and providing the leverage upon which reasons for different courses of action operate. Thus, whilst life chances are not deterministic, they 'strongly condition what type of Social Actor the vast majority can and do become' (Archer 2000, p. 285). Second, structure is argued to be mediated by social actors primarily through affecting their 'constellation of concerns' in relation to the natural, practical, and social orders of reality. This mediation manifests and takes shape through a process of reflexive internal conversation, which then results in chosen courses of action.

Archer challenges the conflations within contemporary social theory that attribute social phenomena either entirely to the influence of structure (e.g. structuralism) or agency (e.g. rational agent models), or, as in the case of structuration theory (Giddens 1979), collapses the two. In response to these deterministic and individualistic approaches, the morphogenetic approach: 'shows (a): how human agency is socially mediated but is irreducible to social norms, and (b) how any account of human agency must include emotional and normative factors as well as any reference to rationality' (Cruickshank 2003, p. 4). It acknowledges the historicity and objectivity of the circumstances of social structure, its consequent impacts on life-chances and the potential for agential reflexivity and choice within the options available to them. It addresses subjectivity by acknowledging an agent's personal powers, and considers reflexivity, or the internal conversation, to be the primary medium by which the social world is mediated in action (Archer 2007). Although it recognises social positioning, or the 'differential placement of agents in relation to the distribution of resources', it highlights 'the impossibility of deducing determinate courses of action from such positionings alone' (ibid., p. 13). It thus rejects both determinism and voluntarism in favour of a dialectical, interactionist and mutually constitutive approach to the explanation of social phenomena. It offers the potential to advance anti-categorical approaches to intersectionality, in which discussions of agency tend to be limited to issues surrounding the discursive construction of power (New 2003; e.g. Prins 2006). Instead, this approach centres on and upholds the primacy of practice, a conceptual parallel for the intersectional feminist notion of 'lived experience', which Archer holds 'yields reasoned knowledge nondiscursively' and also 'underlies practical proficiency in the linguistic domain' (2000, p. 151).

Although the lack of a theory of agency has not prevented researchers from exploring how individuals negotiate intersecting oppressions within their experiences (Archer 2000, p. 151), critical realist notions of the structure-agency relationship, such as Archer's three-stage model (Archer 2000) and morphogenetic approach (1996, 2000) can undoubtedly be used to theorise how individuals and groups can be constrained or enabled by structures, and how agency can affect structures in turn. Table 2 summarises the suggestions offered thus far for how critical realism may usefully be applied to intersectionality. It is not meant to be

Table 2 Limitations, gaps, and the conceptual possibilities of critical realism

Intersectionality theoretical limitations and gaps	*Critical realism conceptual tool*
Tendency to collapse theory and experience (Nash 2008)	Depth ontology (Bhaskar 2008)
Focus on individuals to the detriment of structural analysis (Yuval-Davis 2006); structure under-theorized or limited to mathematical tropes (Mehrotra 2010)	Emergence (Bhaskar 1998; Archer 1995); Morphogenetic approach (Archer 1995/2000)
Push to deconstruct social categories and dismiss them as irrelevant (McCall 2005)	Categories as abstractions with real implications: social, political, cultural and economic (Gunnarsson 2011) Concrete universals (Bhaskar [1993] 2008)
Lack of theory on agency (Nash 2008)	Morphogenetic approach, three-stage model (Archer [1995] 2000)
Lack of theory on privilege (Nash 2008)	Transfactuality and absence (Bhaskar [1975] 2008, [1993] 2008)

exhaustive, but is intended as a starting point for identifying some valuable ways in which critical realist philosophy could potentially help to advance the intersectional project.

Critical realism and a positional approach to methodological complexity

Having critically examined the current problems and tensions within intersectionality theory, it is now possible to introduce a new methodological approach to inform research and theory building. To overcome existing limitations, a novel methodological approach is necessary and can be achieved through drawing upon the ontological assumptions within critical realism. This approach attempts to rectify the problematic assumptions and outcomes of the three approaches outlined by McCall (2005) by drawing upon critical realist philosophy to sketch a novel intersectional ontological framework. The development of such an approach can reinvigorate intersectionality theory with the ability to assess how a particular individual's social position is enabled and constrained by generative structural mechanisms, and how these mechanisms operate in regard to particular intersections of wider structural categories, such as race, class, and gender. Of the existing approaches, the treatment of social categories has been taken to be their most prominent feature and lent itself to their names. However, the conceptual tools found within critical realism enable us to not only acknowledge the importance of such categories, but also to extend attention beyond them to that of positionality. This new approach will therefore be referred to as the 'positional' approach, presented here as an augmented conceptual framework to existing intersectionality theory. Its key characteristics are outlined in Table 3 below.

Table 3 Positional approach to methodological complexity in intersectionality

Approach to complexity	*Positional*
Approach to categories	Use as starting point to analyse broader social locations and processes.
Predominant philosophical influence	Critical realist
Key assumptions	Depth ontology, transfactuality, and morphogenetic approach to structure, culture, and agency. Concrete universals.
Key outcomes	Structure = durable relationships that position, constrain and/or enable. Social positioning as a continuous process, negotiated by agency. Marginality not a monolith. Nuanced experiences of privilege and oppression.

From a critical realist positional approach, abstract concepts such as 'women' would be acknowledged to be 'qualitatively different from lived reality', and so could be used as categories of analysis 'without any expectation that they will correspond to [...] lived reality in any clear-cut sense' (Gunnarsson 2011, p. 32). Instead, they will correspond to structural positions. Into each of these positions will be built, 'certain structured interests, resources, powers, constraints and predicaments', instituted by the web of relationships that make up a social structure (Porpora 1998, p. 344). The notion of structural positions within critical realism strongly echoes the intersectional notion of positionality. Aligning the two concepts, a positional approach enables the claim that generative structural mechanisms of oppression and privilege can emerge from the durable yet dynamic intersections of social categories. Such mechanisms position agents in particular social locations in which agency, the force by which we negotiate our positioning, is enabled or constrained in relation to the effects of such privilege and oppression on lived experience. Archer's well-elaborated notions of agency (1995, 2000, 2007) can help to draw feminist theorising away from post-structuralist conceptions of a fragmented, disempowered subject and towards a unified, embodied subject capable of agency (Clegg 2006) and engaged in processes of social positioning. Accordingly, positionality would be understood to influence life-chances (Archer 2000; Anthias 2001b), concrete access to material, economic, political, symbolic and cultural resources (Anthias 2001a, p. 635), and condition the cognitive resources available for conducting the internal conversations, both conscious and unconscious, that influence agent action (Mutch 2004).

A critical realist intersectional ontology, as shown in Table 4, accounts for the various structural forces privileging and disadvantaging individuals, even if events expected to arise from them did not occur or were not recognised (transfactuality). These forces would be understood to be emergent; as such, they adhere to the critical realist conception of emergence (Bhaskar 1998 [1979];

Table 4 Critical realist intersectional ontology

Real	Real generative mechanisms emerge from intersecting structures of domination that serve to position individuals and groups within social hierarchies. These complex and dynamic mechanisms privilege or disadvantage (enable or constrain) agents in relation to social mobility and material, political, social, cultural, and economic resources.
Actual	Enablement or constraint on the basis of positionality impacts people's lives – in particular, by offering or limiting opportunities and choices, and affecting how they are perceived and treated by institutions, groups and individuals.
Empirical	Via their tendencies, privileges and disadvantages are recognized, acknowledged, and understood by individual agents, others, institutions. They may (to some degree) be measurable or quantifiable. They may (or may not) be taken into account and considered in the exercise of agency.

Archer 1995) in which reality is arranged in levels, and something qualitatively new can emerge from a lower level (Danermark et al. 2002). Some key examples of mechanisms emergent from the level of society are racism (discrimination for not belonging to the dominant race), sexism (discrimination for not belonging to the dominant gender or refusing the prescriptions of one's assumed gender), and classism (discrimination for not belonging to the dominant class). Emergence also means that new forces can arise from the historical interactions of other mechanisms. The notion of misogynoir, defined as the hatred of black women and girls (Durham et al. 2013), is an example of such a mechanism, structurally emergent from the interactions of racism and sexism. A realist intersectional ontology would illuminate how, although social categories may be abstract constructions, they serve to define real relationships of power from which causal mechanisms emerge. Moreover, these mechanisms can in some cases exist unactualised, or be actualised but unrecognised by actors, groups and institutions. Subsequently, research can identify how intersectional forces are perceived (or not) by individual agents and wider social structures. This opens research methodology to explore intersectional forces on the three levels of reality Bhaskar identified, as well as the emergent levels within them (1998 [1979]).

This article has argued that intersectionality has thus far been shaped predominantly by philosophical roots in positivist and hermeneuticist perspectives. From a positivist perspective, prediction is desired, categories are treated as fixed and their intersections conceptualised as separable and calculable (Nash 2011, p. 461; Mehrotra 2010). From a hermeneuticist perspective, social categories are to be deconstructed and rejected, and what is instead sought is 'the constitution of subjectivity within discourse' (New 2003, p. 65 c. f. Weedon 1997, p. 163) with a focus on identity as metonym for how this subjectivity is constructed. In contrast, a critical realist perspective would distinguish between theory and experience, analytically separate categories from the lived experiences of the people to whom they refer and be aimed primarily towards causal explanation, not prediction. Categories would be seen as abstractions and actors as their referents, occupying dynamic, non-deterministic structural positions that constrain or enable them, in concert or in conflict, in intersecting ways. It would reject the additive approach that places oppression as the sum total of multiple categories of discrimination in favour of an approach that understands these categories as mutually shaped by, and shaping, each other (see Yuval-Davis 2006; Walby et al. 2012). Seeking links between the macro and the micro (Mole 2012), it would acknowledge and attend to the fluid nature of intersections and categories as they impact identities and agency, but recognise that the social meanings and conditions attached to categories are structurally emergent and therefore, more durable over time. This conceptual framework thus offers the potential answer Nash's call (2011) to advance intersectional theory and research by enabling it to more effectively explain the nature of structures of domination, as well as how they are connected and replicate themselves.

Conclusion

Critical realism offers intersectional theory an alternative ontological framework that has the potential to remove it from the quagmire of a growing critique that has the potential to obscure and constrain its contribution. This article has helped to illustrate the manner in which the scope and explanatory power of intersectionality theory is limited by implicit philosophical assumptions stemming from roots in positivist and hermeneutic traditions. It argues that critical realism contains the conceptual tools necessary to augment intersectionality theory and rectify some of its problematic limitations. Building on existing feminist critiques of intersectionality, the foundations for a novel approach to intersectional complexity, one that takes critical realism as its predominant philosophical influence, has been proposed. This critical realist positional approach moves away from, on the one hand, inter- and intra-categorical conceptions of discrete and intersecting social categories, and on the other, the popular anti-categorical approaches that reject categories altogether. Instead, categories can be taken as abstract starting points with durable social meaning from which to explore broader structural inequalities as well as dynamic processes of positionality and agency. Using critical realist tools to develop intersectionality theory in this way would enable its advancement beyond discussions of identity and towards the original aims of the intersectional and realist projects of dismantling structures of social oppression, and promoting emancipation and human flourishing.

Note

1 This chapter was originally published as Angela Martinez Dy, Lee Martin, and Susan Marlow (2014) Developing a Critical Realist Positional Approach to Intersectionality, *Journal of Critical Realism*, 13:5, 447–466, DOI: 10.1179/1476743014Z.00000000043. © Taylor & Francis Ltd, http://www.tandfonline.com. Reprinted by permission of the publisher.

References

Acker, J. 2000. "Revisiting Class: Thinking from Gender, Race and Organizations." *Social Politics* 7(2): 192–214.

———. 2006. "Inequality Regimes: Gender, Class, and Race in Organizations." *Gender & Society* 20: 441–464.

Ahmed, S. 2012. *On Being Included: Racism and Diversity in Institutional Life*. Durham and London: Duke University Press.

Anthias, F. 2001a. "New Hybridities, Old Concepts: The Limits of 'Culture'." *Ethnic and Racial Studies* 24(4): 619–641.

———. 2001b. "The Material and The Symbolic in Theorizing Social Stratification: Issues of Gender, Ethnicity and Class." *British Journal of Sociology* 52(3): 367–390.

——— 2002. "Beyond Feminism and Multiculturalism: Locating Difference and the Politics of Location." *Women's Studies International Forum* 25(3): 275–286.

———. 2006. "Belongings in a Globalising and Unequal World: Rethinking Translocations," in *The Situated Politics of Belonging*, eds. N. Yuval-Davis, K. Kannabiran and U. Vieten. London: Sage.

———. 2008. "Thinking Through the Lens of Translocational Positionality: An Intersectionality Frame for Understanding Identity and Belonging." *Translocations: Migration and Social Change* 4(1): 5–20.

Anthias, F., Yuval-Davis, N. 1992. *Racialized Boundaries*. London: Routledge.

Archer, M. 1995. *Realist Social Theory: The Morphogenetic Approach*. Cambridge: Cambridge University Press.

———. 2000. *Being Human: The Problem of Agency*. Cambridge: Cambridge University Press.

Bhaskar, R. 2008 [1975]. *A Realist Theory of Science*. 2nd Edition. London: Verso.

———. 1998 [1979]. *The Possibility of Naturalism*. 3rd Edition. London: Routledge.

———. 2008 [1993]. *Dialectic: The Pulse of Freedom*. 2nd Edition. London: Routledge.

Bordieu, P. 1977. *Outline of a Theory of Practice*. Cambridge: Cambridge University Press.

Bowleg, L. 2008. "When Black + Lesbian + Woman ≠ Black Lesbian Woman: The Methodological Challenges of Qualitative and Quantitative Intersectionality Research." *Sex Roles* 59(5–6): 312–325.

Brown, T., Heggs, D. 2005. "From Hermeneutics to Poststructuralism to Psychoanalysis," in B. Somekh and C. Lewin (eds.) *Research Methods in the Social Sciences*. London: Sage.

Butler, J. 1990. *Gender Trouble: Feminism and the Subversion of Identity*. New York and London: Routledge.

——— 1998. "Merely Cultural." *New Left Review* I(277): 33–44.

Carbin, M., Edenheim, S. 2013. "The Intersectional Turn in Feminist Theory: A Dream of a Common Language?" *European Journal of Women's Studies* 20(3): 233–248.

Clegg, S. 2006. "The Problem of Agency in Feminism: A Critical Realist Approach." *Gender and Education* 18(3): 309–324.

Combahee River Collective. 1977. *A Black Feminist Statement From The Combahee River Collective*. [online] Available at: http://www.feministezine.com/feminist/modern/Black-Feminist-Statement.html. [Accessed 22 Jan 2013].

Cooper, F. R. 2005. "Against Bipolar Black Masculinity: Intersectionality, Assimilation, Identity Performance, and Hierarchy." *U.C. Davis Law Review* 39: 853–904.

Crenshaw, K. 1989. "Demarginalizing The Intersection Of Race And Sex: A Black Feminist Critique Of Antidiscrimination Doctrine, Feminist Theory And Antiracist Politics." *The University of Chicago Legal Forum*: 139–167.

Cruickshank, J. 2003. 'Introduction,' in J. Cruickshank (ed.) *Critical Realism: The Difference it Makes*. London: Routledge.

Danermark, B., Ekström, M., Jakobsen, L., Karlsson, J. C. 2002. *Explaining Society: Critical Realism in the Social Sciences*. London and New York: Routledge.

Davis, A. 1981. *Women, Race and Class*. New York: Random House.

Davis, K. 2008. "Intersectionality as Buzzword: A Sociology of Science Perspective on What Makes a Feminist Theory Successful." *Feminist Theory* 9(1): 67–85.

Dhamoon, R.K. 2011. "Considerations on Mainstreaming Intersectionality." *Political Research Quarterly* 64(1): 230–243.

Durham, A., Cooper, B.C., Morris, S.M. 2013. "The Stage Hip-Hop Feminism Built: A New Directions Essay." *Signs* 38(3): 721–737.

Fleetwood, S. 2004. "An Ontology for Organization and Management Studies," in S. Fleetwood and S. Ackroyd (eds.) *Critical Realist Applications in Organisation and Management Studies*. London: Psychology Press.

Frankenberg, R. 1993. *White Women, Race Matters: The Social Construction of Whiteness.* Minneapolis: University of Minnesota Press.

Geerts, E., van der Tuin, I. 2013. "From Intersectionality to Interference: Feminist Onto-Epistemological Reflections on the Politics of Representation." *Women's Studies International Forum* 41(3): 171–178.

Giddens, A. 1979. *Central Problems in Social Theory: Action, Structure and Contradiction in Social Analysis.* Berkeley and Los Angeles: University of California Press.

Gunnarsson, L. 2011. "In Defence of The Category 'Woman'." *Feminist Theory* 12(1): 23–37.

Hancock, A. 2007. "When Multiplication Doesn't Equal Quick Addition: Examining Intersectionality as a Research Paradigm." *Perspectives on Politics* 5(1): 63–79.

Haraway, D. 1988. "Situated Knowledges: The Science Question in Feminism and the Privilege of Partial Perspective." *Feminist Studies* 14(3): 575–599.

Harding, S. 1991. *Whose Science? Whose Knowledge? Thinking from Women's Lives.* Milton Keynes: Open University Press.

———. 1986. "The Instability of the Analytical Categories of Feminist Theory." *Signs* 11(4): 645–664.

Hill Collins, P. 2000 [1990]. *Black Feminist Thought.* 2nd Edition. New York, NY: Routledge.

hooks, b. 1981. *Ain't I a Woman: Black Women and Feminism.* Boston, MA: South End Press.

Hurtado, A. 1989. "Relating to Privilege: Seduction and Rejection in the Subordination of White Women and Women of Color." *Signs* 14(4): 833–855.

Letherby, G. 2003. *Feminist Research in Theory and Practice.* Buckingham, Open University Press.

Maier, M. 1997. "Invisible Privilege: What White Men Don't See." *The Diversity Factor* 5(4): 28–33.

McCall, L. 2005. "The Complexity of Intersectionality." *Signs* 30(3): 1771–1800.

McIntosh, P. 1989. "White Privilege: Unpacking the Invisible Knapsack." *Peace and Freedom* July/August: 10–12.

McNay, L. 2000. *Gender and Agency: Reconfiguring the Subject in Feminist and Social Theory.* Cambridge: Polity.

Mehrotra, G. 2010. "Toward a Continuum of Intersectionality Theorizing for Feminist Social Work Scholarship." *Affilia* 25(4): 417–430.

Mole, K. 2012. "Critical Realism and Entrepreneurship," in K. Mole (ed.) with M. Ram *Perspectives in Entrepreneurship: A Critical Approach.* Houndmills: Palgrave MacMillan.

Mutch, A. 2004. "Constraints on the Internal Conversation: Margaret Archer and the Structural Shaping of Thought." *Journal for the Theory of Social Behaviour* 34(4): 429–445.

Nash, J. 2008. "Re-Thinking Intersectionality." *Feminist Review* 89: 1–15.

———. 2011. "'Home Truths' on Intersectionality". *Yale Journal of Law and Feminism* 23(1): 445–470.

New, C. 2003. "Feminism, Critical Realism and the Linguistic Turn," in J. Cruickshank (ed.) *Critical Realism: The Difference it Makes.* London: Routledge.

———. 1998. "Realism, Deconstruction and the Feminist Standpoint." *Journal for the Theory of Social Behaviour* 28(4): 349–372.

Oleksy, E. 2011. "Intersectionality at the Cross-roads." *Women's Studies International Forum* 34(4): 263–270.

Porpora, D. 1998. "Four Concepts of Social Structure," in M. Archer, R. Bhaskar, A. Collier, T. Lawson and A. Norrie. *Critical Realism: Essential Readings*. New York, NY: Routledge.

Prins, B. 2006. "Narrative Accounts of Origins: A Blind Spot in the Intersectional Approach?" *European Journal of Women's Studies* 13(3): 277–290.

Walby, S., Armstrong, J., Strid, S. 2012. "Intersectionality: Multiple Inequalities in Social Theory." *Sociology* 46: 224–240.

Yuval-Davis, N. 2006. "Intersectionality and Feminist Politics." *European Journal of Women's Studies* 13(3): 193–209.

7 Agency and ontology within intersectional analysis

A critical realist contribution[1]

Sue Clegg

Introduction

This article will explore one of the most important and influential currents within contemporary feminist analysis, namely, intersectionality. Intersectional analysis was developed by black women scholars who identified important absences, both political and theoretical, in feminist and other strands of anti-racist and critical theory (Crenshaw 1989). The success of intersectional theory has been in its bringing together of activist political concerns with post-structuralist sensibilities. As Kathy Davis (2008, p. 74) argues, intersectional theory has been remarkably successful in overcoming the apparent incompatibilities between these two projects.

It takes up the political project of making the social and material consequences of the categories of gender/race/class visible but does so by employing the methodologies compatible with the post-structuralist project of deconstructing categories, unmasking universalism, and exploring the dynamic and contradictory workings of power.

This is a seductive combination. Davis has argued that the ambiguities and contradictions within intersectional theory, rather than being a problem, are the source of its productivity. In this article, I will explore some of these contradictions and tensions, and suggest that while they do indeed contribute to the theory's popularity, they limit its explanatory potential.

Pointing to the gaps and slippages within intersectional theory is not new (Anthias 1998). However, I argue that we can draw on critical realism, notably, the work of Margaret Archer (1995, 1996, 2000, 2007, 2012), as a resource to reconceptualise what the research projects of intersectional theory might be. Intersectional theory is productive of numerous research questions at different levels of analysis but rather than celebrating, as Davis does, the blurring of distinctions between different projects and analytical levels, I suggest that critical realism offers a way of unpacking them. The challenge faced by intersectional analysis is that analytical distinctions between structure and agency, and between culture and agency, are elided. By equivocating between experiences of oppression and the structures that produce them, the historicity of emergence is collapsed.

This is particularly the case in post-structuralist and other anti-categorical accounts in which, as pointed out by Angela Martinez Dy, Lee Martin and Sue Marlow, 'notions of positionality or structural discrimination are often collapsed into the concept of "identity"' (2014, p. 454, ch. 6 this volume, p.149). Notions of identity are insufficient to the analytical task of providing accounts of the contextual conditions and structural components that engender (or inhibit) them. Along with other authors (Walby, Armstrong and Strid 2012; Martinez Dy, Martin and Marlow 2014; Gunnarsson 2017, ch. 8 this volume) I will argue that critical realism has much to offer. In particular, it avoids elisions between structural processes and the identity work of persons: in Archerian terms (1995), between structurally emergent properties (SEPs), culturally emergent properties (CEPs), and the emergent properties of people (PEPs). Critical realism challenges linguistic notions of identity and offers an account of 'being human' (Archer 2000) and of the *sui generis* powers of persons (the PEPs), not just of social structures. I will argue that such an account of agency is important to sustain the normative intent of intersectional analysis and the political projects that underpin it.

Accordingly, the article is structured in four parts: the first deals with the emergence of intersectional theory and its antinomies and elisions. The second introduces some of the key concepts from critical realism, with a specific focus on morphogenesis. The third involves an analysis of agency, since personal and corporate agency are central to understanding why intersectional theory matters. Finally, I will reprise why I think that critical realism is a better theoretical resource than post-structuralism, notwithstanding the many important insights feminist post-structuralist theorists have contributed to the analysis of the intersections between gender, race, class and other markers of structural and cultural difference.

Intersectional theory

In order to make sense of the current debates about intersectionality, it is necessary to locate the particular historical circumstances within which the term came into usage. Intersectionality is not so much a unified theory as a series of concrete socio-political problems and situations that require analysis. It can be seen as extending the research programme that flowed from initial feminist interventions across the disciplines in the late 1960s. As Heidi Safia Mirza (2009, p. 3) succinctly puts it in her introduction to a special issue of *Race Ethnicity and Education* on black and postcolonial feminisms:

> Women, who are collectively defined as 'black' or 'Asian' in official policy or practice have multiple experiences in terms of their age, sexuality, disability, religion or culture. Thus, it is argued racism, patriarchy, social class and other systems of oppression simultaneously structure the relative position of these women at any one time creating specific and varied patterns of inequality and

> discrimination. It is the cultural and historical specificity of inequality that black, postcolonial and anti-racist feminists stress as important in developing a more holistic intersectional approach to mainstream feminist analysis.

Presented as such, this might seem uncontroversial, but the particular circumstances in which intersectionality came to be seen as a necessary corrective is indicated in the reference in the last sentence to 'mainstream feminist analysis'. From the early days of second-wave feminism there had been debates about the tensions between the idea of 'women' as a unified political subject, and the increasingly voiced lived realities of experiences of difference and other forms of oppression not simply based on gender. These views challenged mainstream feminist theory and gave rise to a perception that feminism was universalistic in its orientation, based on a false generalisation from white women's experiences, which was identified as a weakness both analytically and politically.

This was never a simple story; the women's movement was nothing if not fractious, and vigorous debate emerged about forms of difference based on sexuality, race, class and other categories of oppression and how to theorise them. The general critique was that 1970s feminism had essentialised and generalised from middle-class white women's experiences (Segal 1987, 1999). This was always problematic as the argument fails to distinguish between the political demands of new corporate agents (groups of women) agitating against particular forms of oppression, and identity as a woman. What made this so potent in feminism was the role of the personal (David 2003) and the practice of 'consciousness raising' as a way of going from the personal to the political. This meant that direct personal experience and identity were valorised in ways not found in other radical political projects of the left. It was not an issue in the same way, for example, in class politics (except in its Lukácsian formulation) since class is not assumed to be a unitary identity, although of course one of the criticisms many feminists made against class politics was that it *de facto* represented the interests of white, and often skilled and organised, men.

At its worst, the formulation of the 'personal is political' reduced to forms of bitterly fought identity politics. The charge of unconscious privilege was levelled at white middle-class women who had undoubtedly dominated many early women's groups (Rowbotham 1990). These strains have re-emerged in popular usages of intersectionality (Williams 2013) despite post-structuralism's theoretical break with universalism and 'experience'. The tensions between universalism as a strategy and the necessity of attention to difference reoccur over and over again. For example, in her book *Sexual/Textual Politics: Feminist Literary Theory* Toril Moi (1985) did much to theoretically destabilise the category of woman while insisting on its strategic political importance (cf. Moi 1999), while more recently Gunnarsson (2011, ch. 4 this volume, 2017, ch. 8 this volume) has defended the category of women and the importance of research that deals with the distinctive powers and properties of gender, race and class.

The need to theorise differences between women as well as the nature of women's oppression, therefore, did not begin with the coinage of the term intersectionality, but what it did, according to Davis, was give it a 'novel twist'

(2008, p. 72). As early as 1974, for example, the Manifesto of the Combahee River Collective began '[a]s black feminists and lesbians who know that we have a very definite revolutionary task to perform' and they went on to describe the major systems of oppression as 'interlocking' (Combahee River Collective 1977). The term intersectionality, coined by Kimberlé Crenshaw (1989), was an attempt to concretely theorise these experiences and to show how they worked. What Crenshaw, an academic lawyer, did in articulating 'intersectionality' was to draw attention to the tendency for gender and race to be treated as separate categories, with the result that black women were marginalised in both feminist and anti-racist theory and politics. She argued that:

> Because the intersectional experience is greater than the sum of racism and sexism, any analysis that does not take intersectionality into account cannot sufficiently address the particular manner in which black women are subordinated.
>
> (1989, p. 140)

She made her case through a meticulous analysis of the ways in which black women are erased within anti-discrimination law. Her key example was of a law case brought against General Motors, alleging that the seniority system perpetuated discrimination against black women. Prior to the Civil Rights Act, General Motors had not hired black women, it had hired white women, so the ruling argued that the company was not discriminating on the basis of sex. At the same time the court recommended that their claim be considered with another case as part of a general race discrimination claim, thus denying the relevance of gender. Other cases similarly denied remediation to black women as black women; thus, white women in effect became the default plaintiffs of cases of sex discrimination, while black men took priority in cases of racial discrimination.

Crenshaw was also critical of mainstream feminist theory. She argued that despite having drawn on black women's history, most notably through references to Sojourner Truth's famous words 'Ain't I a Woman?' (Crenshaw 1989, p. 153), white feminists had failed to take account of the needs, interests and experiences of black women when articulating their political demands and in theorising the position of women. Another example of this, much debated in the 1970s, was the theoretical attention paid to women's relegation to the private sphere of the home, but these debates had little to say about black women's history and the ways they were denied a 'home'. Crenshaw (1989) was similarly critical of the ways anti-racist politics and theory failed to address gender and the specificity of black women's experiences.

Since 1989, intersectionality has become a widely used term, and Davis (2008) has persuasively argued that the ambiguity of the term has allowed the interests of both generalist and specialist feminist theoreticians to come together with those of activists. Nira Yuval-Davis (2006), however, points out that intersectional analysis arrived on the European scene from the US without much effect on policy makers. She argues, furthermore, that the 'triple oppression' approach was especially problematic as there 'is no such thing as suffering from oppression "as Black", "as a woman", "as a working class person"' (2006, p. 195). Rather, she and other theorists have pointed to the different ontological bases of each social division, irreducible and distinct from one another (see also Anthias 1998). It is important to notice, therefore, that from the beginning, a number of different sorts of arguments were being adduced: about historically sedimented structures of multiple oppressions, about experiences and identities, about black women as political subjects and the ways their specific issues could be addressed in theory, how feminist and anti-racist theory itself failed to address the particular intersections of race, gender and other forms of oppression, and about the political conclusions that can be made from these different forms of analysis. The breadth of arguments that can be encompassed under the heading of intersectionality and the additive effect of different sorts of arguments make elision particularly problematic.

These problems are compounded by what Martinez Dy, Martin and Marlow (2014) describe as, on the one hand, the feminist empiricist tradition which treats race, class and gender as additive effects, and, on the other, the hermeneutic tradition which concentrates on experiences and anti-categorical notions of identity. As they point out, both these traditions risk omitting 'that which may be unexercised, unactualised, or unobserved' (2014, 452) and exclude an ontology of 'transfactuality'. Along with Martinez Dy, Martin and Marlow (2014) and Gunnarsson (2011, 2017) (see also Walby, Armstrong and Strid 2012), I draw on concepts from critical realism that bring greater clarity to the notion of intersectional explanation, and that also allow us to make analytical distinctions between structure and agency in theorising intersectionality. I will argue that intersectional analysis is better understood not as a singular theory but as a research programme spanning a number of disciplines. I am not, however, presenting a unified critical realist version of intersectionality, since there is no unitary object to be investigated. The questions posed in the debates on intersectionality operate across different time periods, at different analytical levels, and are amenable to different normative conclusions. The analysis of historically specific intersections requires paying attention to structural and cultural properties as well to the operation of individual and collective agency. It makes no more sense, however, to reduce structural problems to individual experience than it does to think that experience can be deduced from structure, which is why I suggest that Archer's morphogenetic approach has much to offer.

Critical realism and morphogenetic analysis

Critical realism offers a series of theoretical concepts that are central to the possibility of doing sociological work in general, a role Roy Bhaskar (1975) described as under-labouring. Bhaskar (1975, 1979) provides a powerful analysis of the inadequacies of both idealism and positivism. In their place he argues for a depth ontology in which the domain of the real encompasses not only experiences (our sensory perceptions of things) and events (actual occurring things) but also underlying mechanisms. These often non-observable mechanisms are nonetheless real and Bhaskar argues that it is they that produce the world of events that we come to experience in the here and now. Explanation involves the identification of underlying mechanisms that operate transfactually in the open systems confronted in doing social science, which has methodological implications. Andrew Sayer (1992), in his book *Method in Social Science*, provides insight into the process of retroduction, 'a mode of inference in which events are explained by postulating (and identifying) mechanisms which are capable of producing them' (1992, p. 107). In particular, he describes the process whereby we need to abstract from the particularities of the concrete situation and exclude those things that have no significant effects in order to isolate and concentrate on the things that do. This form of abstraction and the reconstitution of the concrete is particularly important, as we shall see, when confronted by increasingly extended lists of the numbers of possible intersections (Yuval-Davis 2006). The recognition of the need for a depth ontology is crucial in resolving some of the analytical and methodological problems that have beset research on intersectionality (Martinez Dy, Martin and Marlow 2014).

Equally important, however, given that historicity is equally crucial for understanding the ways multiple structures of oppression operate, is Archer's argument about the historicity of emergence. Archer (1995) is the key theorist of a morphogenetic approach to analysing social life, developed to ground her explanatory methodology.

> The 'morpho' element is an acknowledgement that society has no pre-set form or preferred state: the 'genetic' part is a recognition that it takes its shape from, and is formed by, agents, originating from the intended and unintended consequences of their activities.
>
> (1995, p. 5)

In keeping with the rejection of both idealism and positivism that underpins all critical realism, Archer develops a critique of their sociological manifestations in the form of downward, upward and central conflations of structure and agency. Instead, she argues the need for analytical dualism. Upward conflation involves viewing society as no more than the aggregate of the behaviour of individuals (Archer 1995, p. 4), whereas downward conflation reifies society and reduces individual action to societal determination (1995, p. 3). Central conflation involves a denial of the separability of structure and agency since every aspect of structure is activity dependent, a position endorsed by social theorists such as Anthony Giddens and involving, according to Archer (1995, pp. 60–1), an elisionist rather than an emergentist ontology. Archer argues that conflationary analysis effectively confines itself to a sociology of the present, in which structure is only evident in its present enactments.

In contrast, her morphogenetic approach is fundamentally about historicity. It is based on the necessity of analytically distinguishing between structure and agency and their separate emergent, irreducible and autonomous causal properties. Time becomes the key to understanding how structural conditioning at time 1 and sociocultural interaction at time 2 to time 3 results in structural elaboration (morphogenesis) or structural reproduction (morphostasis) at time 4.

Analytical dualism is the methodological principle whereby the relationship between structure and agency can be analysed over space and time. The key features of the model are historicity, emergence and mediation based on the real powers of structurally emergent properties (SEPs), culturally emergent properties (CEPs) and the emergent properties of people (PEPs). Crucially, this approach allows us to explore restructuring over time and insists on the irreducible and continuing significance of agency as well as structure.

> All structural properties in any society are continuously activity dependent. Nevertheless, it is possible to separate 'structure' and 'agency' through analytical dualism and to examine their interplay in order to account for the structuring and restructuring of the social order. Fundamentally, this is possible for two reasons. Firstly 'structure' and 'agency' *are different kinds of emergent properties* … Secondly, and fundamental to the workability of this explanatory methodology, 'structure' and 'agency' operate diachronically over different tracts of time because: (i) structure necessarily pre-dates the action(s) that transform it and (ii) structural elaboration necessarily post-dates those actions.
>
> (Archer 2012, p. 52, original emphasis)

This is key if we are to make sense of the structuring at time 1 that confronts black women (and other actors) with conditions not of their own choosing and upon which they reflexively act. It is clear from studies that the structuring conditions at time 1 are multiple and, moreover, if we are thinking in terms of both race and gender, that some areas are deeply resistant to change. We can identify a *long durée* in terms of reproduction with periods of morphostasis in relation to gender relations of power, for example. The outcome is not preordained, but our explanations as to why the outcome is change rather than stasis depend on looking at the structuring conditions and at individual and collective, or what Archer (2000) calls corporate, agency.

Archer (1996) not only takes into account structural properties and emergence, but also takes culture seriously, introducing an analytically important distinction between Cultural System and the Socio-Cultural. The Cultural System refers to the existing intelligibilia: the ideas that can be expressed at any one time (whether these are actually expressed or not). The logical relations between these elements within the system can be analysed through the formal features of the system, namely those of contradiction, change, mutual reinforcement (complementarities) and reproduction. The Socio-Cultural refers to how ideas map onto relationships between people – in other words, how ideas are taken up and mobilised. To simply reduce the former to the latter would be a form of epistemic fallacy, since it reduces culture to our understanding of it. Socio-Cultural elaboration at time 2–3 at the cultural level involves paying attention to both the Cultural System and the Socio-Cultural, which again can result in either morphogenesis or morphostasis.

Analytical dualism offers a valuable resource for thinking about intersections because it prises open the connections between structure and agency, and thus opens them up for explanatory accounts. Conflationary analysis is especially problematic in intersectional theorising where structures of oppression are seen as instantiated in the 'doing' of race and gender and other forms of oppression. For example, West and Fenstermaker (1995) make valuable criticisms of mathematical metaphors in feminist theory, of which, of course, the intersection is one. Their solution, however, is to propose an ethnomethodological approach in which 'the "objective" and "factual" properties of social life attain such status through the situated conduct of societal members' (1995, p. 19). Effectively, different forms of oppression are analysed simultaneously by looking at how they are achieved through the ongoing activity of actors in the present. This is a form of central conflation, since neither structure nor agency can be thought of independently of one another. What we have instead is continuous reproduction in present time. The historicity of emergence is lost in this account, and with it, the potential for explanatory analysis, since structure is dissolved into repeated contextual enactments.

This lack of analytical distinction also presents major problems for sustaining analytically useful categories such as women, since of course 'woman' is never instantiated in isolation from other social properties; hence, the charge of essentialism against early feminists who used the term 'women/woman' in their accounts of women's oppression. However, in a carefully argued critical realist account, Gunnarsson (2011) defends the category of women, pointing out that the starting point of feminist theory is to show how women are oppressed and exploited '*by virtue of the fact of their being women*' (2011, p. 24). Drawing on the work of Sayer (1992), she argues that abstract categories such as gender, race and class are essential for theorisation of structures of oppression that do not reduce to the level of the lived reality of individuals. When we use the term women we are referring to an abstraction as part of an explanatory account, and crucially:

> critical realists apply a 'causal criterion' for ascribing a distinct reality to something … If something has an impact on the world that is irreducible to the causal effects of other entities we can talk of it as a distinct reality, *even though this reality is wholly premised on its relationship with other things.*
>
> (Gunnarsson 2017, p. 118, original emphasis)

The critical realist account of explanation and the morphogenetic approach allow us to address the issue of separate but entangled processes in a way that does not lead to central conflation. This ability to hold structure and agency analytically separate is essential to address the multiple forms of oppression and exploitation that Crenshaw identified, since although at the level of lived experience the concrete realities of race, class and gender co-exist, we need to be able to separate structure and agency to account for stasis and change over time.

Social theory needs to wrestle with understanding the multiple determinations of the concrete by employing necessary abstraction and accounting for the unseen. For this reason, critical realists utilise unifying non-deterministic categories as well as recognise the reality of mechanisms, not just events. In addition, the significance of historicity would be common ground for many intersectional theorists, although not necessarily under the terms considered above. Before further considering the potential explanatory power of morphogenetic analysis, however, I want to introduce Archer's concept of agency, since this is highly distinctive and marks a break with post-structuralist theories of identity on which much intersectional analysis rests (Davis 2008).

Agency

Central to Archer's (2000) theory of agency is the assertion of the primacy of practice rather than language, and her insistence that people have *sui generis* properties and powers that are not reducible to either those of structure or culture. In doing so she breaks with the disembodied subject of 'modernity's man', critiquing how '[t]he metaphysics of modernity … adduced a model of instrumentally rational man who could attain his ends in the world by pure *logos*, a rationality working through the formal manipulation of linguistic symbols to generate truth' (2000, p. 23). Instead, in her book *Being Human: The Problem of Agency*, she elaborates a theory of the potentiality of active human agents, whose properties and powers are emergent from our relations with the environment and with relative autonomy from both society and biology.

> The properties and powers of the human being are neither seen as *pregiven*, nor as *socially appropriated*, but rather these are emergent from our relations with our environment. As such they have relative autonomy from biology and society alike, and causal powers to modify both of them.
>
> (2000, p. 87, original emphasis)

By insisting on the primacy of practice – Marx's 'continuous practical activity in a material world' (Archer 2000, p. 122) – and the importance of the embodiedness of human being, as a species being with natural potentials, Archer develops a theory of the conditions for the emergence of the self in its necessary relations with the environment. In doing so she distinguishes between concepts of the self that are necessarily social, and a sense of the self that is not – so that while there are discursively produced subjectivities, there is also an embodied sense of self continuous through the history of a particular life. She argues that a coherent account of the development of agents and social actors needs to be grounded in this nondiscursively formed continuous sense of self. This is a decisive break with the linguistic dominance found in post-structuralist theorising and acts to ground Archer's account of what it means to act in the world.

Archer's model of personal and social identity is one in which individual and collective agents have the resources to act creatively in the world, thus creating conditions for transformation and change as well as social stasis. She theorises the ways in which people come to be able to act reflexively through her notion of the 'internal conversation', which is essential to how humans come to make (always fallible) judgements about the conditions in which they find themselves and deliberate about possible courses of action. She argues that human beings are fundamentally evaluative in their relations with reality, and that the 'inner conversation' is critical in understanding how human beings come to make commitments.

The 'inner conversation' is how our personal emergent powers are exercised on and in the world – natural, practical and social – which is our triune environment. This 'interior dialogue' is not just a window on the world, rather it is what determines our being in the world, though not in times and circumstances of our choosing. Fundamentally, the 'inner conversation' is constitutive of our concrete singularity. However, it is also and necessarily a conversation about reality. This is because the triune world sets us three problems, none of which can be evaded, made as we are. It confronts us with three inescapable concerns: with our physical well-being, our performative competence and our self worth (2000, p. 318).

In keeping with her morphogenetic approach Archer elaborates how the 'me' in the present – 'the conditioning me' at time 1– becomes at time 2 the conversational 'I', whereby possible future projects are reviewed for the 'you' at time 3. The 'I' reflexively monitors its ultimate concerns. Human beings in this account are strong evaluators, with a range of personal powers, who confront their triune environment and who perforce possess embodied knowledge, practical knowledge and discursive knowledge. Reflexivity and the internal conversation are the means by which human beings can come to commit to their central concerns.

Not all forms of reflexivity are the same, and based on her empirical work Archer (2007, 2012) distinguishes between communicative, autonomous, meta and fractured reflexivity (although historically and cross-culturally there may be more). 'Communicative reflexives' remain anchored in the natal social context of their birth families; 'autonomous reflexives' adopt strategic stances towards constraints and become upwardly socially mobile; 'meta-reflexives' are 'contextually incongruous' and '*subversive* towards social constraints and enablements, because of their willingness to pay the price of the former and to forfeit the benefits of the latter in the attempt to live out their idea' (Archer 2007, p. 98, original emphasis); whereas 'fractured reflexives' are people who are unable to form and act on their central projects or cares. Her view of humans includes an elaboration of the importance of both first- and second-order emotion. It is a misapprehension on the part of some feminists, for example, in Nelson's (2003) contribution to a protracted debate about the value of critical realism for feminist economics, that critical realism excludes such matters (Clegg 2013).

Human beings come to reflexively define their central commitments through the internal conversation and this in turn forms the basis for developing corporate agency.

Organised interest groups represent the generation of a new emergent property amongst people (a PEP), whose power is the very special punch they pack as far as systemic stability and change are concerned. Only those who are aware of what they want, can articulate it to themselves and others, and have organised in order to obtain it, can engage in concerted action to reshape or retain the structural and/or cultural features in question. These are termed 'Corporate Agents': they include self-conscious vested interest groups, promotive interest groups, social movements and defensive associations. (Archer 2000, p. 265)

I have argued elsewhere (Clegg 2006) that Archer's concepts give us a powerful basis for theorising agency in feminism and for breaking both with the unified subject of modernity and the post-structuralist problematic of dissolving the political subject of feminism. While post-structuralist analysis has successfully documented aspects of unfixity and fragmentation in terms of social identity, it lacks the theoretical resource to explain the powerful sense of self that it ends up negating. This is because, despite the seeming openness in post-structuralism at the level of ontology, offered by the *and/and* formulation rather than *either/or* (Davies 1997, 2004), post-structuralism's fundamental ontological claim involves the primacy of the discursive and denial of a prediscursive self.[2] With these distinctions in mind, it is now possible to return to the central theme of this article, namely, critical realism as a resource for theorising the multiple intersections to which intersectionality refers.

Intersectional theory and critical realism

I have argued elsewhere (Clegg 2006, p. 2012) that there is often much commonality at the level of concrete analysis between theorists from different traditions. While there is overlap in terms of substantive analysis, critical realism rejects the Nietzschean legacy of post-structuralism and the idea that the individual subject is a fiction, that the will to power is constitutive of identity and reality, and that science itself has no special epistemological significance. Post-structuralism has offered intersectional theorists many useful methodological tools, but these are not the preserve of post-structuralist analysis. Attention to the significance of the discursive is not unique to post-structuralism; critical realism pays attention both to the discursive and the critical deconstruction of categories. In taking issue with specific pieces of research, it is often the ontological status of the claims being made that are being challenged and not the specific empirical arguments or the data presented.

Intersectional theory, as we have seen, resonated powerfully because the substantive situations its analysis sought to address are of immense importance for sociological theory, and it seemed to successfully align competing strands of feminist theory. However, as indicated, the danger in intersectional analysis is that analytical distinctions between structure and agency, and between culture and agency, are elided;[3] additionally, in simultaneously talking about both the experiences and the structures of oppression, the historicity of emergence is collapsed. This is particularly problematic where positions are argued that appear to be about structural and cultural forms of inequality (in Archerian terms: the operation of the SEPs and CEPs at time 1), but where these are then reduced to the question of multiple identities. Yuval-Davis (2006) gives a particularly apposite example of this kind of reasoning in the report of the Working Group on Women and Human Rights. She highlights how the report begins with structural concerns that 'structure the relative positions of women, races, ethnicities, classes and the like' (2006, p. 197), but is transmuted into a concern with specific identities. This slippage allows no space in which to consider how actors engage with structural conditions over time, reflexively engaging with the structural conditions at time 1 in order to commit to projects that may or may not result in morphogenesis. In this instance, the example is policy, in which the ability of people to come to evaluations and act upon their concerns is central. Therefore, the elaboration of particular identities may or may not have salience in the formation of particular social movements or alliances (or in Archerian terms, the exercise of corporate agency).

Thinking about historically sedimented structures of multiple oppressions presents a series of contexts that are suited to morphogenetic analysis at both the cultural and social level. A critical realist reading of Crenshaw's General Motors example could be that constraints in the ideational cultural system at time 1, implied by the legal separation of 'race' and 'gender', are elaborated and challenged at the socio-cultural level at time 2, as actors challenge this separation by insisting on the specificity of their oppression as 'black women' through attempts to seek remediation in court. Crenshaw identifies black women as previously unrecognised corporate actors; as such the ways their activities have led to changes in law and other institutions over time is clearly important. Equally important are questions regarding what has not changed, and the nature of structural constraints. The issue is not the elaboration of intersectional theory as a unitary set of propositions but of the specification of clear problems that can be analysed in ways that show how particular intersections operate over time. Historicity is, therefore, key to the argument.

The challenge for critical realist analysis is to bring the analytical lens that it affords to existing work on intersectionality, with the aim of clarifying what the claims might be, and also to mobilise critical realism as a resource for nascent research projects that explore specific instances of how intersections are operating. From a critical realist perspective, there is an important role for research that looks at the operation of specific mechanisms, in particular geohistorical locations.

> As long as we are clear that an analysis of for instance gender on its own terms relies on an abstraction of some processual parts from an infinitely complex social whole …, it is desirable that some theorists engage in 'separatist' theoretical explorations of what precisely this 'gender' (or 'race', 'class' 'sexuality') is, in certain geohistorical locations. Otherwise there is a risk that we reproduce unreflected notions of their ontologies.
>
> (Gunnarsson 2017, p. 123)

In other words, not all analysis undertaken from a critical realist perspective will be *of* intersections, but the philosophical clarity underpinning the work will mean that the work is capable of contributing to the wider research programme. The work of identifying particular mechanisms is grounded in a general philosophical model of explanation in the social sciences, based on the twin ideas of 'retroduction' and 'retrodiction' (Bhaskar 1986, p. 68). Theoretical explanation is retroductive and involves identifying and analysing underlying causal powers and mechanisms, and the entities that possess them. Retrodiction is the study of concrete phenomena through analysis of the multiple causal forces operating in the messy open systems of the social world. Retrodiction is of particular significance for intersectional analysis because it involves charting how different forms of oppression create 'specific and varied patterns of inequality' (Mirza 2009, p. 3), drawing on our knowledge of the multiple mechanisms at play in order to reconstitute the concrete.

As Davis (2008) points out, the political aims influenced by the idea of multiple oppressions, on the one hand, and post-structuralism, on the other, appeared to share the common goal of deconstructing the unified concept of woman. But post-structuralism, at its extreme, deconstructs all sorts of difference, including those that gave rise to the need to theorise intersectionality in the first place. The danger is that the structures and experiences referred to by Crenshaw and Mirza are reduced to the merely discursive and to the fluidity of unfixed identities. However, this presents particular problems for sustaining the idea of agency in the critical realist sense, which is necessary in order to understand and theorise the collective mobilisation involved in political projects. This problem is produced within post-structuralism by a deconstruction of the subject such that agency and voice are reduced to subjectification, the ongoing process of producing a 'self' that lacks ontological status.

This is illustrated in the arguments of Bronwyn Davies (1997, 2004), where, following Foucault, she describes the unfixity of the subject as the ongoing process of the constitution of the 'self'. While she defines the subject as fictional (note the scare quotes around 'self'), she nonetheless recognises the power of these fictions as central to the feminist project of bringing about change. So, the central contradiction that Davis (2008) identifies with movement activists is, in Davies's account, glossed over into a feminist subject discursively brought into being. What is important to note from a critical realist perspective is that, in this account, the powers accorded to PEPs disappear from view as a subject to be analysed at the empirical and philosophical level, while distinctions between epistemic and judgemental relativism (see Smirthwaite and Swahnberg 2016) are simply collapsed.

In order to meaningfully address issues of identity, we need a proper theory of persons. This is central to the task of analysing experiences and identities from a critical realist perspective. This would allow us to tease out people's concerns in their relations with the natural, practical and social order, to consider how the causal powers of human beings come to be exercised, and how as strong evaluators people come to understand the salience of race and gender, for example, as key aspects (or not) of their personal, and in some circumstances, political identity. This is not a simple or singular exercise and involves understanding how people come to deliberate on their circumstances and reflexively identify themselves (or not) as, say, a black woman. In relation to the emergence of new political subjects, critical realism would suggest that it is within the context of people's emergent powers and possibilities that the development of corporate agency can be understood.

Furthermore, an analysis of social movements and the conditions under which they flourish is essential. In the exchange between Sandra Harding (1999, 2003), from a standpoint theorist perspective, and Tony Lawson (1999, 2002), from a critical realist perspective, Harding makes important arguments about why powerful insights are produced by differently positioned groups of actors. Harding's account of why feminists historically chose to struggle on the epistemological front is one such explanatory account, but that does not foreclose the ontological argument about the stratified nature of reality as emphasised by Lawson. In some of the writing on intersectionality, corporate agency has been strategically deployed not to argue the case for sectional interests (specifically the interests of black women or women of colour), but to extend the case towards the development of a more universal set of claims about social justice. Patricia Hill Collins (2004) in her book *Black Sexual Politics* argues that she is dealing with a local manifestation of more general global phenomena and extends the commitment to social justice to all human beings. So, the sorts of corporate agents she imagines are defined not only in terms of their personal characteristics, but by virtue of their values and commitments to social justice.

These commitments are best analysed within a view of social science which is alive to human values and flourishing. Concerns with social justice constitute a key element of critical realist thinking. An important part of critical realism's Bhaskarian legacy is the connection between critical realism and concerns with human emancipation (Bhaskar 1986). Bhaskar argued that if we can identify the underlying mechanisms that are producing injustice or suffering, then we can show under what conditions it could be otherwise. In these circumstances, the argument becomes that *ceritus paribis* (other things being equal) we should change it.

Sayer in his book *Why Things Matter to People* (2011) deconstructs and shows the inadequacy of the fact/value separation that has plagued much philosophy and social-scientific thinking. This separation is closely related to the historically gendered separation between reason and emotion (Clegg 2013) and the denial of a relation between the two. This dichotomisation and its detrimental consequences have been the target of much feminist scholarship (e.g. Boler 1999), and Archer (2000) has argued that emotions are important for the personal commitments people make to the things that matter to them and are thus central in understanding human agency. Sayer's (2011) naturalistic grounding of claims about the conditions for human flourishing are important for the broader political projects articulated by Collins (2004) and others. They are not the only theorists to do so; critical realists share much common ground with other sorts of critical theory. Normative reasoning and conclusions are central to any political praxis as is the power of deconstruction, and I am not arguing that critical realists have the only claim to these traditions. In *Bodies That Matter* Judith Butler (1993, p. 30), for example, argues that:

> To call a presupposition into question is not the same as doing away with it; rather, it is to free it from its metaphysical lodgings in order to understand what political interests were secured in and by that metaphysical placing, and thereby to permit the term to occupy and to serve very different political aims.

Although Butler eschews an explanatory account of how these metaphysical lodgings came to exercise their hold, the emancipatory logic is clear. I am claiming, however, that radical politics, and this includes the motivating force behind all intersectional theory, is better served by analyses that can impute agency to actors. The tensions between post-structuralist accounts of selfhood as subjectification (Davies 1997, 2004; Carbin and Edenheim 2013) and the aspirations of activists for a better world cannot be simply reduced to the charge of essentialism against the early women's movement (although there are examples of this in speech and writing designed to mobilise). Nor is it to deny that many analyses of particular situations were inadequate because they failed to take account of the complexity of the ways structural features of race, class and other oppressions operate. Explanatory analysis is difficult and always incomplete. However, substantive analyses would be better if not hobbled by inadequate accounts of structure and agency, and the flat ontologies of both post-structuralism and empiricism.

This is why a morphogenetic account is important: it neither reduces society to individual experience, nor experience to society. Furthermore, and most importantly, it does not conflate the two in an endless and amorphous present. Rather, it offers the analytical tools to analyse the historicity of emergence. All this means nothing, however, if our theory of persons is too thin to account for, first, our capacity to act in the world and, second, our reasons as strong evaluators, powered by first- and second-order emotions and reflexivity, for doing so (Archer 2000). Of course, there are differences between critical realists in relation, for example, to the relative importance of habitual action and reflexivity and how to theorise these. No theory is or can be complete, but because I am not a judgemental relativist I think some theories are better than others. Critical realism both acts as an under-labourer for science and, as we have seen in Archer's case, offers substantive propositions about the nature of the internal conversation and situated reflexivity. It brings both of these benefits to the analysis of intersectionality, enhancing the possibilities for its research programme. A philosophical approach that cannot adequately theorise human agency and the possibilities for corporate agency seems inadequate to the task of both analysis and politics. Articulating agency and exploring historical emergence and the morphogenetic cycle can work to ground radical normative aims. While Davis's (2008) argument about the productivity of intersectionality as a research programme is sociologically insightful, a research programme underpinned by a philosophy that clearly explicates its relation to human practice has even more potential.

Notes

1 This chapter was originally published as: Sue Clegg (2016) "Agency and Ontology within Intersectional Analysis: A Critical Realist Contribution", *Journal of Critical Realism* 15(5): 494–510, DOI: 10.1080/14767430.2016.1210470. © Taylor & Francis Ltd, http://www.tandfonline.com. Reprinted by permission of the publisher.
2 With the new materialist turn the discursive has lost its central place in post-structuralist quarters of feminist theory. Yet, the deconstructionist stance towards the subject is retained, although now its fluid characteristics are held to be due to more material kinds of processes.
3 For an explicit argument against such distinctions, see Carbin and Edenheim 2013.

References

Anthias, F. 1998. "Rethinking Social Divisions: Some Notes Towards a Theoretical Framework." *Sociological Review* 46 (3): 505–35.

Archer, M. S. 1995. *Realist Social Theory: The Morphogenetic Approach*. Cambridge: Cambridge University Press.

———. 1996. *Culture and Agency: The Place of Culture in Social Theory*. Cambridge: Cambridge University Press.

———. 2000. *Being Human: The Problem of Agency*. Cambridge: Cambridge University Press.

———. 2007. *Making our Way through the World: Human Reflexivity and Social Mobility*. Cambridge: Cambridge University Press.

———. 2012. *The Reflexive Imperative in Late Modernity*. Cambridge: Cambridge University Press.

Bhaskar, R. 1978 [1975]. *A Realist Theory of Science*. Brighton: Harvester Press.

———. 1979. *The Possibility of Naturalism: A Philosophical Critique of the Contemporary Human Sciences*. Brighton: Harvester Press.

———. 1986. *Scientific Realism and Human Emancipation*. London: Verso.

Boler, M. 1999. *Feeling Power: Emotions and Education*. London: Routledge.

Butler, J. 1993. *Bodies That Matter: On the Discursive Limits of 'Sex'*. London: Routledge.

Carbin, M., and S. Edenheim. 2013. "The Intersectional Turn in Feminist Theory: A Dream of a Common Language?" *European Journal of Women's Studies* 20 (3): 233–48.

Clegg, S. 2006. "The Problem of Agency in Feminism: A Critical Realist Approach." *Gender and Education* 18 (3): 309–24.

———. 2012. "On the Problem of Theorising: An Insider Account of Research Practice." *Higher Education Research and Development* 31(3): 407–18.

———. 2013. "The Space of Academia: Privilege, Agency and the Erasure of Affect," in C. Maxwell and P. Aggleton (eds.) *Privilege Agency and Affect*, pp. 71–87. Basingstoke: Palgrave Macmillan.

Collins, P. H. 2004. *Black Sexual Politics: African Americans, Gender and the New Racism*. New York: Routledge.

Crenshaw, K. 1989. "Demarginalizing the Intersection of Race and Sex: A Black Feminist Critique of Antidiscrimination Doctrine, Feminist Theory and Antiracist Politics." *The University of Chicago Legal Forum* 1989 (1): 139–68.

David, M. E. 2003. *Personal and Political: Feminisms, Sociology and Family Lives*. Stoke-on-Trent: Trentham Books.

Davies, B. 1997. "The Subject of Post-structuralism: A Reply to Alison Jones." *Gender and Education* 9 (1): 271–83.

———. 2004. "Introduction: Poststructuralist Lines of Flight in Australia." *International Journal of Qualitative Studies in Education* 17 (1): 1–9.

Davis, K. 2008. "Intersectionality as Buzzword: A Sociology of Science Perspective on What Makes a Feminist Theory Successful." *Feminist Theory* 9 (1): 67–85.

Gunnarsson, L. 2011. "A Defence of the Category 'Women'." *Feminist Theory* 12(1): 23–37.

———. 2017. "Why We Keep Separating the 'Inseparable': Dialecticizing Intersectionality." *European Journal of Women's Studies* 24(2): 114–27.

Harding, S. 1999. "The Case for Strategic Realism: A Response to Lawson." *Feminist Economics* 5(3): 127–33.

———. 2003. "Representing Reality: The Critical Realism Project." *Feminist Economics* 9(1): 151–9.

Lawson, T. 1999. "Feminism, Realism and Universalism." *Feminist Economics* 5(2): 25–59.

———. 2002. "Ontology and Feminist Theorizing." *Feminist Economics* 9(1): 119–50.

Lindner, U. and D. Mader (eds.) Forthcoming. *Critical Realism meets kritische Sozialtheorie: Erklärung und Kritik in den Sozialwissenschaften*. Bielefeld: Transcript Verlag.

Martinez Dy, A., L. Martin, and S. Marlow. 2014. "Developing a Critical Realist Positional Approach to Intersectionality." *Journal of Critical Realism* 13 (5): 447–66.

Mirza, H. S. 2009. "Plotting a History: Black and Postcolonial Feminisms in 'New Times'." *Race Ethnicity and Education* 12 (1): 1–10.

Moi, T. 1985. *Sexual/Textual Politics: Feminist Literary Theory*. London: Methuen.

———. 1999. *What Is a Woman? and Other Essays*. Oxford: Oxford University Press.

Nelson, J. 2003. "Once More, With Feeling: Feminist Economics and the Ontological Question." *Feminist Economics* 9 (1): 109–18.

Rowbotham, S. 1990. *The Past is Before Us: Feminism and Action since the 1960's*. Middlesex: Penguin.

Sayer, A. 1992. *Method in Social Science*. London: Routledge.

———. 2011. *Why Things Matter to People: Social Science, Values and Ethical Life*. Cambridge: Cambridge University Press.

Segal, L. 1987. *Is the Future Female? Troubled Thoughts on Contemporary Feminism*. London: Virago.

Segal, L. 1999. *Why Feminism?* Cambridge: Cambridge University Press.

Smirthwaite, G., and K. Swahnberg (2016). "Comparing Critical Realism and the Situated Knowledges Approach in Research on (In) Equity in Health Care: An Exploration of their Implications." *Journal of Critical Realism* 15(5): 476–93.

The Combahee River Collective. 1977. "The Combahee River Collective Statement." Accessed 1 August 2014. http://circuitous.org/scraps/combahee.html. Previously published in Home Girls: A Black Feminist Anthology (New York: Kitchen Table, Women of Color Press, 1983), ed. B. Smith.

Walby, S., J. Armstrong, and S. Strid. 2012. "Intersectionality: Multiple Inequalities in Social Theory." *Sociology* 46(2): 224–40.

West, C., and S. Fenstermaker. 1995. "Doing Difference." *Gender & Society* 9(1): 8–37.

Williams, Z. 2013. "Are You too White, Rich, Able-bodies and Straight to be a Feminist?" *The Guardian*, 18 April.

Yuval-Davis, N. 2006. "Intersectionality and Feminist Politics." *European Journal of Women's Studies* 13(3): 193–209.

8 Why we keep separating the 'inseparable'

Dialecticising intersectionality[1]

Lena Gunnarsson

Introduction

What precisely do we mean when we say that something intersects with something else? Whether it be used narrowly so as to depict the intersection between different axes of power and identity categories, or broadly so as to include an infinite range of possible ontological intersections between levels and dimensions of reality, intersectionality gives rise to the question of the exact nature of intersection itself. Disputes about the character of intersection often pivot around the tension between separateness and inseparability, an ambiguity that can arguably be seen as constitutive of intersectional analysis. When Kimberlé Crenshaw (1991), who coined the term 'intersectionality', argued that gender must be analysed as intersecting with for instance race, so that gendered identities be seen as intrinsically racialised, the very term 'intersectionality' at the same time implies that the entities intersecting are distinct from one another in some way – otherwise they could not intersect.

For the most part intersectionality scholars in action treat categories like gender, race and class as somehow both separable and inseparable. However, when the issue of separability versus inseparability is explicitly addressed, it is often played out in terms of a polarisation between those emphasising the inseparability of intersectional categories (the 'anticategorical' approach in Leslie McCall's [2005] famous formulation) and those maintaining the need to separate them (the 'intercategorical' approach). For instance, I recently attended a seminar set up as a transversal dialogue between two intersectionality scholars seeking ways of bridging their opposed positions in this in/separability dispute (Lundberg and Strid, 2014).

In this article I take issue with the either/or thinking that underpins what I see as an unnecessary and unproductive polarisation in the debate over the in/separability of intersectional categories. Drawing on Roy Bhaskar's dialectical critical realist philosophy, I argue that we can think of intersectional categories as both separate and unified, an argument that actualises the question of what it actually means for something to be distinct or separate as opposed to inseparable or unified with something else. I begin by introducing Bhaskar's conceptualisation of reality's differentiations and interconnections. Giving some examples of ways of arguing in different areas of feminist thought that seem to be premised on a view of separateness and inseparability as mutually exclusive, I show how Bhaskar's dialectic, centring round the figure of unity-in-difference, can counter unproductive dualisms between separateness and unity. I go on to examine some examples of how intersectional theorists, broadly defined, address the theme of in/separability, taking issue with accounts emphasising *either* separability or inseparability and developing my own view on the in/separability dilemma. While the notion of intersection is mostly used to characterise the relations between different identity categories or power relations, I include the relation between different ontological levels, which is also paramount in intersectional debates.

Dialectical critical realism

Dialectical critical realism was developed by the British philosopher Roy Bhaskar (2008 [1993]) as part of the broader school of critical realism, which brings ontological issues to the fore of social meta-theory, challenging both positivism and postmodernism (Bhaskar, 1997 [1975], 1998 [1979]; Dy et al., 2014, ch. 6 this volume; Gunnarsson, 2011, ch. 4 this volume, 2013, 2014; McCall, 2005; Sayer, 1992, 2000; Walby et al., 2012). Bhaskar defines dialectics as 'the art of thinking the coincidence of distinctions and connections' (2008 [1993], p. 180). What in particular distinguishes realist dialectics from other kinds of dialectical philosophies is its pronounced standpoint that the reason why we need to *think* dialectically is because *reality* is dialectically structured, via different modes of unity-in-difference whereby things have both points of identity with one another and points of divergence. Such coincidence of difference and unity may be constellated in a variety of ways, ranging from the necessary tensions built into our existence to historically accumulated splits between things that are fundamentally unified, such as humanity's exploitative separation from the nature that sustains it (Gunnarsson, 2013, 2014).

The initial reason why I was long ago attracted to critical realism generally and dialectical critical realism specifically was precisely this non-absolutist approach to distinctions and relationality, which is anchored in the view of reality as a stratified and differentiated whole whose elements are both intrinsically connected and relatively autonomous from one another.[2] I was frustrated with what I saw as a tendency among many feminist theorists to challenge atomistic and dualistic modes of making distinctions by altogether denying separability, since this move in fact reproduces the atomist's basic view of reality: either things are absolutely separate and autonomous, or they cannot be separated at all. This mode of reversal can be seen in the way that some feminist theorists argue against the distinguishability of ontology from epistemology (Barad, 2003, 2007; Hekman, 2010; see Gunnarsson, 2014). It can be identified in the posthumanist scepticism towards separating the human from the nonhuman (e.g. Hird and Roberts, 2011, p. 109), and in many neo-materialists' reluctance to delimit the social from the natural (e.g. Davis, 2009, p. 67; see Gunnarsson, 2013). Similarly, the deconstructionist approach to the subject is characterised by a tendency to deny the relative autonomy (and, hence, realness) of the subject, on the grounds that it is constituted by processes outside of itself (e.g. Butler, 1999 [1990]). While this move is often seen as a radical challenge to the atomist view of the subject as self-contained, as I argue elsewhere it in fact replicates its absolutist notion of autonomy (Gunnarsson, 2014; cf. Alcoff, 2006). Finally, the fact that gender coalesces with other power relations and identity categories has led some scholars to 'completely reject the separability of analytical and identity categories' (McCall, 2005, p. 1771; e.g. Butler, 1999 [1990]; Spelman, 1990; see Gunnarsson, 2011).

This emphasis on inseparability is an understandable reaction to rigid modes of separation, which deny co-constitution, fluidity and mutual transformation. We might indeed interpret these kinds of interventions as a matter precisely of emphasis, rather than as a complete rejection of distinctions. What supports such a reading is the fact that all the authors mentioned above, who explicitly deny the possibility of separating ontology from epistemology, the social from the natural, the subject from its constitutive context and gender from other intersectional categories, at the same time make use of such distinctions in their writing. However, even if it is just a matter of accentuation, the tendency shared by atomist and anticategorical theorists to emphasise either separateness or inseparability is problematic in itself, since it easily reproduces absolutist and undifferentiated notions of difference as well as unity.

Dialectical critical realism takes issue *both* with accounts that obscure the co-enfoldment of phenomena *and* with claims that phenomena cannot be at all separated if they have intrinsic ties to one another. If applied to the relation between epistemology and ontology, these can be seen as both separate and 'constellationally unified' (Bhaskar, 2008 [1993], p. 114). As Alan Norrie highlights in his work on dialectical critical realism, ontology and epistemology are co-enfolded in one another in the sense that 'knowing is … a subset of being, and the study or theory of being (onto-*logy*) is already epistemically committed' (2010, p. 17, emphasis in original), but they must nevertheless be distinguished since one cannot be collapsed into the other; they are different things.

On the dialectical critical realist view, being is an interconnected, open-ended whole, whose different parts and dimensions are both intrinsically connected and relatively autonomous from one another, due to processes of differentiation, stratification and emergence. Reality has a structure to it, but is also a processual becoming, and neither the structuredness nor the fluidity of being are absolute but become meaningful in relation to one another. Bhaskar's figure of dialectical totalities conveys that something can, however paradoxical it may sound, be both part of something else and separate from it, as in the case of knowledge being both part of and separate from reality, and of humanity being both part of and different from nature (Bhaskar, 2008 [1993]; Gunnarsson, 2013, 2014). What underpins all these kinds of dualities is the notion of unity-in-difference, which challenges what I see as the most basic and problematic of all dualisms, that between separateness and inseparability itself (cf. Kirby, 2008).

The unclear meaning of 'inseparability'

I begin my examination of ways of dealing with the in/separability of intersectional categories by shortly turning to a statement by Judith Butler, which exemplifies a line of thought that is equally ambiguous and influential (cf. e.g. Brown, 1997; Geerts and van der Tuin, 2013). Although Butler is rarely labelled an intersectional theorist, she does address intersectional issues, and the anticategorical intersectionality identified by McCall owes much to the deconstructionist approach to gender and the category 'woman', of which she is an important representative. In *Gender Trouble* Butler states:

> If one 'is' a woman, that is surely not all one is … gender intersects with racial, class, ethnic, sexual, and regional modalities of discursively constituted identities. As a result, *it becomes impossible to separate out 'gender'* from the political and cultural intersections in which it is invariably produced and maintained.
>
> (1999 [1990], p. 6, emphasis added)

What does Butler mean with this statement about the impossibility of separating out 'gender'? At first glance the claim seems valid. As highlighted by Wendy Brown, who represents a similar line of thought, gender, ethnicity, class, etc. are not 'discrete units' (1997, p. 86) that we can disentangle in a clear-cut way. If understood in this basic sense, however, Butler's statement appears trivial; it would arguably be difficult to find someone who did not agree. We could also interpret it as a stronger claim against any kind of separation of categories. In this case, though, Butler seems to engage in a performative contradiction, in that while stating that gender cannot be separated from other modalities, she nevertheless separates them in this very statement. If gender were not in some sense separable from the other relations she lists, there would simply be no need for Butler to call them by different names (cf. Jónasdóttir and Jones, 2009).

The ambiguous meaning of Butler's statement raises the question of what we mean when we say two things are separate or distinct from one another, an issue that is in my view too rarely raised by theorists. Some authors arguing against separability seem to apply the implicit criterion that for things to be separable their discreteness must be tangible. For instance, as part of her argument against the category 'women', Elizabeth Spelman highlights the impossibility of pointing to a particular 'woman part' of herself that is not also a 'white part' (1990, p. 134). Although Brown's line of reasoning is more sophisticated than Spelman's hyper-empiricist mode of arguing, she seems to display a similar concern with the tangible, when highlighting that 'we are not fabricated as subjects in *discrete units* by … various powers' (1997, p. 86, emphasis added). I find it difficult to discern the sense of these kinds of statement. Of course, we cannot identify discrete woman, white and middle-class (or other) 'parts' or 'units' in a person. I doubt that anyone arguing in favour of the separability of gender, race and class would be ready to base their claim on such a premise.

From a critical realist perspective, something's existence as separate from something else is premised neither on the possibility of distinguishing it as a tangible unit, nor on the kind of absolute autonomy that precludes co-constitution and intra-connection. Instead, critical realists apply a 'causal criterion' for ascribing a distinct reality to something (Bhaskar, 1998 [1979], p. 12). If something has impact on the world that is irreducible to the causal effects of other entities we can talk of it as a distinct reality, *even though this reality is wholly premised on its relations with other things*. For instance, we can talk of the human subject as a distinct entity, that has a reality outside of the relations that are also, paradoxically, inside it, in that they constitute it. This is because by means of its *emergence*[3] from its constitutive relations, the subject has its own distinct properties and powers, which cannot be inferred from the relations through which it is constituted. When applied to intersecting categories, this perspective allows for a separation between gender, race, class, etc., despite the fact that these ongoingly co-constitute one another and are seamlessly unified in concrete subjects and social processes. They can be seen as relatively autonomous since the characteristics and impact of one cannot be derived from or explained solely in terms of the properties of the others.

The intersectional in/separability tension is sometimes dealt with by means of a distinction between the different *levels* of social reality. For instance, although Brown states that the 'powers of subject formation are not separable in the subject itself' (1997, p. 86), she also highlights that these powers are different in kind and, consequently, require 'distinctive models of power' (1997, p. 87). For her, this amounts to a paradox that creates problems for intersectional theorising. By contrast, Nira Yuval-Davis (2006), who represents a more realist–materialist intersectional approach, seems to see a clearer separation between the different levels of intersectional relations as a way out of the in/separability dilemma. She shares the view that intersectional categories cannot be separated in concrete subjects and experiences but argues they ought to be separated on the deeper structural level where 'each social division has a different ontological basis, which is irreducible to other social divisions' (2006, p. 195). At this level, she holds class to relate to 'economic processes of production and consumption'; gender to 'a mode of discourse that relates to groups of subjects whose social roles are defined by their sexual/biological difference'; sexuality to a discourse 'relating to constructions of the body, sexual pleasure and sexual intercourse'; and ethnic and racial divisions to 'discourses of collectivities constructed around exclusionary/inclusionary boundaries' (2006, p. 201). Yuval-Davis's way of solving the problem of inseparability versus separateness is thus to argue for a vertical separation of levels, so as to then argue for horizontal separations on the level of ontological basis, while claiming inseparability on the level of concrete identity and experience.

Although I elsewhere make a similar argument (Gunnarsson, 2011, 2014), as will be clear throughout the article my way of dealing with the in/separability tension differs somewhat from Yuval-Davis's. To begin I want to complicate her claim that 'the ontological basis of each of these divisions is autonomous'

(Yuval-Davis, 2006, pp. 200–201), by stressing that even if analysed on the deepest level of abstraction, I doubt that we can think of economic, gendered, sexual and racialised relations as absolutely independent from one another. I am unsure how starkly Yuval-Davis's claim about autonomy should be interpreted. What seems certain, though, is that many will interpret such a claim as one about *absolute* autonomy, in turn provoking one-sided arguments about inseparability. This highlights the need for anti- and intercategorical theorists alike to be clearer about what they actually mean by 'separate', 'autonomous' and associated terms.

Intra-action and 'processification'

In order to affirm the inter-permeation of the different dimensions of intersectionality, some theorists prefer to use the term 'intra-action', rather than 'interaction', to depict their interplay (Egeland and Gressgård, 2007; Geerts and van der Tuin, 2013; Lykke, 2010, 2011). In the field of feminist theory the term 'intra-action' was introduced by Karen Barad, who states that 'in contrast to the usual "interaction", which assumes that there are separate individual agencies that precede their interaction, the notion of intra-action recognises that distinct agencies do not precede, but rather emerge through, their interaction' (2007, p. 33). Barad takes issue with '[t]hingification – the turning of relations into "things"' (2003, p. 812), stressing the ontological priority of relations over the entities they produce. Nina Lykke judges the Baradian notion of intra-action to fit well with many intersectional researchers' 'agreement that intersectional interplays between categorisations should be analysed as mutual and intertwined processes of transformation and not as a mere addition of gender, class, ethnicity, race, sexuality and so on' (2010, p. 51).

Interestingly, Bhaskar (2008 [1993]) also uses the term 'intra-action' in his dialectical work. In addition, there is an interesting affinity between Barad and Bhaskar in that they both adopt realist worldviews (in Barad's case Niels Bohr's agential realism). There is also a crucial difference, though, associated with the theme of either/or versus both/and thinking that is central in this article. The same kind of either/or thinking that sustains the dualism between separateness and inseparability can be identified in the way that Barad emphasises the processual roots of entities *at the cost* of their relative autonomy and stability. A closer look at her formulations about intra-action reveals an underlying temporal dualism between the product and agent of intra-action. For Barad, 'distinct agencies do not precede, *but* rather emerge through, their interaction' (2007, p. 33, emphasis added). From the Bhaskarian perspective things can instead be *both* a product of intra-actions *and* precede, be the point of departure of, new inter- and intra-actions. Even if something is a product of intra-active processes, it may have a relatively stable existence *as* product – or 'thing' if you like – from the point of view of which it then inter/intra-acts with other dimensions of reality. We do not need to replace thingification with 'processification'. Instead, I suggest we think of the entities in the world as multifaceted in character, being simultaneously products, producer and process.

The theme of things versus processes is intimately linked to that of in/separability, inasmuch as things are commonly thought of as bounded whereas processes are not. A statement in Evelien Geerts and Iris van der Tuin's intersectional intervention, drawing on Barad's work, highlights this link: 'The idea that patterns are constantly evolving, and that different patterns intra-act instead of merely interacting with one another … generating an assemblage that is holistic – i.e., *not separable* – is one of Barad's onto-epistemological key points' (2013, p. 176, emphasis in original). Here the emphasis on processual intra-action leads to an emphasis of inseparability. Although the formulation 'instead of *merely* interacting' suggests there might be aspects of unbounded intra-action *as well as* interaction between relatively delimited entities, Geerts and van der Tuin go on to state that 'the concept of interaction stands for a traditional atomist ontology' (2013, p. 176), seemingly wanting to throw it out altogether. Whereas the intersectional theorists drawing on Barad's work (Egeland and Gressgård, 2007; Geerts and van der Tuin, 2013; Lykke, 2010, 2011) seem to suggest we use the term 'intra-action' to denote all kinds of intersectional relations, as I read him Bhaskar instead sees intra-action as *one* kind of interplay between phenomena. Sometimes, when the interplay has little internal impact on the phenomena in interplay, the term 'inter-act' might be more adequate. This multifaceted view of how things relate to one another is one of the strengths of the dialectical critical realist ontology, which could be drawn on in intersectional analysis.

Seeing boundedness and boundlessness as two interdependent aspects of the tissue of being works as a remedy against tendencies to get stuck in debates about whether gender, race, class, etc. are separate or not. Bearing in mind that there are many modes as well as degrees of connection and distinction, we can put our energy into more precise theorisations of how different power processes work for and against each other in different spatio-temporal locations and for different subjects. What, in various geohistorical locations and on different levels of abstraction, is the precise inter- or intra-active relation between structures like male dominance, heteronormativity, racism and capitalism? To what extent are they independent from one another and to what extent co-constitutive and intra-active, in the past and in the present? Do they support or contradict one another, or both?

This kind of analytical endeavour was commonplace at the time when feminist theorists were more structurally oriented, even though the term intersectionality was not yet invented (Lykke, 2010). For instance, an important topic in discussions among Marxian feminists was the exact relation between capitalism and patriarchy, including how they co-constitute versus conflict with one another (Hartmann, 1979). On one hand, capitalism is fundamentally entangled with patriarchy in the way, for instance, that it is premised on a gender-based division of labour based on women's subordination to men. Also, capitalism is inherently patriarchal and misogynist in that it necessarily underprivileges the reproductive practices on which it depends and cannot by itself provide the means needed to protect and support the agents of reproduction. On the other hand, in a historical perspective capitalism's centring of the individual has been central for the emergence of the women's movement and in this sense it has constituted a challenge to male dominance. In addition, capitalism's need for an increased supply of workers has challenged the structure of male dominance in that it enabled/-s women to enter the labour market. Rather than making a case here for the exact nature of these intersections, my point is to illustrate that all these kinds of intersectional interrogations can be fruitfully informed by the guiding thread offered by the dialectical theme that unities-in-difference can be *differently* constellated.

Structures and subjects

I now want to turn more focused attention to the relation between the different *levels* of intersectional analysis, complicating further the somewhat messy picture of crisscrossing separabilities and inseparabilities. Like the relation between categories of gender, race, class, etc., this relation is characterised by the kind of unity-in-difference that is, as I see it, bound to generate theoretical confusion and unnecessary polarisation unless approached from a dialectical 'both/and perspective'.

As noted above, Yuval-Davis emphasises the need to distinguish ontological levels that in her view are often confused in intersectional theorising (cf. Dy et al., 2014). She states that in contemporary literature identities, 'the individual and collective narratives that answer the question "who am/are I/we"', are 'often required to "perform" analytical tasks beyond their abilities' (2006, p. 197). In her view, a crucial task of intersectional studies is to examine the *relationships* between structural positioning, identity and political values, but this is 'impossible if they are all reduced to the same ontological level' (2011, p. 160). Here it is interesting to note that whereas some intersectional theorists see the connections between levels as an argument against separating them, for Yuval-Davis it is the fact that they relate *to* one another that motivates their separation.

An important strength about Yuval-Davis's account is that she makes a case not only for an analytical separation between different aspects of reality but highlights that this need is due to an ontological distinction. This departs from the common strategy of solving the in/separability dilemma by claiming to make only an analytical distinction between things that are *really* indistinguishable (e.g. Fraser, 1998, p. 12, 15). From a realist perspective, instead, the reason why analytical distinctions make sense and are efficient means for grasping reality is because they accord with a differentiation in being itself.

However, again, Yuval-Davis's claim about separability is characterised by some lack of clarity, which opens up for anti-separative critique. Sumi Cho, Kimberlé Crenshaw and Leslie McCall (2013) take issue with what they see as an upsurge of intersectional work distancing itself from a preoccupation with identities and subjectivities in order to focus on structural inequalities. They are concerned about the division between structural power and identity on which this debate is premised, suggesting that 'the opposition between identity and power is itself a rigid and nondynamic way of understanding social hierarchy' (2013, p. 797). Although they do not refer to Yuval-Davis's work, it is not far-fetched to assume that what they have in mind is the kind of intersectional writing of which Yuval-Davis is a leading figure.

The way that the respective perspectives of Yuval-Davis and Cho et al. become positioned in relation to one another here illustrates how the tendency to see inseparability and separateness as mutually exclusive creates an otiose polarisation. Both Yuval-Davis, with her emphasis on separateness, and Cho et al., with their claim about inseparability, are in my view right. Communication would work smoother, though, if they could also affirm the other side of the picture. In my view, Cho et al.'s argument draws a lot of its strength from contrasting itself against a largely 'invented target', to borrow Andrew Sayer's expression (2000, p. 68). What it challenges is 'the *opposition* between identity and power', but I believe it is hard to find a theorist arguing for the existence of such an opposition, whereas many would claim they are different things and must thus be analytically distinguished. Opposition denotes a sense of conflict and mutual exclusion; by contrast, a mere distinction between identity and structure is a premise for analysing how they enable one another and interact in mutually transforming ways.

Cho et al.'s intervention resembles Maria Carbin and Sara Edenheim's post-structuralist argument about the relation between the different levels of intersectionality. They take issue with how some intersectional theorists frame the division between 'structuralist' and post-structuralist perspectives in terms of their respective focus on structures versus subjectivity/agency. Against this, they argue that post-structuralism constitutes a challenge to the very '*binarism* between structure and agency', on which this scheme is in their view based (Carbin and Edenheim, 2013, p. 241, emphasis added). Similarly to Cho et al.'s charge of 'opposition', this formulation is problematic in that it confuses the act of identifying 'two analytical levels' (Carbin and Edenheim, 2013, p. 241) with the institution of a *binarism*, a term that connotes a dualistic opposition that is not necessarily entailed by a distinction. As I highlight elsewhere (Gunnarsson, 2013, 2014), there is a remarkable lack of clarity in much feminist work as to the difference between mere *distinction* or *difference* on the one hand and *dualism* or *binary* on the other, indicated by the fact that they are often used interchangeably (e.g. Hird and Roberts, 2011, p. 109). In their conventional usage, dualisms or binaries refer to the kind of absolute separation which ignores any interconnection and mutual constitution between the two terms in question, while distinction simply means that two things are not the same. Conflating these different kinds of difference easily makes us see distinctions as such as the problem. This is troublesome for, as highlighted by Yuval-Davis (2006), it is only by distinguishing phenomena that we can honour their respective irreducible constituencies and examine their interrelation, thereby avoiding that one is subsumed under the logic of the other.[4]

Abstraction and the continued need for 'separatist' theory

Intersectional theorists often take issue with more conventional modes of discrimination analysis, which tend to reify categories like 'Black' and 'woman' in a way that ignores how they are (co-)constituted through historically formed processes of power. As Catharine MacKinnon highlights, any analysis which obscures the hierarchies underpinning raced and gendered categories 'mirrors the power relations that form hierarchies that define inequalities rather than challenging and equalizing them' (2013, p. 1023). How, then, are we to think of the relation between categories and the social processes underpinning them? Floya Anthias makes clear that we cannot circumvent the analytical tension implied in this relation:

> Arguably one danger with the notion of intersections is found in constructing people as belonging to fixed and permanent groups. ... This undermines the focus on social processes, practices and outcomes as they impact on social categories, social structures and individuals. This is further complicated by the fact that, despite the danger of seeing people as belonging to fixed groups, groups do exist at the imaginary or ideational level as well as the juridical and legal level.
>
> (Anthias, 2008, p. 14)

While it is common to think of categories in terms of 'groups', it is important to bear in mind that this is not the only meaning of categories. Intersectional theory deals with group categories such as whites, women, gays and middle-class, but also with the relational categories of race, gender and class, which are constitutive of these groups as well as supported by the categorical divisions on which groups are based. Whereas categories are an indispensable tool for representing the patterns and structuredness that is such a pervasive part of reality, as expressed in the grouping of people and the distribution of resources along these lines, they are less fit to do the job of grasping the ultimately processual-practical character of power relations, which tends to eschew categorical delimitations. As soon as we refer to these processes by means of abstract categories like gender, race and class, claiming they intersect, it is easy to lose sight of the full picture of how these relational structures are processually constituted. However, against some pessimistic accounts (e.g. Brown, 1997), I do not think that this impossibility of perfect representation is a reason for seeing intersectional categorisations as inherently problematic. This is the way language works, and we need not despair because we cannot get the full picture in one particular statement or study, as long as we are clear about our partiality and imperfection (Gunnarsson, 2011; Sayer, 1992).

For many intersectional theorists abstracting one category from concrete reality while putting others aside amounts to a violation of the complexity of reality, in which, as Anthias puts it, 'classes are always gendered and racialised and gender is always classed and racialised and so on' (2008, p. 13). Appreciating the *relative* ontological autonomy of intersecting categories as well as our always necessarily partial epistemological outlook, we need not come to this conclusion, though. As long as we are clear that an analysis of for instance gender on its own terms relies on an abstraction of some processual parts from an infinitely complex social whole (Jónasdóttir, 1994), it is desirable that some theorists engage in 'separatist' theoretical explorations of what precisely this 'gender' (or 'race', 'class', 'sexuality') *is*, in a certain geohistorical location. Otherwise there is a risk that we reproduce unreflected notions of their ontologies. As Sylvia Walby, Jo Armstrong and Sofia Strid state, similarly drawing on critical realism, there is a need to 'systematically address the ontological depth of each of the inequalities' (2012, p. 231), so that their dynamic can be 'made more available for analysis' (2012, p. 236; cf. Dy et al., 2014). Whether we conceive of gender as, for instance, an effect of the reiterative enactment of norms organised by a heterosexual discursive matrix (Butler, 1999 [1990]) or as a historically shaped social–organic practice involving flows of erotic and caring powers (Jónasdóttir, 1994) will significantly affect the intersectional analysis of any concrete situation.

Within the field of intersectionality studies Anthias and Yuval-Davis have begun to draw the contours of a promising dialectic between separatist and intersectional theorising, by mapping the different ontological bases of social divisions (Anthias, 1998, 2008; Anthias and Yuval-Davis, 1992; Yuval-Davis, 2006). Separatist modes of theorising need not be carried out within an intersectional framework, though, but theorists of gender, race, class, sexuality respectively should in my view feel free to focus on specifying the dynamics of each of these relations, thereby creating platforms for intersectional theorists to further the analysis of their interplay. One problematic consequence of one-sided claims about inseparability is that they tend to stand in the way of such in-depth separatist theorising of the *specificity* of racial, gendered, classed and sexual power dynamics.

Before concluding I shall point to a final way in which my way of dealing with the in/separability tension differs from Yuval-Davis's approach, which on the whole has crucial affinities with my own realist take on intersectionality. Whereas Yuval-Davis has figured as my prime example of an intersectional theorist highlighting the need for analytical distinctions, she takes an anti-separatist stance when it comes to concrete experiences of oppression. She rejects the classical formulation that Black women suffer from 'triple oppression', as Blacks, women and members of the working class, basing this on the fact that 'in concrete experiences of oppression, being oppressed, for example, as "a Black person" is always constructed and intermeshed in other social divisions' (2006, p. 195; cf. Anthias and Yuval-Davis, 1983). Although I concur that concrete experiences are complexly formed wholes that are difficult to divide into neat categories, I do not agree that talking about someone as oppressed specifically as Black, woman or working class is necessarily an 'attempt to essentialise "Blackness" or "womanhood" or "working classness"' (Yuval-Davis, 2006, p. 195). Sometimes it does make sense to think of somebody as oppressed by virtue of her racial identity rather than her gender, although this racial identity is concretely articulated only in mediation with gender and not altogether separable from it. When Hannah Arendt said 'If one is attacked as a Jew, one must defend oneself as a Jew' (in Bernstein, 1996, p. 21), she had no difficulty abstracting Jewishness from the concrete complexity of experience and identity and such abstractions would make no sense unless they had some bearing on reality. As I argue elsewhere (Gunnarsson, 2011), we can think of for instance 'womanhood' in other terms than a reified attribute, namely as an abstraction that points to that dimension of a woman's situation that is produced via her positioning in a socially produced gender structure, a position that intra-acts with other social positions but which nevertheless has its own irreducible properties (cf. Alcoff, 2006).

It seems to me that Yuval-Davis seeks to escape the ontological ambiguousness of reality by making a somewhat too clear-cut separation between the level of structural ontological basis, where it is possible to separate neatly between different categories, and the level of identity and experience, where such separations are totally impossible. I think this is making it too simple. In fact, this is an example of how too sharp a separation in one place tends to be accompanied by a neglect of differentiation on another level. It is because any concrete identity or experience has points of intrinsic interconnection with each of the ontological bases that Yuval-Davis lists (rather than being altogether separable from them) that it sometimes makes sense to distinguish between how these different ontological bases are articulated in a concrete situation.

I think we need to take a humble stance towards our analytical tools, recognising that their way both of splitting up and holding the world together are never perfect, ultimately because of the processual character of reality. The structure, stratification and differentiation of reality make it viable as well as necessary to make the kind of distinctions in which human language excels. However, structuredness and boundedness exist only in dialectic with processes and flows, and these are difficult to grasp with analytical categories. Hence there can never be a perfect fit between knowledge and being. What also characterises analytical language and thinking is its aversion to paradox and I think this lies behind much of the either/or thinking that I have mapped in this article. If we as intersectional theorists could accept the tensions and imperfections that are necessarily involved in theorising, due to the clumsiness of the linguistic categories that we are bound to use, I think some of the conflicts among us might be recognised as largely semantic in kind.

Conclusion

Dialectical thinking is remarkably absent from contemporary feminist theorising. Magnus Granberg notes that whereas '[d]ialectics was once seen as the major alternative to positivist approaches; perhaps presently post-structuralism and its offshoots in gender, postcolonial and intersectional studies have usurped this position' (2013, p. 2). Peculiarly enough, while dialectics offers tools for transcending malestream dualisms, for many post-structuralist thinkers, in particular those influenced by Gilles Deleuze, dialectics is instead understood as part and parcel of the dominant western tradition and associated precisely with the kinds of dichotomous thinking that it challenges (Braidotti, 2011 [1994]). Against these anti-dialectical currents, in this article I have sought to demonstrate the usefulness of Bhaskar's dialectical critical realism for intersectional purposes, focusing on how tendencies in intersectional studies to emphasise either the separability or inseparability of categories can be challenged by the dialectical insight that difference and unity are not mutually exclusive but two coexisting aspects of most relations. The strength of the dialectical critical realist perspective is that it offers analytical tools for challenging both atomist separations and conflationist accounts which overemphasise connectedness and inseparability at the cost of differentiation and stratification.

As part of my argument I highlighted that it is often unclear what authors mean when claiming that something is impossible to separate from something else. Given that all kinds of theorising are largely based on the making of distinctions and connections of different kinds, I call for more systematic reflections about this epistemological-ontological issue. For intersectionality theory this is of particular importance, inasmuch as many conflicts within the field pivot around the issue of in/separability. Most intersectional theorists seem to work with an implicit notion of intersectional categories as somehow both separate and inseparable, while emphasising only one pole in this duality when being more explicit about the issue of in/separability. I hope I have been able to furnish some of the implicit dialecticians with a theoretical structure that can work against this kind of either/or thinking, since it in my view produces somewhat artificial conflicts among theorists, which stand in the way for dealing with the more substantial and politically pressing issues of intersectionality.

Funding

This research is part of the project 'Feminist Theorizings of Intersectionality, Transversal Dialogues and New Synergies', supported by the Swedish Research Council.

Notes

1 This chapter was originally published as Lena Gunnarsson, "Why we keep separating the 'inseparable': Dialecticizing intersectionality", *European Journal of Women's Studies* (24, no. 2) pp. 114–127. © 2017, Sage. DOI: 10.1177/1350506815577114.
2 This dialectical theme is present already in traditional critical realism but elaborated in its dialectical adaptation.
3 See Gunnarsson (2013, 2014) for an elaboration of the theme of emergence.
4 See Dy et al. (2014) for a theorisation of the relation between structure and agency in intersectionality, a relation that they hold to be undertheorised in the field.

References

Alcoff, L. M. 2006. *Visible Identities: Race, Gender and the Self.* Oxford: Oxford University Press.

Anthias, F. (1998) "Rethinking social divisions: Some notes towards a theoretical framework." *Sociological Review* 46(3): 505–535.

———. (2008) "Thinking through the lens of translocational positionality: An intersectionality frame for understanding identity and belonging." *Translocations: Migration and Social Change* 4(1): 5–20.

Anthias, F. and N. Yuval-Davis. 1983. "Contextualizing feminism: Gender, ethnic and class divisions." *Feminist Review* 15: 62–75.

Anthias, F. and N. Yuval-Davis. 1992. *Racialised Boundaries: Race, Gender, Colour and the AntiRacist Struggle.* London: Routledge.

Barad, K. 2003. "Posthumanist performativity: Toward an understanding of how matter comes to matter." *Signs* 28(3): 801–831.

———. 2007. *Meeting the Universe Halfway: Quantum Physics and the Entanglement of Matter and Meaning.* Durham, NC: Duke University Press.

Bernstein, R. 1996. *Hannah Arendt and the Jewish Question.* Cambridge, MA: MIT Press.

Bhaskar, R. 1997 [1975]. *A Realist Theory of Science.* London: Verso.

———. 1998 [1979]. *The Possibility of Naturalism.* London: Routledge.

———. 2008 [1993]. *Dialectic: The Pulse of Freedom.* London: Routledge.

Braidotti, R. 2011 [1994]. *Nomadic Subjects: Embodiment and Sexual Difference in Contemporary Feminist Theory.* New York: Columbia University Press.

Brown, W. 1997. "The impossibility of women's studies." *Differences* 9(3): 79–101.

Butler, J. 1999 [1990]. *Gender Trouble: Feminism and the Subversion of Identity.* London and New York: Routledge.

Carbin, M. and S. Edenheim. 2013. "The intersectional turn in feminist theory: A dream of a common language?" *European Journal of Women's Studies* 20(3): 233–248.

Cho, S., K. Crenshaw and L. McCall. 2013. "Toward a field of intersectionality studies: Theory, applications, and praxis." *Signs* 38(4): 785–810.

Crenshaw, K. 1991 "Mapping the margins: Intersectionality, identity politics, and violence against women of color." *Stanford Law Review* 43: 1241–1279.

Davis, N. 2009. "New materialism and feminism's anti-biologism: A response to Sara Ahmed." *European Journal of Women's Studies* 16(1): 67–80.

Dy, A. M., L. Martin and S. Marlow. 2014. "Developing a critical realist positional approach to intersectionality." *Journal of Critical Realism* 13(5): 447–466.

Egeland, C. and R. Gressgård. 2007. "The 'will to empower': Managing the complexity of the others." *NORA. Nordic Journal of Women's Studies* 15(4): 207–219.

Fraser, N. (1998) *Justice Interruptus: Critical Reflections on the 'Postsocialist' Condition.* New York: Routledge.

Geerts, E. and I. van der Tuin. 2013. "From intersectionality to interference: Feminist onto-epistemological reflections on the politics of representation." *Women's Studies International Forum* 41(3): 171–178.

Granberg, M. 2013. "A contextual analysis of Deleuze's critique of dialectics." Unpublished paper, Mid Sweden University.

Gunnarsson, L. 2011. "A defence of the category 'women'." *Feminist Theory* 12(1): 23–37.

———. 2013. "The naturalistic turn in feminist theory: A Marxist-realist contribution." *Feminist Theory* 14(1): 3–19.

———. 2014. *The Contradictions of Love: Towards a Feminist-Realist Ontology of Sociosexuality*. London and New York: Routledge.

Hartmann, H. 1979 "The unhappy marriage of Marxism and feminism: Towards a more progressive union." *Capital and Class* 3(2): 1–33.

Hekman, S. 2010. *The Material of Knowledge: Feminist Disclosures*. Bloomington: Indiana University Press.

Hird, M. and C. Roberts. 2011. "Feminism theorises the nonhuman." *Feminist Theory* 12 (2): 109–117.

Jónasdóttir, A. 1994. *Why Women Are Oppressed*. Philadelphia: Temple University Press.

Jónasdóttir, A. and K. B. Jones. 2009. "Out of epistemology: Feminist theory in the 1980s and beyond," in Jónasdóttir, A. G. and K. B. Jones (eds.) *The Political Interests of Gender Revisited*, pp 17–57. Manchester: Manchester University Press.

Kirby, V. 2008. "Natural convers(at)ions: Or, what if culture was really nature all along?," in S. Alaimo and S. Hekman (eds.) *Material Feminisms*. Bloomington: Indiana University Press.

Lundberg, A. and Strid S. 2014. "A tool to titter. Transversal Dialogue organized by Feminist Theorizings of Intersectionality." *Transversal Dialogues and New Synergies*, 17 June 2014, Örebro University.

Lykke, N. 2010. *Feminist Studies: A Guide to Intersectional Theory, Methodology and Writing*. New York and London: Routledge.

———. 2011. "Intersectional analysis: Black box or useful critical feminist thinking technology," in H. Lutz, M. T. Herrera-Vivar and L. Supik (eds.) *Framing Intersectionality: Debates on a Multi-faceted Concept in Gender Studies*. Farnham: Ashgate, pp. 207–221.

McCall, L. 2005. "The complexity of intersectionality." *Signs* 30(3): 1771–1800.

MacKinnon, C. 2013. "Intersectionality as method: A note." *Signs* 38(4): 1019–1030.

Norrie, A. 2010. *Dialectic and Difference: Dialectical Critical Realism and the Grounds of Justice*. London and New York: Routledge.

Sayer. A. 1992. *Method in Social Science: A Realist Approach*. London and New York: Routledge.

———. 2000. *Realism and Social Science*. London: Sage.

Spelman, E. 1990. *Inessential Woman: Problems of Exclusion in Feminist Thought*. London: Women's Press.

Walby, S., Armstrong J. and Strid S. 2012. "Intersectionality: Multiple inequalities in social theory." *Sociology* 46(2): 224–240.

Yuval-Davis, N. 2006. "Intersectionality and feminist politics." *European Journal of Women's Studies* 13(3): 193–209.

———. 2011. "Beyond the recognition and re-distribution dichotomy: Intersectionality and stratification," in H. Lutz, M. T. Herrera-Vivar and L. Supik (eds.) *Framing Intersectionality: Debates on a Multi-faceted Concept in Gender Studies*, pp. 155–170. Farnham: Ashgate.

Part III

Methodology and methods

Critical realism and empirical research

The third and final section of this reader will relate the philosophical resources that were developed in its previous two sections to discussions about both methodology (here understood broadly as involving reflection on the logics and principles of research/science) and – to a lesser extent – the use of specific methods. In so doing, it examines and aims to demonstrate the value of critical realist philosophy for empirical forms of feminist and gender studies research.

Importantly, the link that the four chapters contained in this section make (whether implicitly or explicitly) between philosophy, one the one hand, and methodology and methods, on the other, cannot – at least in the current intellectual context – be taken for granted. Approaches that actively seek to sever this link have, after all, become increasingly influential throughout the last few decades. Prominent authors like Anthony J. Onwuegbuzie and Nancy L. Leech (2005), Alan Bryman (2007), and Abbas Tashakkori and Charles Teddlie (1998), for instance, have argued in favour of a form of methodological pragmatism (or eclecticism) that – rather than getting bogged down in discussions about the (de)merits of specific philosophical frameworks and their preferred methods – places the importance of the research question centre stage. According to such authors, research/science should be *problem-* or *question*-driven rather than *philosophy-* or *method*-driven. More generally, leaving behind the idea that using certain types of methods/tools (e.g. quantitative or qualitative) should be restricted to proponents of the schools of philosophical thought that are most commonly associated with them (e.g. positivism or interpretivism/hermeneutics) is, according to methodological pragmatists, essential to securing a much-needed 'paradigm peace', pluralising our research practices, and facilitating mixed-methods research.

This orientation – along with the impatience with philosophy which it reflects – has obvious emotional appeal, especially when it is explicitly situated within the longer-term context of the nineteenth-century *Methodenstreit* and its seemingly inexhaustible power to give rise to various methodological rifts, splits, and 'paradigm wars'. Indeed, as Sadie Parr highlights in her chapter in this section, feminist and gender studies authors too have frequently stressed 'the need for a less rigid conception of "method" that allows the researcher flexibility' (p. 267).

An identical (pragmatist and pluralist) perspective appears, at first glance, to be apparent within critical realist philosophical and methodological writings as well. After all, the proponents of critical realism have repeatedly and explicitly repudiated 'scientism', or the methodological naturalist idea that – irrespective of what we study – the methods/tools appropriate for doing so remain the same. As such, they have staunchly opposed the idea that there exists such a thing as *the* (single, universal, and completely context-transcendent) 'scientific method'. Such claims are, however, animated by an altogether different logic than the logic which inheres in the idea that research/science should be exclusively problem- or question-driven. Specifically, critical realists have argued that any severing of the methods/tools we employ from broader philosophical considerations is not just *undesirable* but, more importantly, is ultimately *illusory*. Our methods/tools, they suggest, inevitably presuppose philosophical commitments of various kinds, and it is therefore impossible to detach the problems and questions to which methodological pragmatists have given precedence from accounts (whether explicit or implicit) of being and knowledge.

For example, when we adopt semi-structured interviews as part of our 'anti-naturalist' research strategy, this presupposes that people, as opposed to e.g. (sub-atomic) particles, are knowledgeable and agential, and that – as a result of this – we will be unable to develop reliable forms of knowledge about human behaviour without asking them to shed light on the motivations or forms of reasoning that underpinned their actions. In contrast, if we choose to forego such interviews in favour of 'naturalist' methods/tools that aim solely to identify and record empirical regularities (and which are therefore purportedly more objective) this presupposes either (1) that people, like (sub-atomic) particles, do *not* possess the characteristics of knowledgeability, agency, and so on, or (2) that their possession of such characteristics is in any case without value for our attempts to develop reliable forms of knowledge about human behaviour.

In addition to illustrating that attempts to sever the link between methods/tools and philosophical accounts of being and knowledge are bound to fail, however, these two examples also bring to the fore a second problem with the adoption of a pragmatist methodological orientation; specifically, they highlight the fact that, when we operate 'as if' such a split is possible, this puts us at significant risk of philosophical inconsistency. For instance, if – in our (entirely justifiable) desire to side-step the 'paradigm wars' – we combine methods/tools that presuppose that human beings are irreducibly agential with methods/tools that presuppose that human behaviour, like everything else in nature, is the result of deterministic causal laws, this cannot but result in an incoherent amalgam of competing philosophical positions. While it remains tempting – in the face of more than a century-and-a-half of bickering – to simply 'let a hundred methodological flowers bloom' or endorse the epistemologically-anarchist slogan that 'anything goes' (Feyerabend 2002 [1975]), there are therefore reasons to be concerned about the philosophical costs that will be incurred as a result. Moreover, when our simultaneous use of philosophically incompatible methods/tools produces conflicting results – as it surely will – we are left with a question that is fundamentally insoluble from a methodological pragmatist perspective: how do we adjudicate between the results that were produced by means of 'method/tool A' and 'method/tool B'? Any compelling answer to such questions will be rooted in an explicit account of reality (i.e. an ontological stance) and/or knowledge (i.e. an epistemological stance) and – by extension – it will provide us with a critical evaluation of the methodological pragmatist imperative to 'just get on with it'.

As the four chapters in this section of the reader show, critical realist philosophy serves exactly this critical purpose. In so doing, however, this approach is by no means unique. Rather, in electing to place philosophy centre-stage, it mirrors the more systematic versions of positivism and interpretivism/hermeneutics, which have always maintained that the link between philosophy and our methods/tools should play a prominent role in our research/scientific practices as well.

In contrast with the *naturalism* of positivism and the *anti-naturalism* of interpretivism/hermeneutics, however, critical realist philosophy proposes a *critical naturalism*. This philosophico-methodological position, like the positions that were discussed in the previous two sections of this reader, involves both a *negation* – in this case, a negation of the 'either/or' logic that inheres in the existing naturalism/anti-naturalism problematic – and a *synthesis*, here in the form of a principle of *methodological unity-in-difference* that has the distinctive 'both/and' logic of dialectical thought built into it. The various philosophical strands that, when they are woven-together, form the whole that is methodological unity-in-difference require some initial untangling and further explanation before (1) they can be re-entwined, and (2) their relevance and value to the areas of feminist and gender studies theory and praxis can be fully demonstrated. Specifically, to engage in this untangling and explanation it will be necessary to return – once more – to the concepts of *ontological depth* and *emergence/ontological stratification*.

The critical realist claim that being is characterised by depth, for instance, provides research/science with a general logic of investigation/explanation that contrasts with the emphasis on induction and/or deduction which characterises traditional approaches to this topic; specifically, the idea that real causal powers/mechanisms produce actual and empirical events suggests that – while both conventional modes of inference like induction and deduction and less conventional modes of inference like abduction have a role to play – it is *retroduction* that is of greatest significance to research/science. In short, retroduction refers to the creation of models of causal powers/mechanisms that, if they were to exist and act in the postulated manner, would account for the event (or phenomenon) with which our investigation is concerned. As such, rather than attempting to subsume some event/phenomenon of interest – e.g. sex- and gender-based violence, or some specific instance of it – under a deterministic/probabilistic causal law (whether through induction, deduction, or their combination) retroductive logic encourages researchers/scientists to 'work back' from an event/phenomenon to its causal conditions of possibility.

This process and the broader importance of retroduction for forms of research with a specifically feminist or gender studies orientation are fleshed out in Amber Fletcher's chapter, which brings these abstract critical realist claims to bear on a concrete case study that is centred on the lives of female Canadian farm workers. For now, however, it is worth noting two things in particular. First, the stress that critical realist philosophy places on retroduction is consistent with questions on which feminist and gender studies authors have – historically speaking – placed great emphasis as well. When social reproduction theorists (e.g. Bhattacharya 2017) pose questions about the (informal/unpaid) reproductive labour that is required for (formal/paid) employment to take place, for instance, they are – in typical retroductive fashion – 'working back' from an event/phenomenon to its causal conditions of possibility. As such, any potential contribution of critical realist philosophy to feminism and gender studies is much better understood in terms of *clarifying*, *legitimising*, and *reinforcing* the role of a mode of inference that is already established than it is in terms of *introducing* it. Second, and more generally, it is also worth noting here that it is the pivotal role that retroduction plays in capturing the depth of being that substantiates the 'unity' that is inherent to the aforementioned principle of methodological unity-in-difference.

If it is the critical realist claim that being has depth that provides a basis for the 'unifying' idea that retroduction is of primary importance to (feminist and gender studies) research, however, it is emergence/ontological stratification that provides the primary impetus for incorporating 'difference' into the principle of methodological unity-in-difference.[1]

In short, emergentism (whether specifically critical realist in orientation or otherwise) claims – first – that there exist real differences between the varied types of 'stuff' that make up being in its entirety. Second, it argues that these differences result from the relational organisation of parts into causally and taxonomically irreducible wholes. For example, a water molecule has any number of features (e.g. the power to extinguish fires, the property of liquidity) which its component parts (hydrogen and oxygen atoms) clearly do not. Emergentist philosophy commonly suggests, however, that the process which brings about these holistic causal/taxonomic properties occurs throughout the entirety of being. Reality can therefore be understood as consisting of an indeterminate number of levels, all of which are characterised by irreducible properties. As these levels remain existentially dependent or build on pre-existing levels of reality for their existence (i.e. the irreducible features of a water molecule do not simply erase those of the hydrogen and oxygen atoms which make it up but depend on them for its existence), being in its entirety may be understood as *stratified*; or, in other words, it may be understood in terms of a principle of *ontological unity-in-difference* that arguably gets us all the way from (subatomic) particles to people and politics in a philosophically-coherent and non-reductionist manner.

Within critical realist philosophy, this *ontological* principle is then paired with the aforementioned *methodological* principle of the same name. The latter of these, in turn, is rooted in Bhaskar's multifaceted claim that 'it is the nature of the object that determines the form of its possible science' (1998, p. 3). This statement aims to get across – among numerous other things – that the appropriate methods/tools for a particular discipline are dependent on the nature of what it studies. For instance, if it is true – and critical realist philosophy suggests it is – that people possess the broad range of emergent properties that are most commonly described by means of terms like 'agency', then it only makes sense for researchers/scientists to use e.g. semi-structured interviews to enquire into their reasons for acting a certain way. In contrast, if we extend the use of this method/tool – one that is clearly of significant value to the study of both people and politics – to engage in research on (sub-atomic) particles, this effort is ill-fated from the start; no matter how much any hapless (but heroic!) scientists/researcher may try, after all, the silence of their object of study is unlikely to be anything but abiding. While a range of additional considerations should guide our methodological practice as well – e.g. the specific aim(s) of our research, the stage of the research process in which we find ourselves, the kind of research which is most useful at the current stage of our discipline's development, and a whole host of epistemological considerations – this 'fit' between the *nature of what we study* and *the methods/tools we use to study it* is therefore invariably an essential consideration. Indeed, endorsing the use of a particular method/tool before taking this fit into consideration (i.e. an *a priori* endorsement) is, from a critical realist philosophical perspective, tantamount to subscribing to the idea that the methodological cart should always and everywhere be placed well ahead of the horse.

Such claims mark a clear contrast between critical realism and scientistic approaches. This is the case, primarily, because they are rooted in the competing idea that real, emergent differences in the nature of what researchers/scientists study will require them to adopt different types of methods/tools. As a result, critical realist philosophy paves the way for an unmistakably pluralistic methodological orientation. The sort of methodological pluralism that it grounds, however, is not at all the same as the kind that was discussed above. Rather, critical realism champions a kind of methodological pluralism that is persistently attentive to its object(s) of study and – by encouraging us to pay systematic attention to the presuppositions of our methods/tools – actively counters the risk of philosophical inconsistency to which methodological pragmatism remains wilfully blind. Such philosophical risk-taking in the name of a methodological pluralist cause – and, more broadly, in the name of 'paradigm peace' – is especially disconcerting because it is so unnecessary; after all, critical realist philosophy *also* provides researchers/scientists with a rationale for the adoption of a substantially pluralistic methodological approach. Rather than remaining entirely 'untethered', however, this approach is fastened to the ground by means of ontological and epistemological positions like those that were developed in the first two sections of this reader. As opposed to an unprincipled, opportunistic, or uncritical methodological pluralism, critical realist philosophy therefore provides research/science with a basis for what Danermark et al. (2002, 152) have helpfully referred to as a *critical* methodological pluralism.

It is its broader philosophical stance as well which sets critical realist reflections on methodology/methods apart from the parameters of the existing naturalism/anti-naturalism debate. While it mirrors approaches like positivism and interpretivism/hermeneutics in affirming the important role of philosophy, for instance, it negates both (1) the *naturalist* idea that there is (or at least can/should be) an essential unity of methods between different (natural, social, etc.) scientific disciplines, and (2) the *anti-naturalist* idea that there exists a fundamental, irreconcilable methodological divide between *explanation* (within science) and *understanding* (within the humanities).

While the former of these positions has been discussed at some length, the latter requires some further clarification; in particular, what is in need of explanation is how the critical realist critique of scientism differs from the dualistic anti-naturalist emphasis on the methodological contrast between studying particles and people or politics. To do so, it is essential to begin by noting that – while anti-naturalists have sought to defend the autonomy of understanding/the humanities from encroachments by explanation/the sciences – they have also tended to implicitly universalise an (essentially positivistic) understanding of what it means to 'do' science; specifically, they have commonly left intact the assumption that science means scient*ism*. Not only does such an understanding drastically underestimate the methodological variety that actually characterises disciplines like physics, chemistry, and biology, however, the merits of scientism as an account of science are also – for reasons that were discussed above – extremely debatable.

In fact, if it is true – as critical realist philosophy claims – that the fit between the nature of what we study and the methods/tools we use to study it should always be at the forefront of our minds when we develop our research design, this allows us to both *reclaim* and *rethink* research/science. Specifically, it allows us to *reclaim* science from persistent efforts by proponents of positivist philosophy to monopolise the meaning of this term and *rethink* it by rooting the epistemological dialectic which characterises this practice in critical realist concepts like ontological depth, transfactual causality, emergence/ontological stratification, structure, referential detachment, etc. This strategy is, however, strikingly different from the anti-naturalist strategy of defending the autonomy of understanding and the humanities. In contrast with this approach, for instance, the critical realist 'game plan' rejects the idea that the human/social/cultural domain cannot be studied in accordance with 'scientific methods' in favour of the idea that – while there are many different types of useful knowledge and many different types of useful tools/methods – all of being/reality is susceptible to scientific investigation. As such, the critical naturalism which its advocates favour avoids the problematic, dualistic consequences – both philosophical and methodological in nature – that have long plagued anti-naturalist/humanistic work. Moreover, this anti-dualistic methodological orientation is further reinforced by the abovementioned fact that critical realist philosophy explicitly rejects the (positivist) idea that it is its use of a specific *method/tool* which provides research/science with its unity; rather, critical realism suggests that it is the primacy of retroductive *logic* within research/science – whether focused on the 'natural' or the 'human/social/cultural' domain – that plays this unifying role.

The final section of this reader – or rather, the four chapters which it contains – examine and demonstrate the value of these abstract claims for empirical forms of feminist and gender studies research. While concepts like critical naturalism, methodological unity-in-difference, and critical methodological pluralism do not make an appearance in every chapter, all are situated within the broader philosophico-methodological context that they provide.

The first chapter, by Amber Fletcher, discusses the relevance of retroduction and abduction to feminist and gender studies research, and – as mentioned – is centred on a case study that is concerned with the lives of female Canadian farm workers. The second chapter, by Michiel van Ingen, draws on critical realist claims about ontological depth, emergence/ontological stratification, and transfactual/mechanismic causality to argue that the (broadly defined) constructivist orientation of much *Feminist Security Studies* (FSS) work 'is incapable of providing this [*International Relations*] sub-field with adequate philosophical grounding' (p. 225). This is the case, he argues, because the analytical framework that results from adopting this orientation is both 'incapable of providing a basis and rationale for the kind of integrative, interdisciplinary research that is required to do justice to the events and phenomena with which *FSS* is concerned' and 'ill-suited to grounding empirical forms of feminist research' (p. 238). Such claims are rooted in the idea that constructivist *FSS* authors – like many proponents of the cultural turn – have adopted a one-dimensional focus on discourse/meaning that is both anthropocentric and premised on a unidirectional understanding of causality. Moreover, van Ingen's chapter suggests that constructivism is 'plagued by persistent theory/praxis inconsistencies' (p. 226). In contrast, it claims that 'critical realist philosophy – especially its *emergentist/stratified ontology* and *power-/mechanism-based understanding of causality* – does pave the way for interdisciplinary research' (p. 226); this is the case, in short, because – contra constructivism – it 'paves the way for an approach to *FSS* that is multi-dimensional, anti-anthropocentric, premised on a multidirectional understanding of causality, [...] and able to effectively avoid theory/praxis inconsistencies' (p. 226).

The third chapter, by Sadie Parr, is rooted in research that was carried out with a group of women who were receiving intensive family support to help address their family's 'anti-social behaviour'. More generally, it explores the questions and normative/political dilemmas that arise when researchers/scientists seek to marry the common feminist concern with documenting and/or amplifying the experience, knowledge, and understanding of unheard/silenced/labelled/marginalised women with critical realist claims about judgmental rationalism (i.e. the idea that some accounts of reality are explanatorily better than others).

Parr explicitly acknowledges that her chapter does not provide an 'easy answer' to these questions (p. 263). This should not come as a surprise, as arguably there just are no easy answers available to us; or rather, the easy answers that are provided by dismissive, hubristic approaches to securing the authority of researchers/scientists and approaches which urge the wholesale, indiscriminate valorisation of 'women's voices' are – for both epistemological and normative/political reasons – highly dubious. Instead, an approach that allows for greater epistemological nuance, complexity, and mutuality seems required. This is, of course, exactly what critical realist philosophy aims to provide by means of (1) its dialectical understanding of the epistemological process that lies at the heart of research/science, and (2) its 'holy trinity' of ontological realism, epistemic relativism, and judgmental rationalism.

The final chapter, by Wendy Sims-Schouten, develops a methodological approach for Critical Realist Discourse Analysis (CRDA). In so doing it draws on interviews with Dutch and English mothers and focuses on the varied accounts they provide of motherhood, female employment, and day-care. As Sims-Schouten stresses, CRDA 'views non-discursive factors [...] as causal mechanisms that operate alongside discursive factors' (p. 280); that is to say, it 'is informed by the anti-anthropocentric view that discourse does not constitute or create our world independently but, rather, that it *co*-constitutes the realities that we experience' (p. 280). As such, Sims-Schouten argues that the critical realist resources on which her chapter draws to ground this approach are invaluable exactly because they allow researchers/scientists 'to side-step the age-old structure/agency and materialism/idealism (or constructivism) dualisms in favour of an approach that conceives of these as dialectically co-constituted' (p. 291). Like van Ingen's chapter, then, this chapter maintains that critical realist philosophy provides crucial resources 'for researchers who wish to avoid *both* the anthropocentric social constructionist tendency to reduce all dimensions of our existence to discourse *and* biological reductionism or materialist determinism' (p. 291).

Note

1 Primary, but not only; for instance, Bhaskar's original formulation of critical realist philosophy stressed the existence of ontological, epistemological, methodological, and relational differences between the natural and social/cultural/human sciences (1998 [1979], especially Chapter 2).

References

Bhaskar, R. 1998 [1979]. *The Possibility of Naturalism: A Philosophical Critique of the Contemporary Human Sciences*, third edition. London: Routledge.

Bhattacharya, T. 2017. "Introduction: Mapping Social Reproduction Theory," in T. Bhattacharya (ed.) *Social Reproduction Theory: Remapping Class, Recentering Oppression*, pp. 1–20. London: Pluto Press.

Bryman, A. 2007. "Barriers to Integrating Quantitative and Qualitative Research." *Journal of Mixed Methods Research* 1(1):8–22.

Danermark, B., M. Ekström, L. Jakobsen and J. C. Karlsson. 2002. *Explaining Society: An Introduction to Critical Realism in the Social Sciences*. Abingdon, Oxon: Routledge.

Feyerabend, P. 2002 [1975]. *Against Method*, third edition. London and New York: Verso.

Onwuegbuzie, A. J. and N. L. Leech. 2005. "On Becoming a Pragmatic Researcher: The Importance of Combining Quantitative and Qualitative Research Methodologies." *International Journal of Social Research Methodology* 8(5):375–87.

Tashakkori, A. and C. Teddlie (1998) *Mixed Methodology: Combining Qualitative and Quantitative Approaches*. Thousand Oaks, London, and Greater Kailash I: Sage Publications.

9 The reality of gender (ideology)

Using abduction and retroduction in applied critical realist research

Amber J. Fletcher

Introduction

Feminist theory and research have a long history of ontological debate. Feminist scholars have worked diligently to dismantle essentialist discourses that seek to naturalise women's supposed inferiority through references to the body. Such discourses have – historically speaking – taken many different forms, from the sexist phrenology of the 1800s to contemporary statements like the infamous 2017 'Google memo'.[1] Considering the emphasis on anti-essentialism in feminist work, it is not surprising that post-structuralist thought has so powerfully influenced feminist thinking over the past few decades. The anti-categorical, anti-essentialist emphasis of post-structural theory has clearly provided useful tools for challenging dominant discourses about gender and sex, including the view of gender and sex as natural dualisms of opposites (e.g. Butler 1990). Taken to their logical endpoint, however, post-structuralist approaches can also result in a dismantling of the subject, a rejection of intentionality and agency (Clegg, 2016, ch. 7 this volume), and an inability to speak about the reality of gendered experiences of oppression. Further, post-structuralist approaches do little to inform empirical feminist research, mostly because they deny validity and reality to the lived experiences of 'subjects' (Scott 1991).

In contrast, critical realism – a philosophy of science originating in the work of Roy Bhaskar (2015, 2008) and developed further by authors like Margaret Archer (e.g. 2010, 1995), Andrew Sayer (e.g. 1992, 1997, 2000), Andrew Collier (e.g. 1994) and others – arguably has much to offer empirical feminist research. For instance, critical realism combines *ontological realism* (the idea that reality exists, at least for the most part, independently of individual human understandings of it) and *epistemological relativism* (the idea that all claims are socially produced and historically/geographically situated). It therefore assigns an important role both to empirical data and to critical engagement with observers' explanations of data. Furthermore, because of its assertions about social reality, particularly its claims about the multi-layered nature of this reality, critical realism *does* allow us to attribute a reality to gendered experiences of oppression. Indeed, it helps us conceive of gender as a causal mechanism that produces very real effects in everyday life (Gunnarsson 2011, ch. 4 this volume).

Despite its usefulness, however, critical realism has unfortunately remained under-utilised within feminist research (Gunnarsson, Martinez Dy, and van Ingen 2016). This under-utilisation is reflected in the continuing dominance of post-structuralism and has resulted in a reluctance on the part of some feminists to speak of ontological reality. More generally, however, its persistent marginalisation is due to the relative lack of methodological guidance offered by critical realism itself. Although critical realism has been well developed at a philosophical level there remains a lack of empirical work that clearly demonstrates its utility for informing methodological practices (for exceptions, see Edwards et al. 2014; Fletcher 2017; Lennox and Jurdi-Hage 2017; Parr 2015, ch. 11 this volume; Yeung 1997). This challenge extends to the small (but growing) literature on critical realism, feminism, and gender, in which most attention has been paid to ontological and epistemological questions (e.g. Gunnarsson 2011, 2017, ch. 8 this volume; Holmwood 2001; New 2005; Sayer 2000) but far less to methodological applications.

This chapter therefore aims to demonstrate the methodological value of critical realist philosophy as a framework for empirical feminist research. Drawing on a study of Canadian farm women, it will argue that the adoption of a critical realist approach facilitates useful engagements with the reality of gender in everyday life. Building on a recent article that describes the basic process of using critical realism in this study (Fletcher 2017) the chapter will elaborate on how the processes of abduction and retroduction were used to identify gender ideology[2] as a key causal mechanism. In particular, it will emphasise the usefulness of two critical realist tenets for gender research: first, the often-under-emphasised tenet that social beliefs and values have causal power and, second, the often-obscured processes of abduction and retroduction. It will show how, taken together, these aspects of critical realist philosophy allowed for the identification of gender ideology as a social, but highly causal, mechanism that shaped gender relations in everyday life.

The usefulness of critical realism for gender research

The term 'gender' is used in a variety of ways, depending largely on the ontology that is adopted. Perhaps the most common usage is to describe behaviours and attributes expected of men and of women – in this conceptualisation, men and women are viewed as dichotomous groups linked (biologically, socially, or both) to similarly dichotomous sexed bodies. Alternatively, gender can be viewed as an identity that is potentially detached from sexed bodies (i.e., gender identity) or as a performance of that identity (e.g. gender expression).

Regardless of definition and ontological perspective, gender relations are complex and multifaceted; they involve material, discursive, and ideological dimensions. Materially, gender is visible in the different roles played (or performances enacted) by people within a given society, in the way people are positioned and treated based on their perceived gender (or lack thereof), and in the way rights and resources may be differentially allocated along gendered lines. These material gender relations are shaped and reinforced at an ideological level and become manifested in discourses that proclaim and reinforce particular 'truths' about gender relations. The term gender ideology therefore describes a set of social beliefs that naturalises and engrains particular gender relations in the social world; or, as Lorber (1994, p. 30) notes, it both refers to 'the justification of gender statuses, particularly their differential evaluation' and involves a neutralisation of criticisms 'by making these evaluations seem natural'.

Currently dominant ideologies and discourses not only naturalise gender roles for women and men but they also naturalise the very idea of gender as a dualism of opposites which positions non-binary or transgender individuals as deviant or 'abnormal'. This chapter will use the term *gender* as a practical shorthand for this complex matrix of material, ideological, and discursive factors. However, in the empirical study discussed here, it was *gender ideology* – more specifically – that appeared as the most relevant causal mechanism in the context of Canadian farm women's lives. The purpose of this chapter is therefore not to argue that one particular formation or definition of gender is more accurate than others. Rather, it identifies gender ideology *itself* as a mechanism that produced and naturalised a particular set of gender relations in the lives of the participants, thereby raising the possibility that gender ideology operates similarly as a naturalising mechanism for different gender relations in other contexts.

While most feminist analyses – this chapter included – emphasise the social origin of gender, biological essentialist explanations of gender relations have persisted in both academic and social discourse. While these have argued that gender differences are determined primarily by biophysical differences between men and women, scholars in a range of disciplines have cogently disputed such claims (e.g. Blinkhorn 2005; Fine 2010). In light of the persistence of these problematic (and sometimes blatantly sexist) bio-essentialist discourses it is no surprise that many feminist scholars have embraced post-structuralist thought, which helpfully exposes how gender binaries become naturalised through discourse. In so doing, however, post-structuralist feminism also commits what Bhaskar (2015, p. 133) has referred to as the 'epistemic fallacy': the reduction of ontology to epistemology. If sex, gender, and even subjectivity are not real but merely the result of fluctuating discourse-power relations, it becomes impossible for feminists to argue that (gendered) experiences are the product of some structure that can be not only identified but also changed (Downs 1993). The post-structuralist rejection of any kind of non-discursive reality (that possesses powers/properties that are not provided by discourse itself) can thus make it difficult to claim knowledge of – and to challenge – gender inequality throughout the social world. At best, gender equality becomes something to be worked at rather atomistically, one discursive formation at a time.

Critical realist philosophy provides an important intervention into this debate between biological essentialist and post-structuralist views on gender, allowing us to assert a reality to diverse experiences of gender inequality without resulting in the kind of essentialism to which many feminists have objected. Its combination of *ontological realism* and *epistemological relativism*, for instance, suggests that the social world and social relations are real, but that this reality is variously explained and interpreted. In addition to this, critical realism favours the idea of *judgmental rationality*: the idea that it is possible, at least in principle, to evaluate the adequacy of contrasting/competing explanations and interpretations. The goal of critical realist research is therefore to identify the most accurate of these explanations/interpretations, to dismantle problematic understandings, and – more generally – to develop 'explanatory critiques' (discussed below) that support emancipatory efforts to create a better world.

From this perspective, explanations must move beyond the realm of the empirical (i.e., events as experienced and interpreted by embodied, socially/culturally situated human beings) to the relatively enduring, structural causes of these events at a deeper level of reality – the level of real causal mechanisms (Bhaskar 2008). Critical realism therefore subscribes to the idea of ontological depth; specifically, it distinguishes between (1) the *empirical* level of events as experienced through human understanding and perception, (2) the *actual* level, which comprises the totality of events, including those that we are unable to experience directly, and (3) the level of the *real*, of structures and their causal mechanisms that, when triggered, produce events at the other two levels. Although structures and causal/generative mechanisms are often conflated, in his postscript to *The Possibility of Naturalism* Bhaskar clarified that casual mechanisms are the particular powers held by a structure, which cause it to potentially have an effect on the world. The same causal power may be held by multiple different structures, either alone or in combination with other mechanisms, but all exist at the level of the real (Bhaskar 2015).

Because reality is characterised by depth, human beings only experience causal mechanisms (if we experience them at all) at the level of their empirical effects. Indeed, because causal mechanisms generally operate outside of (experimentally) closed systems, where they interact with other mechanisms to create contingent outcomes, people's experiences are always mediated by the different conditions in which they live their lives. Furthermore, no single individual can experience the empirical effect of a causal mechanism in its entirety; rather, the effects of a mechanism may manifest differently (or not at all) depending on various social conditions. In line with this depth ontology, critical realism asserts the existence of two dimensions of knowledge that roughly correspond with epistemology and ontology, respectively (Danermark et al. 2002): the transitive and intransitive. The transitive dimension is the realm of changing knowledge about (social) objects, while the intransitive is the realm of relatively stable phenomena that knowledge claims seek to explain.

In the openness of social systems and across the multiple strata or layers of reality, objects can combine to form new entities which have powers that are irreducible to those of their components – these are referred to by critical realists as 'emergent powers' (Danermark et al. 2002). The principle of emergence, as well as the quest to identify causal structures and mechanisms, sets critical realism in opposition to methodologically individualist approaches like rational choice theory, which reduce social phenomena to an aggregation of individual acts. In a similar way, both biological essentialist and interpretivist explanations reduce gender to what can be experienced at the empirical level. From a biological essentialist perspective, gender relations are the direct result of observable and relatively permanent sex differences. For interpretivists, gender relations are understood through, for example, individual experiences of sexism. Interpretivism is commonly relativistic in treating all viewpoints as equally valid; for many interpretivists, 'reality' is in the eye of the beholder.

In contrast, instead of reducing what is real to what we can observe (i.e., the primacy of experience), Bhaskar argued for the primacy of ontology. He argued, for instance, that

> it is because sticks and stones are solid that they can be picked up and thrown, not because they can be picked up and thrown that they are solid (though that they can be handled in this sort of way may be a contingently necessary condition for our *knowledge* of their solidity).
>
> (2015, p. 25)

In a similar way, we may know about gender inequality through individual experiences at the empirical level (e.g. individual women's experiences of sexism), and even by the accumulation of various gendered experiences at the actual level (e.g. documented trends of gendered violence and pay inequity). It is not these individual experiences or social trends, however, that cause gender inequality in the first place. Contrary to interpretivism, critical realism argues that it is not the collection of experiences as such that make up the reality of gender. Rather, this approach asserts that there is something deeply structural that *causes* both these individual experiences and social trends. The critical realist strategy of explanatory critiques therefore aims to identify and expose the nature of the causal structures that produce gender inequality in everyday life, with the ultimate goal of promoting positive social change.

Beliefs and values as causal

One of the most useful tenets of critical realism for gender analysis is its claim that social beliefs and values are real and can be causal (i.e., they can have an effect in the world) (Bhaskar 1998). Indeed, as Bhaskar points out,

> for the critical realist, everything is real, everything, which is a causal agent, is real. Thus, for a critical realist, beliefs [...] are also, in virtue of being causally efficacious, real. For critical realists, language is real, mathematics is real, materiality is real; whatever has a causal effect is real and that gives a critical realist a maximally inclusive ontology.
>
> (2017, p. 49)

Importantly, this ontology includes social structures and their causal powers. Critical realists conceive of social structures as 'transfactually efficacious' (i.e. active, irrespective of any outcome at the level of empirical patterns of events) as well as 'irreducibly historical', in the sense that they are bounded by space and time (Bhaskar 2015, pp. 123–24). Social mechanisms can also be characterised as intransitive because – although they do not exist independently of knowledge as such, and knowledge about them has the power to shape and transform them (Bhaskar 2015, p. 169) – they do usually exist outside of our knowledge of them as scientists/researchers. In this way, the transitive dimension (knowledge about social objects) and the intransitive dimension (relatively stable phenomena to which that knowledge aims to refer) are both distinct *and* interconnected. Similarly, social objects (e.g. beliefs and values) can be both causal *and* epistemic (Bhaskar 1998); in other words, social objects have an ontological or intransitive existence that gives them the power to causally affect events, but they also have an existence in the epistemic or transitive realm of representation. While social objects may therefore be represented in a way that does not encompasses their (full) ontological reality (Bhaskar 1998), partial or false understandings still have causal powers. After all, when people act upon their beliefs and values, these actions may have an effect in the social world.

In this way, critical realism facilitates critical engagement with systems of belief, including ideologies. In fact, given its resonances with Marxist thought, the proponents of this approach have commonly stressed the power of ideology and its ability to shape social relations, even though ideologies are false or partial representations of the way things actually are at an ontological level. According to Bhaskar, identifying a false belief about an object can allow us to negatively evaluate the source of that false belief; this is referred to as the theory of explanatory critiques, and is what makes critical realism both emancipatory and critical (Bhaskar 1998). Just as false beliefs can exist about the natural world, this approach suggests that it is possible for social objects to be represented falsely or incompletely. As this chapter will argue, such is the case with gender. Beliefs about gender are both causal social objects and are commonly false.

Identifying causes through abduction and retroduction

Critical realists suggest, first, that the real consists of the realm of structures and causal (i.e., generative) mechanisms, and second, that these produce specific patterns of actual and empirical events. These patterns may be characterised by so-called 'demi-regularities', or event regularities that – in contrast to what has commonly been assumed by (neo-)positivists – are both restricted in range and 'also somewhat partial and unstable' (Lawson 2003, p. 79). The 'demi' in demi-regularities hence refers to the fact that, in the open systems of the social world, patterns are never fully invariant: there will always be exceptions, resulting from situations in which a causal mechanism has either not been triggered at all or its effects have been altered/cancelled out by counteracting mechanisms. For example, a survey showing that 80% of people hold a belief is not the same as a survey showing that 100% of people hold that belief, but it is still a notable pattern that is worth investigating. In quantitative research, demi-regularities may appear as statistical trends. In qualitative research, demi-regularities may take the form of themes in our interview or focus group data, as well as any other forms of social data we may analyse.

Although such data should always inform our analyses, critical realist philosophy suggests that we cannot stop at simply describing it. Rather, abduction and retroduction are necessary if we are to infer and reason from our data (especially the demi-regularities it documents) to the causal mechanisms that provide its basis. Unfortunately, the methodological literature on critical realism has lacked clarity with regard to the difference between abduction and retroduction, perhaps due to the many ways in which abduction has been defined. For instance, abduction has been described as a basic cognitive process of explanation similar to 'common sense' (Shank 1998); as the use of reasoning to produce a summative description of a situation (Olsen 2007); and, drawing on the work of Charles Peirce, as a mode of logical inference that moves from events to theory to explain social phenomena (Bertilsson 2004). The last of these definitions supports the idea that abduction and retroduction involve essentially the same logical process, aimed at explaining empirical phenomena by identifying their causal structures and mechanisms.

Critical realist philosophy, in contrast, tends to separate out both the abductive and retroductive processes themselves and the different functions they serve. In their book on critical realism in the social sciences, Danermark et al. (2002, p. 205) describe abduction as a process of 'inference or thought operation' which suggests 'that a particular phenomenon or event is [to be] interpreted from a set of general ideas or concepts'. This definition is consistent with the important role of pre-existing theory in critical realist research. Retroduction, in contrast, is understood as employing the *results* of abduction (theoretical description and analysis of empirical phenomena) to 'reconstruct the basic conditions for these phenomena to be what they are' (Danermark et al. 2002, p. 80). From this perspective, abduction is the use of theory to cast new light on the phenomenon under investigation, allowing us to see it from a different angle, while retroduction builds on this theoretical explanation to think through the causal mechanisms that would cause the explanation to hold.

Furthermore, while abduction draws on different theories or concepts to answer 'what' questions (e.g. 'what is happening here?') retroduction moves us to a deeper level of reality in order to answer the 'why' questions (e.g. 'why is this happening?'). From this perspective, retroduction uses the tools of abduction – for example, theoretical thought experiments about what the phenomenon would look like under different conditions (Bhaskar 2015) – but adds a vertical movement from empirical data to theory and back again, with the ultimate goal of identifying the causal mechanisms that cause the data to be what they are. It is this move from one level of reality to another, therefore, that distinguishes the retroductive from the abductive process. Importantly, this movement also distinguishes retroduction from empiricist uses of induction and deduction, which either test hypotheses by using empirical data (deduction) or use empirical data to produce hypotheses or generalisations (induction); both of these modes remain at the empirical level of reality and therefore lack the ontological depth and vertical movement that critical realist philosophy suggests is necessary.

In one of the few texts to address the abduction/retroduction distinction directly, Thora Bertilsson (2004) critiques critical realism by arguing that it ultimately reduces abduction to a creative process while retroduction is positioned as a logical and scientific one. This, Bertilsson (2004, p. 385) argues, has the effect of privileging (social) scientific explanations without considering their power to constitute or shape the social world. She writes that 'retroduction becomes favoured as logical thought-operation and as the height of scientific inquiry, but it now appears as a discrete – transitive – act: it carries no long-term consequences as to world constitution'. Thus, 'science has no real practical consequences; it merely "is"' (Bertilsson 2004, p. 386). However, this critique does not consider the fact that scientific explanations – like other systems of explanation, beliefs, and values – exist within the causal realm, and that the transitive dimension can therefore shape the intransitive dimension (Bhaskar 2015). Beliefs, in other words, can causally affect the events or phenomena that scientists investigate. To assert a distinction between abduction and retroduction based on the level of reality at which they operate is therefore not to privilege one mode of reasoning over the other. Rather, it is simply to acknowledge the importance of both in the overall process of explanatory critique.

The sections that follow will build on the critical realist claim that systems of belief and explanation (whether scientific or 'common sense') can have a powerful causal effect in the social world. Drawing on the aforementioned study of farm women, the discussion will illustrate the processes of abduction and retroduction to demonstrate their power in analysing gender ideology as a real causal mechanism.

The Saskatchewan Farm Women Study

The Saskatchewan Farm Women Study (SFWS) was a predominantly qualitative research project conducted in the Canadian prairie province of Saskatchewan. The project examined the impact of neoliberal agricultural policy on the working lives of farm women, as well as farm women's adaptive responses to policy changes. The methods used included 30 in-depth interviews with farm women, three key informant interviews with agricultural leaders, use of national statistics from the Census of Agriculture, and analyses of historical reports and parliamentary transcripts documenting two policy changes that affected Canadian agriculture. Both policy changes had a dramatic impact on farmers' lives, and both exemplify tenets of a neoliberal policy paradigm. The first policy change was the erosion and eventual elimination of a popular grain transportation support, known colloquially as the 'Crow Rate', throughout the late 1980s and early 1990s. The Crow elimination is an example of neoliberal deregulation aimed at aligning federal policy with international trade agreements. The second policy change was the 1990 implementation of Plant Breeders Rights (PBR), a form of intellectual property right on seed varieties. PBR exemplified the more recent neoliberal trend of 'new constitutionalism' – the reorientation of government policy towards facilitating corporate profit-making and capital accumulation (Gill 1998; McBride 2011).

The SFWS was guided from the outset by theories from the field of feminist political economy (FPE), which highlights the gendered dimensions of broader political-economic structures (see, for example, Bakker 2007; Bezanson and Luxton 2006; Rai and Waylen 2014; Vosko 2002). In particular, FPE encourages us to connect social trends, such as the gendered division of labour, to political and economic systems and structures that shape people's work in various ways.

Neither of the two policy cases, at the time of their implementation, were portrayed as having possible gendered impacts. The SFWS was (and still is) one of very few studies to examine the gendered impacts of neoliberal agricultural policy in Canada. A major goal of this study was therefore to explore (1) whether 'gender neutral' policies like agricultural transport and seed policy in fact have gendered impacts in everyday life, and (2) what those potential impacts were in the context of the study. Critical realism was selected as the guiding philosophy of the study because of its potential for identifying causal mechanisms and grounding an explanatory critique. In a recent article (Fletcher 2017) I described my application of critical realist philosophy to demonstrate its utility as a framework for applied feminist research. In the section below, I will expand on this earlier article to provide a more detailed discussion of the abductive and retroductive processes involved. The results included the identification of two key causal mechanisms that were shaping the lives of farm women and men in Canadian agriculture: gender ideology (the main focus of this chapter) and corporatisation. Finally, the importance of gender ideology as a causal mechanism will be described and discussed.

Applying abduction and retroduction in the SFWS

Analysis of the interview transcripts and documents revealed several notable demi-regularities. The first set of these demi-regularities pertained to women's work – specifically, the marginalisation of women's farm work and their motivations for working off-farm. Although all but one of the participants was actively engaged in farm work of some type, and many of the participants regularly performed a wide variety of tasks, the most commonly named role (mentioned by 20 of the 29 participants) was a variant of 'helping out' – for example, acting as 'hired hand' or 'hired man', 'employee', 'go for', or 'assistant'. The qualitative data showed that, with only a few exceptions, men were viewed as the main farmers, while women's work was portrayed as peripheral. One participant summarised this trend by saying:

> A lot of times the men take all of the responsibility for the financial planning and dealings and that type of thing and other times the women are doing it, but it's still not really their decision at the end of the day.

Another participant commented: 'We're, kind of, behind the lines supporting what they're doing on the front'.

Like nearly half of Canadian farmers many of the farm women held off-farm employment in addition to their farm duties (Statistics Canada 2017). The women in the SFWS also performed the overwhelming majority (89%) of unwaged domestic and caregiving work within their respective households and families. To find out why women were working off-farm in addition to their many other tasks, particularly while reporting heavy workloads and stress, I used a questionnaire with a quantitative Likert-type question (0 = not at all a factor; 6 = the most significant factor). In light of the financial challenges that many family-farms experience, and in light of women's already heavy responsibilities at home and on the farm, I expected that off-farm work was done mostly out of financial necessity. Therefore, my expectation was that 'earn money to support the farm operation' would be most highly rated as a motivation. However, to my surprise, the most highly rated reason for working off-farm was 'personal goals and self-fulfilment' (average score of 4.13), followed by earning money for household needs (average score of 4.08), and earning money for 'wants' or luxury items (3.42). Earning money to support the farm was, in fact, the least significant motivator, with an average score of only 2.05.

Another interview question added more complexity to the findings: despite the emphasis on personal goals as a motivator, when asked about their ideal working conditions in a world where money was not an issue, 10 out of the 20 women working off-farm indicated that they would choose to amend their current working conditions. Their preferred options included, in particular, ones that would have allowed them to reduce hours at their off-farm job or (in a few cases) to quit their off-farm job to focus entirely on farm or household work.

The second set of significant demi-regularities pertained to changes in the political-economic structure of agriculture more broadly. Participants often spoke of the increasing power of others (variously construed as corporations, government, or actors unknown to the participants) over the economic conditions of agriculture. In particular, the women reported an overarching experience of lost control over the conditions of production, market prices, and input costs.

When asked about changes in seed policy, one participant stated that the system is 'just taking the power and control away from farmers so much [that] it gets to the point where you've got [farmers] backed into a corner'. Loss of control was also linked to the aforementioned two policy changes, although the policies were not seen as the only causal factors. Participants noted, for instance, that the Crow elimination had increased their costs of production and that this policy change had driven the dual trends of farm-size growth and rural depopulation, as farmers adapted to the increased financial pressure either by increasing the size of their farm or leaving it entirely. The implementation of PBR, they reported, had also limited what farmers could and could not do with their seed, while facilitating capital accumulation for the makers of those seed varieties. These findings were supported not only by the existing literature on corporatisation in agriculture (e.g. Baines 2017; Epp and Whitson 2001; Kuyek 2007) but also by my document analyses, which demonstrated the increasing presence and power of private and corporate actors in the policymaking process (Fletcher 2013).

Abduction

Once these demi-regularities were identified in the data, the process of abduction allowed me to interpret them in a more abstract way by drawing on existing explanations and theoretical concepts. As mentioned, abduction in critical realist thought involves moving from (thick) description to a theoretical interpretation of the circumstances under study. Indeed, abduction draws on *existing* theoretical frameworks and concepts to help answer questions about 'what is happening here?' Through FPE theory, it became apparent that Saskatchewan family farming is structured by a highly gendered division of labour, with a tendency for 'feminised' tasks to be less recognised or valued. Tasks involving more direct contact with crops and machinery are more likely to be performed by men and are more likely to be seen as 'real' farming. Despite their importance, tasks frequently performed by women – such as picking up parts for machinery, moving workers or equipment from field to field, bookkeeping and accounting, and cooking large meals for hired farm workers – were less likely to be seen as central to farming (Fletcher 2013). Although FPE theory works best with waged/formal rather than unwaged/informal work, agricultural forms of labour cannot be so easily distinguished. Nonetheless, FPE's concern with the *value* of unwaged work (e.g. Luxton 2006) is useful when it comes to questions about the value (or lack thereof) that is assigned to differently 'gendered' tasks. FPE concepts therefore proved to fruitful resources for explaining what was happening in the data.

However, according to Meyer and Lunnay (2013), abduction also 'involves analysing data that fall outside of an initial theoretical frame or premise'. This observation applied in the SFWS findings as well. The question of women's motivations for doing off-farm work, for instance, required further explanation beyond what was possible with FPE concepts. With its focus on political-economic context an FPE analysis would consider how the structural conditions of agriculture – the on-going pressure of balancing unpredictable market prices with rising input costs, the increasing demand for profit by large corporations in the agri-food chain, and the 'get big or get out' imperative – interact with existing gender roles to shape work patterns in gendered ways. If (as I had expected) the major motivator for women taking off-farm work was to support the farm financially, such an analysis would have been sufficient. But this was not the case. Although political-economic structural factors may help explain why earning money for household items was an important driver of women's off-farm work these do not readily explain the women's strong emphasis on personal choice and self-fulfilment.

Insights from liberal feminist theory facilitated, but did not complete, the abductive interpretation of this particular demi-regularity. A liberal feminist perspective draws attention to issues of choice, rights, and equality, while also engaging critically with institutionalised inequality and underrepresentation (Tong 2009). In the current context, such a perspective would highlight women's under-representation as farm operators in Canada (according to the 2016 Census of Agriculture, only 29% of Canadian farm operators are women) and situate (as well as critically evaluate) Canadian agriculture as a male-dominated profession. Indeed, considering the emphasis that the women themselves placed on choice and self-fulfilment as a motivation for their off-farm employment, it would not be unreasonable to conclude that these forms of employment are the product of their agential responses to the male-dominated nature of farming. In an industry that marginalised them and discounted their contributions, women simply make choices: they seek autonomy and fulfilment off the farm.

While this explanation is useful, however, it is also insufficient to explain other important demi-regularities; for example, if women are working off-farm as a response to the male-dominated nature of agriculture, why are Canadian farm men also working off-farm at an almost equal rate (Statistics Canada 2006)? Further, when asked about their ideal work arrangements in a hypothetical situation where money is not an issue, why did half of the women report that they would choose a different arrangement than the one that was currently in place?

Both questions point to the continuing relevance of financial factors and, by extension, broader political-economic structures in agriculture. It was worth asking, therefore, if the demi-regularity of 'lost control' also shaped women's work choices and, if so, how? While liberal feminist theory usefully attunes us to the possibility of choice by emphasising the importance of agency (albeit within certain constraints), another theoretical perspective was necessary to explain what was truly happening. From a critical realist perspective, treating choices as simply neutral and free is to ignore social emergence, reducing these choices to individualised and atomistic components by ignoring the structural conditions that shape them. Indeed, while the combination of liberal theory's agential focus and FPE's structural analysis arguably provides a more complete interpretation of the forces shaping women's lives, the adoption of a critical realist perspective suggests that this may only provide us with an actualist analysis (i.e., an analysis that connects empirical experiences and observed events to broader trends at the level of the actual). Outstanding questions remain about the origins of these forces. What causal mechanisms actually *drive* the trends of gendered work roles and decreasing control over production? The use of retroduction was therefore needed to identify the mechanisms causing these trends to occur.

Retroduction

In critical realist philosophy, the goal of retroduction is to answer the 'why' question: 'why do we have data that suggest X exists?' (Olsen 2007). As Bhaskar (2015, p. 12) put it, retroduction involves 'building a model [...] of a mechanism, which if it were to exist and act in the postulated way would account for the phenomenon in question'. Retroduction therefore aims to identify causal mechanisms or structures in the intransitive realm by asking questions about what needs to exist (causally) for empirical events to occur as they have. In this way, retroduction requires a back-and-forth movement from the data – especially any demi-regularities they may record – to the mechanism(s) that help explain them. From this perspective, structures (whether these are social, physical, or whatever) possess inherent powers and liabilities that cause them to act, or have the potential to act, in certain ways (Psillos 2007). Depending on contextual conditions, these powers and liabilities may or may not be triggered (Brown et al. 2002); if they are, they become actualised and may have empirical effects.

Caroline New (2005, ch. 3 this volume) explains how this approach relates to gender by building on Collier's (1994) discussion of actualism. She suggests that a structural critique of gender inequality must dig deeper than analyses that simply link individual experiences to gendered trends. An actualist explanation, she shows, would simply move from the empirical to the level of the actual, thereby attributing women's experiences of gender inequality to larger social trends that extend beyond the individual. While this is of significant importance, actualist analyses do not help us to explain what mechanisms are ultimately producing these trends. Furthermore, while New (2005, ch. 3 this volume) argues that biological sex difference is a low-level, base mechanism that helps cause gender orders, she clarifies that sex is only one of many causal factors that co-produce gender orders; therefore, gender cannot be seen merely as a direct effect (or simple expression) of sexed bodies. New argues that sex does not determine gender, nor is gender reducible to sex. Unfortunately, New's philosophical discussion does not explain *how much* of gender is attributable to sex. From the critical realist perspective she adopts this is in fact a question that can only be answered by empirical research. The following section therefore describes how I came to the conclusion that gender ideology, as opposed to biological sex, was the key causal mechanism in the SFWS.

The retroductive movement discussed here began with the unexpected finding about women's motivations for working off-farm (i.e., personal goals and self-fulfilment). Although research on Canadian farmers' motivations for off-farm employment is very limited, existing findings from the Census of Agriculture (Jetté-Nantel et al. 2011) suggest that income variability and risk management (i.e., financial factors) may increase off-farm work. In other words, in an agricultural environment marked by both financial and climatic uncertainty, farmers may seek off-farm employment for added security and income stability. Such motivations fall within the scope of FPE analyses and help to explain the decisions of Canadian farmers generally in response to a context of financial uncertainty. However, since over 70% of farmers in Canada are male (Statistics Canada 2017), even the limited research that exists on off-farm work motivations may primarily reflect farm men's perspectives. Indeed, although the SFWS focused on women, several participants mentioned that their husbands were working off-farm primarily for financial reasons. This finding reflects the aforementioned positioning of men as the 'main farmer', as the one ultimately responsible for the farm's financial success or failure.

This financial explanation, however, provides only a partial explanation for farm *women's* motivations for off-farm work. While farmers generally lack control over the political-economic structures that shape agriculture, women experience a type of 'double disconnection' – they are disconnected from control at both the political-economic level and at the level of the farm itself. In this context, off-farm work provides women with fulfilment, with a locus of control outside of the farm. Their employment decisions thus cannot be simplistically reduced to either financial factors or individual choices, but rather exemplify an agential response that is structured by both the aforementioned *political-economic* mechanisms and *gendered* mechanisms. For the remainder of this chapter, I will focus on discussing the gender-specific findings, as these are most pertinent to the focus of this volume.

The SFWS findings highlight the existence of a rigid, gendered division of labour rooted in binary gender ideology. Specifically, gender ideology helps to (re)produce gendered divisions of labour on Canadian family farms by asymmetrically attributing value to tasks that are marked masculine or feminine and socialising those identified as (wo)men into the associated tasks, thereby reinforcing the conditions that marginalise women in agriculture. These conditions become engrained, and certain roles are understood as the 'natural' domain of (wo)men. This was evident in some of the women's discourses about (wo)men's roles in agriculture, illustrating the internalisation of ideology as a causal mechanism. One woman, for example, stated that, 'Most women I know live in their heart, most men live in their head, and it gives you a totally different perception'. Another participant argued that women are inherently more detail-oriented than men, stating that 'I think that's how we were made. That's why man can't live alone'.

In line with New's (2005, ch. 3 this volume) argument that bodies constitute a low-level mechanism for gender relations, several farm women did suggest that their work roles – and their associated disconnection from the farm – were linked to their disproportionate responsibility for childcare. In a discussion about the gendered division of labour, one woman stated that, 'I think, initially, it's because the men take the main role of farmer, and I think also because most women have children, and they do most of the childcare'. However, as argued above, the gender relations observed in the SFWS are insufficiently explained by drawing attention to biological reproduction alone, nor does childbirth necessitate disproportionate responsibility for childcare or indicate an inability to farm. Gendered work roles are the product of an emergent phenomenon that, while it presupposes sexed bodies, is also irreducible to them.

Although some participants attributed gender roles to biological factors, others spoke only of the roles themselves without attributing cause. Despite some expressions of frustration about the demands of these roles, few participants challenged or questioned the gendered division of labour on their farms. With the exception of a single female farmer who identified as a feminist, gender roles in farming were largely accepted as pre-given and unchangeable. These trends are summarised in one participant's statement that

> farm men … they have more on their shoulders because of keeping the machinery going. And, on the whole, I think making most of the decisions, the marketing of the grain, you know the hauling it in – don't get me wrong, farm women are definitely important too, but those tasks … the farm women can't do.

In contrast, many of the other women in the study were involved in marketing and grain hauling.

Unlike interpretivist approaches, which suggest that people's contrasting/competing accounts of reality are equally valid, critical realism employs the aforementioned principle of judgmental rationality to engage critically with existing explanations of a phenomenon, irrespective of whether these explanations have been provided by our participants or other researchers. Judgmental rationality – as opposed to judgmental relativism (Lawson 1999) – is based on the premise that, because there exists a real (and relatively independent) world which has particular powers and properties, some explanations are more effective than others. Although it would have been possible to stop the analysis by attributing gender relations to biological sex differences or some kind of natural order this would not have allowed me to explain the additional themes of political-economic control and women's detachment from farm control.

Through judgemental rationality, it is possible to see the operation of gender ideology in the internalisation of gender roles as normal and unchangeable. Importantly, women do exercise agency in their off-farm work and other pursuits. However, the on-going portrayal of some farm activities as something women 'can't do' serves to reinforce their disconnection from agriculture, which could be a potential site of fulfilment for women under different conditions (e.g. if women were more frequently socialised to become farmers). As liberal feminist theory reminds us, women are not simply passive victims; they are agents who make choices in response to their reality. However, this reality is shaped by political-economic structures and the causal mechanisms of gender ideology. These causal mechanisms serve to reinforce the demi-regularities of women's disconnection and their agency-seeking off-farm, which, in turn, reinforces the further masculinisation of Canadian agriculture observed in this and other agricultural contexts (e.g. Clarke and Alston 2017).

Conclusion

In this chapter I have suggested the usefulness of critical realism as a framework for empirical feminist research. Using concrete examples from a study of

Canadian farm women's work and experiences with neoliberal policy change, I have sought to both clarify and demonstrate the utility of abduction and retroduction as analytical processes when it comes to identifying causal mechanisms. Two key demi-regularities were identified in the data: first, farm women's motivations for off-farm employment were identified primarily by means of a quantitative, Likert-type question, which was then supplemented by qualitative insights on the marginalisation of women's work; second, the study identified a qualitative theme of 'lost control' that was experienced by farmers generally with regard to their conditions of agricultural production.

In critical realist research, abduction aims to interpret such findings by referring to existing theory and concepts. In my own abductive process, I employed insights from FPE theory and, to a more limited extent, liberal feminist theory, to interpret the findings in a way that answers the question: 'what is going on here?' Building on these abductive insights, my retroductive analysis moved from the empirical data that I gathered to the identification of causal mechanisms, guided by questions that focused on 'why' events occurred as they did. This retroductive process resulted in the identification of two causal mechanisms that were held responsible for shaping the lives and work of farm women: gender ideology and corporatisation. While corporatisation acts as a generative mechanism to influence farmers' control and agency, gender ideology shapes farmers' work roles and, by extension, their responses to these events. When these two generative mechanisms are combined they shed light on a context that is characterised by the 'double disconnection' of farm women from farm production.

Furthermore, this chapter has suggested that critical realist research on gender can undermine biological reductionism, or the emphasis of some approaches on biological sex as the major cause of gender relations. Such approaches commit the epistemic fallacy by reducing gendered social trends to the biophysical realm of observable sexed bodies, thus disregarding emergence and social causation. Instead, this chapter has built on the critical realist argument that social causes are irreducible to non-social causes, and that systems of belief and explanation (including ideologies) can have powerful causal effects on people's lives. In line with this argument, gender ideology was argued to have strong explanatory power in the empirical study.

While critical realism, in contrast with (neo-)positivism and interpretivism, seeks to identify mechanisms that operate at the deepest level of reality, this aim therefore should not be mistaken for ontological or methodological reductionism. Although sexed bodies may be a 'low level' phenomenon upon which some social beliefs and ideologies are built or justified (New 2005, ch. 3 this volume), complexly gendered societies are emergent from (and hence irreducible to) this level. Moreover, some societies have featured gender systems featuring more than two genders and thus move further from sex as a base mechanism (Cameron 2009). As Bhaskar emphasised, 'because social structures are themselves social products, social activity must be given a social explanation, and cannot be explained by reference to non-social parameters' (2015, p.

38). Because reality is stratified, biological reductionist approaches inevitably exclude the causal power of social objects from consideration.

Gender ideology is such a causal social object. Acting as a mechanism, ideology may (re)produce different gender formations across time and space. Gender ideology itself may therefore serve as a relatively persistent causal mechanism for gender structures, possessing its own causal powers and essential structure. A critical realist approach allows us to assert a reality to gender ideology, and, by extension, to people's experiences of that ideology at the empirical level. However, this approach also allows for critical engagement with both existing scholarly and common-sense explanations of reality. The combination of ontological realism with epistemological relativism may prove useful to feminist scholars by facilitating anti-essentialist analyses that do not succumb to the relativism of interpretivism and the deconstruction of agency and experience found in post-structuralist approaches. By stressing that gender ideology is a social mechanism, furthermore, the critical realist approach developed in this chapter shows that gender ideology is not just intelligible and knowable but that it is also something that can be challenged by means of both explanatory critiques and collective action.

Notes

1 The 'Google Memo' (formally titled 'Google's Ideological Echo Chamber') was a memorandum written by James Damore, an American engineer at Google who was later fired for his comments. The memo drew on controversial biological arguments to justify women's under-representation in the industry, questioned Google's diversity efforts, and accused Google of alienating conservative white men.

2 This chapter focuses on (and engages critically with) one particular formation of gender ideology that has variously been referred to as dualistic/binary, traditionalist, biological essentialist, etc. because, in the study on which it is based, this particular formation was found to affect the lives of the participants. While feminist discussions about whether or not gender *as such* is ideological (as in some gender abolitionist or postgenderist work) are certainly of significant importance, such discussions are beyond the scope of this chapter.

References

Archer, M. S. 2010. "Morphogenesis versus Structuration: On Combining Structure and Action." *The British Journal of Sociology* 61:225–52.

———. 1995. *Realist Social Theory: The Morphogenetic Approach*. Cambridge and New York: Cambridge University Press.

Baines, J. 2017. "Accumulating through Food Crisis? Farmers, Commodity Traders and the Distributional Politics of Financialization." *Review of International Political Economy* 24(3):497–537.

Bakker, I. 2007. "Social Reproduction and the Constitution of a Gendered Political Economy." *New Political Economy* 12(4):541–56.

Bertilsson, T. M. 2004. "The Elementary Forms of Pragmatism: On Different Types of Abduction." *European Journal of Social Theory* 7(3):371–89.

Bezanson, K. and M. Luxton. 2006. *Social Reproduction: Feminist Political Economy Challenges Neo-Liberalism*. Montreal: McGill-Queen's University Press.

Bhaskar, R. 2008. *A Realist Theory of Science*. London and New York: Verso.

———. 1998. "Facts and Values: Theory and Practice/Reason and the Dialectic of Human Emancipation/ Depth,Rationality and Change," in M. Archer, R. Bhaskar, A. Collier, T. Lawson, and A. Norrie (eds.) *Critical Realism: Essential Readings*, pp. 409–44. Abingdon and New York: Routledge.

———. 2015. *The Possibility of Naturalism: A Philosophical Critique of the Contemporary Human Sciences*. fourth edition. London and New York: Routledge.

———. 2017. *The Order of Natural Necessity: A Kind of Introduction to Critical Realism*. edited by G. Hawke. CreateSpace Independent Publishing Platform.

Blinkhorn, S. 2005. "Intelligence: A Gender Bender." *Nature* 438(7064):31–32.

Brown, A., S. Fleetwood and J. M. Roberts. 2002. "The Marriage of Critical Realism and Marxism: Happy, Unhappy or On the Rocks?" in A. Brown, S. Fleetwood, and J. M. Roberts (eds.) *Critical Realism and Marxism*, pp. 1–22. London and New York: Routledge.

Butler, J. 1990. *Gender Trouble: Feminism and the Subversion of Identity*. New York: Routledge.

Cameron, M. 2009. "Two-Spirited Aboriginal People: Continuing Cultural Appropriation by Non-Aboriginal Society," in P. A. Monture and P. D. McGuire (eds.) *First Voices: An Aboriginal Women's Reader*, pp. 200–6. Toronto, ON: Inanna.

Clarke, J. and M. Alston. 2017. "Understanding the 'Local' and 'Global': Intersections Engendering Change for Women in Family Farming in Australia," in A. J. Fletcher and W. Kubik (eds.) *Women in Agriculture Worldwide: Key Issues and Practical Approaches*, pp. 13–22. Abingdon and New York: Routledge.

Clegg, S. 2016. "Agency and Ontology within Intersectional Analysis: A Critical Realist Contribution." *Journal of Critical Realism* 15(5): 494–510.

Collier, A. 1994. *Critical Realism: An Introduction to Roy Bhaskar's Philosophy*. London and New York: Verso.

Danermark, B., M. Ekström, L. Jakobsen and J. C. H. Karlsson. 2002. *Explaining Society: An Introduction to Critical Realism in the Social Sciences*. London: Routledge.

Downs, L. L. 1993. "If 'Woman' Is Just an Empty Category, Then Why Am I Afraid to Walk Alone at Night? Identity Politics Meets the Postmodern Subject." *Comparative Studies in Society and History* 35(2):414–37.

Edwards, P. K., J. O'Mahoney and S. Vincent, (eds). 2014. *Studying Organizations Using Critical Realism: A Practical Guide*. Oxford, UK: Oxford University Press.

Epp, R. and D. Whitson, (eds). 2001. *Writing off the Rural West: Globalization, Governments and the Transformation of Rural Communities*. Edmonton, AB: University of Alberta Press and Parkland Institute.

Fine, C. 2010. *Delusions of Gender: How Our Minds, Society, and Neurosexism Create Difference*. New York: W. W. Norton & Company.

Fletcher, A. J. 2017. "Applying Critical Realism in Qualitative Research: Methodology Meets Method." *International Journal of Social Research Methodology* 20(2):181–94.

———. 2013. "The View From Here: Agricultural Policy, Climate Change, and the Future of Farm Women in Saskatchewan." University of Regina, Regina, SK.

Gill, S. 1998. "New Constitutionalism, Democratisation and Global Political Economy." *Global Change, Peace & Security* 10(1):23–38.

Gunnarsson, L. 2011. "A Defence of the Category 'Women'." *Feminist Theory* 12 (1):23–37.

———. 2017. "Why We Keep Separating the 'Inseparable': Dialecticizing Intersectionality." *European Journal of Women's Studies* 24(2):114–27.

Gunnarsson, L., A. Martinez Dy and M. van Ingen. 2016. "Critical Realism, Gender and Feminism: Exchanges, Challenges, Synergies." *Journal of Critical Realism* 15(5):433–39.

Holmwood, J. 2001. "Gender and Critical Realism: A Critique of Sayer." *Sociology* 35(04):947–65.

Jetté-Nantel, S., D. Freshwater, M. Beaulieu and A. Katchova. 2011. *Farm Income Variability and Off-Farm Diversification in Canadian Agriculture*. Ottawa, ON: Statistics Canada.

Kuyek, D. 2007. "Sowing the Seeds of Corporate Agriculture: The Rise of Canada's Third Seed Regime." *Studies in Political Economy* 80:31–54.

Lawson, T. 1999. "Feminism, Realism, and Universalism." *Feminist Economics* 5(2):25–59.

———. 2003. *Reorienting Economics*. London and New York: Routledge.

Lennox, R. and R. Jurdi-Hage. 2017. "Beyond the Empirical and the Discursive: The Methodological Implications of Critical Realism for Street Harassment Research." *Women's Studies International Forum* 60:28–38.

Lorber, J. 1994. *Paradoxes of Gender*. Yale University: Yale University Press.

Luxton, M. 2006. "Feminist Political Economy in Canada and the Politics of Social Reproduction," in K. Bezanson and M. Luxton (eds.) *Social Reproduction: Feminist Political Economy Challenges Neo-Liberalism*, pp. 11–44. Montreal: McGill-Queen's University Press.

McBride, S. 2011. "The New Constitutionalism: International and Private Rule in the New Global Order," in S. McBride and G. Teeple (eds.) *Relations of Global Power: Neoliberal Order and Disorder*, pp. 19–40. Toronto, ON: University of Toronto Press.

Meyer, S. B. and B. Lunnay. 2013. "The Application of Abductive and Retroductive Inference for the Design and Analysis of Theory-Driven Sociological Research." *Sociological Research Online* 18(1):12.

New, C. 2005. "Sex and Gender: A Critical Realist Approach." *New Formations* 56:54–70.

Olsen, W. 2007. "Critical Realist Explorations in Methodology." *Methodological Innovation Online* 2(2):1–5.

Parr, S. 2015. "Integrating Critical Realist and Feminist Methodologies: Ethical and Analytical Dilemmas." *International Journal of Social Research Methodology* 18(2):193–207.

Psillos, S. 2007. "Causality," in M. Hartwig (ed.) *Dictionary of Critical Realism*, pp. 57–61. London and New York: Routledge.

Rai, S. M. and G. Waylen, (eds). 2014. *New Frontiers in Feminist Political Economy*. London and New York: Routledge.

Sayer, A. 1992. *Methods in Social Science : A Realist Approach*. London: Routledge.

———. 1997. "Critical Realism and the Limits to Critical Social Science." *Journal for the Theory of Social Behaviour* 27(4):473–88.

———. 2000. "System, Lifeworld and Gender: Associational versus Counterfactual Thinking." *Sociology* 34(4):707–25.

Scott, J. W. 1991. "The Evidence of Experience." *Critical Inquiry* 17(4):773–97.

Shank, G. 1998. “The Extraordinary Ordinary Powers of Abductive Reasoning.” *Theory & Psychology* 8(6):841–60.

Statistics Canada. 2017. *Census of Agriculture 2016*. Ottawa, ON: Government of Canada.

———. 2006. “Snapshot of Canadian Agriculture.” Retrieved April 16, 2013 (http://www.statcan.gc.ca/ca-ra2006/articles/snapshot-portrait-eng.htm).

Tong, R. 2009. *Feminist Thought: A More Comprehensive Introduction*. Boulder, CO: Westview Press.

Vosko, L. F. 2002. “The Pasts (and Futures) of Feminist Political Economy in Canada: Reviving the Debate.” *Studies in Political Economy* 68(1): 55–83.

Yeung, H. W. 1997. “Critical Realism and Realist Research in Human Geography: A Method or a Philosophy in Search of a Method?” *Progress in Human Geography* 21(1):51–74.

10 After constructivism

Rethinking *Feminist Security Studies* through interdisciplinary research

Michiel van Ingen

Introduction

The ascent of feminist approaches since the mid-1980s has resulted in a significant challenge to the character and identity of the International Relations (IR) discipline. The vitality and force of these approaches became apparent especially during the fourth (so-called) 'Great Debate'[1] of IR; the debate, that is, between neo-positivist and post-positivist approaches. By siding largely with the latter side, feminist scholars were able to challenge the very foundations of mainstream (or 'malestream') IR. Importantly, this challenge was mounted primarily by stressing the need to adopt distinctly *feminist* methods and epistemological perspectives. It was commonly argued, for instance, that these (1) facilitated greater recognition of the ubiquitous *analytical* significance of sex/gender, and (2) provided a superior basis for explicitly *normative* concerns with dismantling or deconstructing various sex-/gender-based hierarchies and prejudices.

Security concerns played a prominent role in feminist IR from the outset (e.g. Elshtain 1987; Enloe 1988; Peterson 1992; Sylvester 1994; Tickner 1992). Since the start of the third millennium, however, 'there has been a veritable explosion of feminist work in *Security Studies*, to the point where one can now confidently refer to FSS [*Feminist Security Studies*] as a sub-field at the intersections of Security Studies and feminist IR' (Wibben 2010, p. 85; see also Stern and Wibben 2015). Perhaps the most significant advance that has resulted from this development is the fact that FSS authors have successfully problematised sexual- and gender-based violence (SGBV).[2] It is very largely due to their efforts, for instance, that sexual torture, sexual slavery, and (mass) rape are increasingly considered legitimate topics of foreign policy-making. Indeed, the claim that rape is a weapon or tactic of war – which is now 'the refrain of practically all contemporary academic research, political advocacy and media reporting' on this issue (Kirby 2012, p. 798) – has self-evident roots in the feminist IR literature (e.g. Enloe 2000; Hansen 2001).

Such achievements notwithstanding, this chapter will argue that the 'thick' constructivism to which many prominent FSS authors currently subscribe is incapable of providing this sub-field with adequate philosophical grounding.

This is the case, in short, because the textualist framework that results from this form of constructivism is (1) unable to provide a basis and rationale for the kind of integrative, interdisciplinary research that is required to do justice to the events/phenomena with which FSS is concerned, and (2) ill-suited to grounding empirical forms of feminist research.

The focus on constructivism that this chapter adopts may, at first glance, appear to be at odds with the philosophical and methodological heterogeneity of FSS work. Authors like Annick T. R. Wibben have stressed, after all, that FSS scholars 'embrace a variety of epistemological and political positions, all of which shed light on different aspects of the security puzzle' (2010, p. 87). More generally, FSS has commonly been construed as diverse, pluralistic, or eclectic. The current chapter does not intend to simply invert such characterisations; however, it does suggest the need to qualify them considerably by stressing that a philosophico-methodological trend – which will be referred to as the *constructivist consensus* – has become increasingly apparent. It will employ this notion, quite self-consciously, as a practical short-hand which refers to FSS work that has been variously identified as constructivist, post-structural, post-modern, and (more tangentially) post-colonial. While it might reasonably be objected that there exist relevant differences between (as well as within) these approaches, a close reading of the FSS literature reveals that the lines which purportedly divide them have, at best, been inconsistently drawn. Indeed, not only have constructivist FSS authors frequently used the first three of these terms interchangeably (e.g. Leatherman 2011) they also have significantly more in common than separates them.

If this is the case, however, why does this chapter hold the constructivist consensus to be incapable of providing a basis and rationale for integrative, interdisciplinary research? The answer that is provided to this question in the sections below will centre on the one-dimensional focus on discourse/meaning that constructivists – like many proponents of the cultural turn – have adopted; more specifically, it will fasten on their tendency to reduce all types of being to a disembodied form of textualism. This tendency results in an approach that – while it is unable to sustain an account of agency – is both *anthropocentric* and *premised on a unidirectional understanding of causality*. In turn, this ensures that constructivism is (1) plagued by persistent theory/praxis inconsistencies, and (2) ill-suited to grounding interdisciplinary research. In contrast, this chapter will contend that critical realist philosophy – especially its *emergentist/stratified ontology* and *power-/mechanism-based understanding of causality* – does pave the way for interdisciplinary research. In fact, it will argue that this philosophical approach – in direct contrast with constructivism – paves the way for an approach to FSS that is multi-dimensional, anti- or post-anthropocentric, premised on a multidirectional understanding of causality, capable of sustaining a robust account of agency, and able to effectively avoid theory/praxis inconsistencies.

Before developing these arguments, however, it will be necessary to provide an answer to two prior questions. The first of these concerns the importance of theory/praxis (in)consistency and asks why this issue should matter to (constructivist) FSS authors? What, in other words, justifies this chapter's focus on said subject as a basis for critique? The second question relates to the importance of integrative, interdisciplinary research and asks – again – what justifies the chapter's concern with this subject as a basis for critique? A satisfactory answer to these questions must arguably be provided before proceeding to the substance of the argument; after all, without doing so this argument is likely to be dismissed as providing a critique that is rooted in a perspective which is entirely alien to – and therefore simply has no bearing on – constructivism. The next part of this chapter will therefore serve the purpose of side-stepping such verdicts. Its remainder will then proceed by sketching the main tenets of constructivist FSS and arguing (1) that it fails the test of theory/praxis consistency, (2) that it is incapable of providing a basis and rationale for interdisciplinary research, (3) that critical realism does pave the way for such research, and (4) that this approach avoids the theory/praxis inconsistencies which beset constructivist FSS.

On the importance of theory/praxis (in)consistency and interdisciplinary integration

Theory/praxis consistency

Why should theory/praxis (in)consistency be adopted as a criterion when we evaluate the merits of a philosophico-methodological approach? First, it deserves emphasis that an initial answer to this question is provided by many constructivists FSS authors themselves. Wibben's work, for instance, repeatedly stresses that feminist IR 'traverses the practice/theory divide' because (1) it developed out of the practical concerns of activists/campaigners, and (2) it continues to put such concerns centre-stage (2011, p. 111). To the extent that constructivist FSS theorists subscribe to the aim of contributing to feminist practices – whether implicitly or explicitly – an affirmation of the importance of theory/praxis consistency is therefore already present in their work. Indeed, it is because of this that many of the claims that are developed and defended in this chapter can be usefully read as developing an *immanent* critique of constructivist work.

Second, and more generally, theory/praxis (in)consistency is a significant criterion because – if our practical activities contradict our theoretical positions – this likely suggests either (1) that we do not actually hold the beliefs that we say we do, or (2) that our theoretical framework is inadequate or deficient in some manner. The former of these conclusions was drawn by the (African-American) writer and social critic James Baldwin, who disputed the claims of his white countrywomen and men when they asserted that they did not hold racist beliefs. Baldwin famously countered such claims by stating that 'I can't believe what you say […] because I see what you do' (1998 [1966], p. 738). Distinguishing between 'bloodied hands and honeyed tongues' (Khalili 2012, p. 5) in this manner remains an invaluable analytical and political strategy. This chapter's comments on the theory/praxis inconsistencies that suffuse constructivist FSS, however, should be interpreted solely as claiming that the philosophical and methodological positions which its proponents adopt are unequal to the task of grounding FSS as a theoretico-practical project. Indeed, more specifically, these comments should be read as making a case for the (critical) realist claim that – whether we like it or not – 'reality has a habit of biting back' (Norrie 2010, p. 109).

Interdisciplinary integration

Why should an (in)ability to ground integrative, interdisciplinary research be taken into account when we evaluate the merits of a philosophico-methodological approach? There are arguably many valid reasons to do so. First, and most important in the current context, is the fact that narrow forms of *intra*-disciplinarity and (non-integrative/additive) *multi*-disciplinarity have remained the norm in the study of security issues.[3] As a result, *Security Studies* is characterised both by ceaseless accusations of disciplinary reductionism/parochialism/imperialism and a chronic fragmentation of knowledge.[4] This is deeply regrettable, especially for those who – like constructivist FSS authors – aim to clear the way for practical interventions that would help to prevent or alleviate the suffering which results from situations of insecurity. Second, this situation also makes for a sharp contrast with the value that the broader institutional and intellectual context has continued to place on integrative research. As various authors have shown (e.g. Aldrich 2014; Bhaskar et al. 2018; Holland 2013), the ideal of interdisciplinarity has not only persisted in circumstances that are otherwise characterised by endless disciplinary fissures, it has in fact flourished. The *World Health Organization* and *European Commission*, for instance, actively encourage/fund interdisciplinary research (Bhaskar et al. 2018, p. 9), and countless universities have created new centres/institutes or re-organised existing departments into broader schools to attract this funding/promote collaboration. Similarly, recent decades have witnessed the rapid rise of an agenda, of which FSS itself is a manifestation, that advocates the creation of various interdisciplinary areas of study. These range from 'women's, gender, queer and feminist studies' to 'post-colonial and race studies' and – as authors like Rosi Braidotti have highlighted – provide a significant challenge to 'the traditional organization of the university in departmental structures' (2013, pp. 148, 144).

In line with Dominic Holland's position this chapter will argue that such developments 'reflect an explicit recognition – although far from [a] complete understanding – of [both] the interconnected nature of reality' and 'the need to develop forms of knowledge that express this characteristic' (2013, p. ix). Before doing so, however, it will proceed by sketching the main philosophical and methodological tenets of constructivist FSS. While this chapter is plainly not the place to discuss these tenets at any significant length, a number of especially salient constructivist positions are worth briefly examining here to provide context for the second half of this chapter.

On mainstream *Security Studies* and its feminist 'other'

Feminist Security Studies: a sketch of the constructivist consensus

If we are to make reliable sense of the philosophico-methodological orientation that constructivist FSS authors adopt, it must be situated in the broader context from which it emerged. This context includes, most prominently, the hegemonic status that neo-positivism enjoyed in the decades preceding the fourth 'Great Debate'. Constructivist FSS authors have explicitly distanced themselves from this mainstream hegemony by attempting to 'disturb the foundational narratives of IR as well of modernity and modern science' (Wibben 2011, p. 27). As such, they have expressed considerable scepticism about or hostility towards the foundationalism of modernist (philosophy of) science. Caron E. Gentry, for example, states that the 'ontological starting point' of constructivism is 'anti- or non-foundationalist' (2016, p. 24), while Wibben suggests that constructivists should reject the idea of fixed foundations in favour of temporary resting points (or 'hermeneutic anchors') that should be perpetually left open to negotiation/contestation (2011, p. 36).

It is not just the foundationalism of modernist (philosophy of) science, however, to which constructivist FSS authors generally object. Rather, they express scepticism about or hostility towards a wide range of its purported features.

First, constructivist FSS authors commonly understand modernist (philosophy of) science as privileging certain kinds of texts/discourses/narratives and actors over others. They argue, for instance, that mainstream/neo-positivist work systematically excludes the varied roles/voices/experiences/interests/viewpoints/etc. of women from consideration by speaking about combatants, insurgents, etc. almost exclusively in gender-neutral terms. More specifically, they claim that the positivist fixation on science and neutrality has meant that its war stories have – in practice – almost exclusively been about (powerful) men (e.g. Parashar 2016, p. 43; Wibben 2011). As such, mainstream/neo-positivist work is charged with universalising their roles/voices/experiences/interests/viewpoints/etc. to the detriment of a sex-/gender-differentiated account of both personhood and (in)security. Second, constructivist FSS authors frequently accuse mainstream/neo-positivist philosophy of encouraging a disregard for emancipation (e.g. Basini 2016, pp. 177–178; Parashar 2016, pp. 42–43). Its emphasis on separating facts/nature from values/normativity, for instance, is routinely highlighted as a key reason that constructivist IR has continued to be 'sidelined as a political rather than a scientific project' (Wibben 2011, p. 11). Similarly, the positivist emphasis on developing nomothetic generalisations/identifying natural, causal laws is frequently argued to have traditionalist implications. Describing contemporary gender relations as natural, for instance, seems to exempt them from requiring an explanation (ibid., 34), while characterising them as the result of nomothetic processes appears to suggest that they are immutable.

Third, constructivist FSS authors frequently understand modernist (philosophy of) science – as well as some earlier feminist writings on violence/insecurity[5] – of resulting in biological reductionism/determinism or gender essentialism. In fact, their work makes a forceful intervention into the broader feminist debate about essentialism and/in the natural sciences. Wibben claims that this is 'the most fundamental and far-reaching debate among feminists' (2010, p. 88) and suggests that it is rooted in the question of whether 'women and men have underlying, universal essences – a uniquely female or male nature – that is more fundamental than any variations among them' (2010, p. 88; see also Bueno-Hansen 2016, p. 188). She adds, furthermore, that '[f]eminists whose work presupposes such an essence often argue that it is rooted in biology – for them, gender difference follows sex difference' (2010, p. 88). In contrast, such claims – often alluded to in the context of FSS debates by pointing to Francis Fukuyama's (in)famous claim that '[w]hat is bred in the bone cannot be altered easily by changes in culture and ideology' (1998, p. 27) – are comprehensively rejected by contemporary feminist approaches. In so doing, however, these approaches adopt contrasting analytical orientations; while some justify their opposition to gender essentialism primarily by means of *biological/scientific* claims, for instance, others have – instead – prioritised the use of *philosophical*, *normative/political* and/or *empirical* claims and evidence.

In this regard, constructivist FSS work commonly employs empirical evidence to reinforce its philosophical and normative/political claims. In particular, it employs this empirical evidence to highlight that the sheer variety which characterises the behaviour of women and men during situations of insecurity undermines (neo-) positivist claims about the (quasi-)nomothetic processes/causal laws that purportedly govern this behaviour (e.g. Al-Ali and Pratt 2016; Alison 2003; Bayard de Volo 1998; Butalia 2001; Cockburn 2001; Conway 2008; Dietrich Ortega 2012; Ehrenreich 1999; Elshtain 1987; Gentry and Sjoberg 2007; Ibáñez 2001; Ling 2000; Mulinari 1998; Neugebauer 1998; Parashar 2016; Scheper-Hughes 1998; Sharoni 2001). While constructivist authors generally acknowledge that some generalisations appear to stand up to empirical scrutiny relatively well they have therefore concluded that – on the whole – there is very little evidence to suggest that differences between women and men (in terms of their proclivity to engage in violent acts) are biologically determined.[6] Indeed, explanations that invoke the biological makeup of human beings are increasingly received with scepticism or hostility because – it is claimed – these result in stereotyping, de-agentialising, and/ or binaristic narratives.

More generally, constructivist FSS authors tend to steer clear of arguments about gender essentialism that take science as a point of reference. This is the case because, from the philosophical perspective they favour, such arguments – *whether they favour or oppose essentialism* – inevitably succumb to the masculinist or androcentric logic that characterises this practice. Such ideas are rooted in the claim that – if we are to reveal its various biases and 'hidden agendas' (Wibben 2011, p. 37) – science should be read 'as a text' (or discourse). These become discernible, in particular, when the binary oppositions that mainstream work employs are examined. As Gentry explains, feminists 'often look at how binaries [...] operate, in an effort to deconstruct them' (2016, p. 19). This is imperative, she claims, because 'one element is prioritized and valued over the other element' in a binary opposition, and western societies have prioritised 'masculine rationality over feminine irrationality', 'logic over illogic (hysteria)', 'stoic passivity over emotions' and 'resoluteness over flightiness' (ibid.; see also Richter-Montpetit 2016, p. 96; Marhia 2013, pp. 26–27). When constructivists apply this deconstructionist approach to science it commonly leads them to conclude that the rationality, objectivity, universality, neutrality, rigour, etc. which are conventionally associated with this practice are manifestations of a masculinist, androcentric, or anti-feminist logic (e.g. Tickner 2005, especially pp. 2174–2177). Indeed, it leads them to conceive of science as a text or discourse that is rooted in 'the ideas of white males', whose experiences are 'taken as the ideal to be imposed on all others' (Wibben 2011, p. 18).

Similarly, this deconstructionist framework provides constructivist FSS authors with a basis for their claims about the contrast between *feminist* and *scientific* methods. These claims concern a wide range of issues.[7] The most important of these for this chapter, however, is the fact that constructivists frequently maintain that feminist methods enjoin researchers to engage with the *contextual* (or 'relative') nature of lived experience, meaning, and truth (e.g. Cohn 2013; Moser and Clark 2001; Sharoni 2001; Wibben 2011, 2016); or, in other words, they have claimed that their idiographic focus provides a corrective against the (neo-)positivist focus on developing objective, (quasi-) nomothetic generalisations/identifying causal laws. Wibben, for instance, suggests that decontextualisation 'is central to [scientific] approaches striving for objectivity by presenting only what is seen or perceived – without comment or interpretation' (2011, p. 19). In fact, she approvingly quotes Nancy J. Hirschmann's claim that '[c]ontext is what makes meaning possible' and 'meaning makes reality' (ibid., p. 27). Such claims are frequently accompanied by radical efforts to counter decontextualised, a-social/under-socialised, liberal understandings of human beings. As Natasha Marhia argues, liberal humanism portrays human beings as 'stable, bounded subject[s]' and 'autonomous, rational chooser[s]' (2013, p. 26). In contrast, constructivist authors claim that this portrayal (1) has been 'extrapolated from the highly individualistic competitive behavior of Western men in the marketplace' (Tickner 2005, p. 2177), (2) obscures 'the matrices of power through which individuals become socially differentiated' (Marhia 2013, p. 19), and (3) fails to account for how these differentiations 'can function in exclusionary ways' (ibid., p. 22). Hence, liberal humanism is understood as a framework that is unable to account for the fact that an individual's security is 'to a large extent a function of their social situatedness, their location in a web of interpersonal and social relationships [...] and intersecting fields of discourse' (ibid.).

In summary, constructivists FSS authors conceive of modernist (philosophy of) science as a text or discourse that is complicit in the reproduction of gendered prejudices, biases, and injustices. As a result, they have become increasingly sceptical of the idea that 'we can locate anything morally and politically worth redeeming or reforming in the scientific world view, its underlying epistemology, or the practices it legitimates' (Harding in Wibben 2011, p. 18). Importantly, this stance departs from humanist critiques of science, as it rejects their claim that 'the natural and human sciences are fundamentally different' (ibid., p. 32). Wibben's narrative approach, for instance, suggests that one of the main errors of humanism is the fact that it tries to 'redefine rather than dissolve Enlightenment dualisms' (ibid.). Instead, constructivists propose what we might term an anti-dualistic *universalisation of hermeneutics* that 'takes the text (or discourse) as its unit of analysis' (Norris in Gentry 2016, p. 25). In contrast with the scientific emphasis on *facts* and their *verification* and/or *falsification* this approach endeavours to examine the *political effects* of 'adopting one mode of representation over another' (Milliken in ibid.). This aim is, of course, characteristic of significant parts of the broader constructivist literature as well. Indeed, constructivist FSS – in its disavowals of mainstream/scientific methods, dualistic thought, essentialism, foundationalism, modernist/liberal humanism, etc. – has self-evidently mirrored the philosophico-methodological orientation that is now generally associated with the cultural turn.

Theory/practice inconsistencies: constructivist FSS as a compromise formation

This section will argue that the 'thick' textualism which constructivist FSS authors favour results in what critical realists – echoing Freud – refer to as a *compromise formation*. This concept refers to situations in which 'a falsity in theory [is] held in tension with a truth in practice' (Bhaskar in Hartwig 2009, p. xxx) and – as a result – it encompasses a concern with theory/praxis inconsistencies.

The first – and most fundamental – of these inconsistencies results from the abovementioned claim that there is nothing in the scientific worldview that is worth redeeming or reforming. Specifically, it concerns the contradictions that result when constructivist authors' *theoretical* understanding of science is contrasted with their *practical* activities. Like virtually everyone in the (post-) modern world, after all, the lives of these authors are utterly dependent on and completely intertwined with scientific knowledge that has accumulated over the centuries. When they engage in field research, for instance, constructivists are likely to be dependent on the propulsion systems of aircraft, the internal-combustion engines of motor vehicles, and the radio frequencies that link mobile/cell phones. Further to this, it is also worth drawing attention to the fact that the feminist cause to which constructivist FSS authors subscribe has, of course, consistently sought to ensure that women have access to safe, effective, and affordable healthcare, especially sexual and reproductive services. To the extent that these authors subscribe to such initiatives, however, their concurrent commitment to the idea that (medical) science is inherently and unavoidably masculinist, androcentric, or anti-feminist is suffused with theory/praxis inconsistencies; in fact, because their work both *rejects* and *presupposes* a scientific worldview *at the same time* it provides FSS with an incoherent amalgam or 'ensemble' (Bhaskar et al. 2018, p. 59) of competing philosophical and methodological positions.

The same applies to other aspects of the constructivist consensus as well. In particular, it applies to its abovementioned universalisation of hermeneutics. This stance is reminiscent of Ludwig Wittgenstein's claim that truth is an immanent feature of particular 'language games' or 'forms of life' (2009 [1953]) and effectively scuppers metaphysical considerations. The work of constructivist FSS authors has, likely for this reason, stopped short of affirming the reality of non- or extra-discursive 'stuff'. While these authors may well consider this to be among its merits, it deserves emphasis that, as a result, the threat of theory/praxis inconsistencies again looms large.

This is the case because many of these authors have – in practice – continued to base their claims on scientific research. As most constructivists FSS authors have subscribed to the idea that security should be conceived of in broad terms, for instance, they have commonly understood climate change as contributing to insecurity (e.g. Tickner and Sjoberg 2010, p. 203). To the extent that they have accepted scientific evidence about climate change, however, this contradicts their reduction of science to a masculinist, androcentric, or anti-feminist text. Indeed, their concurrent commitment to a negative *theoretical* view and a positive *practical* view of science results in further theory/praxis inconsistencies. These are epitomised by a claim in the work of Nicole Detraz, who – in a critique of state-centric approaches to environmental security – suggests that, '[r]ather than assume that the presence of threats is [an] objective fact, a feminist environmental security discourse' should understand these 'as rooted in perception' (2017, p. 207). Our understanding of climate change has arguably improved, however, exactly because scientists have *transcended* perception; that is to say, we now have greater knowledge of this phenomenon because scientists have developed better accounts of the broader natural world as it is, independent of our opinions, wishes, discursive constructions, etc. In fact, climate change provides us with both a pertinent illustration and a dark omen of the fact that reality has a habit of biting back. Detraz's claims, instead, *presuppose* and *contradict* a scientific worldview *at the same time*. We may infer, therefore, that the analytical framework which she urges us to adopt represses our awareness of this in favour of a compromise formation that – because it encourages us to analyse *perceptions* of climate change rather than its *reality* – is acutely anthropocentric in nature. What is repressed, however, inevitably resurfaces ('bites back') as a theory/praxis inconsistency.[8]

To the extent that constructivist FSS authors subscribe to the idea that climate change is both *real* and a *real problem*, however, an additional issue arises as well. Indeed, more generally, this issue permeates any type of theory that seeks to change the world. Any such theory will require, of course, a robust account of agency. As constructivists seek to radically counter modernist/liberal understandings of human beings, however, they are likely to encounter significant difficulties in sustaining such an account. Specifically, they are likely to encounter exactly the same difficulties that post-structuralists in the broader feminist and gender studies literatures have already experienced. As Sue Clegg notes, '[t]he relationship between post-structuralism and feminism has always been complex' and '[t]ensions over the problem of agency and the grounds of political activism have surfaced at many points' (2006, p. 312). This is the case, she suggests, because post-structuralism contains 'an ontological claim for the primacy of the discursive' (ibid., p. 314). As contemporary feminists have commonly drawn on the works of Michel Foucault and Jacques Derrida, for instance, agency 'is always having to be shoehorned [...] into theories whose impetus and genealogy are profoundly anti-humanist' (ibid., p. 315).[9] The 'death of the subject' (Heartfield 2002) that post-structuralism conjures therefore 'sits uneasily with feminism as an emancipatory project' (Clegg 2006, p. 313). In fact, the theoretical resources that are required to ground a robust account of agency – and hence (in)justice – are simply lacking from this approach. Throughout the broader feminist movement, however, the need for such an account has been clearly recognised. As Clegg stresses, '[t]he emancipatory impulse of feminism, and all radical projects, depends on recognising the possibility that [...] we can do something to change the conditions which continue to generate profound injustices and inequalities' (ibid., p. 323).

While constructivist FSS authors therefore lament the de-agentialising effects of science, the theoretical orientation on which their work commonly draws does not provide us with the resources that are required to overcome this problem. In fact, more forcibly, post-structuralist theory actively *impedes* the development of such resources. An alternative framework is therefore urgently required, and the second half of this chapter will contend that such a framework is provided by critical realist philosophy. This is of importance, however, for reasons that exceed the *normative* aims of feminism; in particular, these include the fact that a robust account of agency is required for its *analytical* purposes as well. This point has repeatedly been made by constructivist FSS authors (e.g. Gentry and Sjoberg 2007, 2015; Moser and Clark 2001) but it has, so far, remained without an explicit philosophical basis. As a result, the FSS literature has exhibited all the 'symptoms' of a compromise formation, especially its tendency to result in persistent theory/praxis inconsistencies. In turn, the prevalence of such inconsistencies illustrates that the philosophical and methodological beliefs that proponents of constructivism hold are inadequate for the purpose of grounding FSS as a theoretico-practical project.

Interdisciplinary integration: constructivist FSS and the fragmentation of knowledge

Why is constructivism ill-suited to grounding interdisciplinary research? To provide an answer to this question it will be necessary to begin this section by providing an outline of the main differences between interdisciplinarity and (1) *intra-disciplinarity*, (2) *disciplinary reductionism*, (3) *multi-disciplinarity*,[10] and (4) *anti-disciplinarity*.[11] These categories have, after all, been used in competing/incompatible ways throughout a wide range of disparate intellectual and institutional contexts. As space is limited, this section will not attempt to reconcile or adjudicate between these uses; rather, it will simply define or understand the above categories to mean the following:

Intra-disciplinarity: research which takes place within a single discipline, studies the subjects/answers the questions/addresses the kinds of problems that are characteristic of this discipline, and uses the tools/methods/modes of analysis that are familiar to or prevalent within it.

Disciplinary reductionism: a philosophical (primarily ontological) position that claims that the subject matter of one discipline is ultimately reducible to the subject matter of another discipline (e.g. psychological entities/processes are nothing but biological entities/processes, biological entities/processes are nothing but chemical entities/processes, etc.).

Multi-disciplinarity: a philosophical and methodological position that claims that interaction and communication between researchers with contrasting disciplinary backgrounds should be promoted to study a subject/answer a question/address a problem. While numerous areas of study are thus provided with 'a seat at the table' by multi-disciplinarity, it remains largely additive, differentiated, and non-integrative in nature because of its focus on multiplicity/heterogeneity.

Anti-disciplinarity: a philosophical and methodological position that claims that researchers should transcend all disciplinary distinctions to study a subject/answer a question/address a problem. Research is understood as a unified endeavour and disciplinary boundaries are argued to be mere conventions or artificial/unwarranted/arbitrary/damaging impositions. In contrast with multi-disciplinarity, anti-disciplinarity is therefore undifferentiated and holistic.

How does *interdisciplinarity* differ from or relate to these categories? It is useful to begin the process of answering this question by highlighting that a number of them can be organised along a continuum, ranging from completely fragmented on the one hand, to fully holistic on the other. In particular, a systematic commitment to *intra-disciplinarity* would result in complete fragmentation, whereas *multi-disciplinarity* allows for interaction and communication between different types of researchers, and *anti-disciplinarity* eliminates disciplinary distinctions and boundaries altogether. From the critical realist perspective that is advanced throughout this chapter, interdisciplinarity should be understood as a philosophico-methodological position that occupies a space along this continuum that is located *in-between* multi-disciplinarity and anti-disciplinarity; more specifically, it occupies a space that does not deny the need for and uses of disciplinary differentiation/specialisation and – simultaneously – allows for the (re)integration of differentiated/specialised knowledge claims. It is because interdisciplinarity is *necessarily* integrative, then, that it amounts to *more* than multi-disciplinary interaction and communication among researchers, and it is because it *necessarily* accepts (or even welcomes) the need for and uses of disciplinary differentiation/specialisation that it amounts to *less* than anti-disciplinarity.

In contrast, interdisciplinarity differs from/relates to disciplinary reductionism in a *contingent* fashion. While it does not deny the need for and uses of disciplinary differentiation/specialisation, after all, it does not follow from this that it also provides *a priori* support for (or fetishises) the existence of every and any kind of discipline. Rather, whether or not the existence of a discipline is warranted is a question that – from a critical realist perspective – can only be answered in an *a posteriori* fashion because it is dependent on the provision of a robust rationale. When such a rationale cannot be provided, therefore, interdisciplinarity is compatible with the specific reduction in question. Contrariwise, it is incompatible with a generalised commitment to such reductions as this produces a deflationary spiral that results in anti-disciplinarity.

If some light has been shed both on the concept of interdisciplinarity itself and the ways in which it differs from and relates to contrasting/competing notions, however, we are now in a position to return to the question that was posed at the start of this section; that is to say, we can now ask why it is that constructivist FSS is ill-suited to grounding interdisciplinary research? As discussed above, my answer to this question will focus on (1) the one-dimensional, textualist focus on discourse/meaning that this approach has adopted, (2) its inability to sustain an account of agency, (3) its anthropocentrism, and (4) its unidirectional understanding of causality.

With regard to the first of these issues, the 'thick' constructivist stance that many prominent FSS authors have adopted has resulted in seemingly all-encompassing forms of textualist monism that are fundamentally incompatible with interdisciplinary research; if the study of being is ultimately reducible to the study of texts/discourses, after all, both disciplinary distinctions themselves and the idea that interdisciplinary (re)integration is required are lacking in any kind of ontological warrant. In fact, from a consistent monist perspective, FSS should be a fully anti-disciplinary endeavour. As Holland has noted (in a different context), if it is true that reality/being is *undifferentiated* 'it is unclear why science should be *differentiated* and why scientific integration is desirable' (2013, p. 47, emphasis mine). In terms of its inability to ground interdisciplinary research, however, this *textualist* monism is not altogether dissimilar to the *physicalist* monism that is favoured by some positivist authors. The proponents of physicalism have argued, after all, that a fully developed form of science would be able to reduce all phenomena – whether these are conventionally described as 'biological', 'psychological', 'social', or whatever – to one set of basic *causal laws* (grounding a unified 'theory of everything') and *entities* (generally understood as 'fundamental' or 'elementary' particles). Such claims are incompatible with interdisciplinarity because, if it is true that all forms of being are ultimately reducible to a set of basic laws and entities, disciplinary distinctions appear – once again – to lack any ontological justification. Indeed, to the extent that positivism is physicalist, the internal logic of this one-dimensional approach suggests – absurdly – that biologists, psychologists, sociologists, etc. should simply retrain as physicists. An analogous criticism applies, however, to the constructivist focus on discourse/meaning; rather than retraining as physicists, this approach suggests – equally absurdly – that researchers of various kinds should retrain as (critical) discourse analysts.

In light of such criticisms, it deserves emphasis that some constructivist authors have countered that their work (1) does *not* involve a textualist monism at all, and (2) does *not* deny the reality of non-/extra-discursive forms of being either. These claims – along with their limitations – can be helpfully illustrated by sketching the outlines of an on-going debate within both FSS itself and the broader feminist and gender-studies literatures.

On one side of this debate are proponents of the view that biology matters in ways that are irreducible to its sociocultural construction. This perspective depends on the second wave feminist distinction between sex and gender, as well as on its attendant notion of sex/gender systems. On the other side are proponents of third wave feminism who have either expressed significant scepticism about or wholly rejected the idea that sex has a reality which is irreducible in this manner.[12] The FSS literature – including its influential constructivist wing – is characterised by significant equivocation about this issue.[13] Nonetheless, third wave feminist thought has clearly made its presence felt. Christine Sylvester (2002), for instance, systematically refers to 'people called women' rather than simply 'women', while Melanie Richter-Montpetit maintains that feminists should transcend 'analytics such as male/female, victim/perpetrator, war/peace, national/international, and power/resistance' (2016, p. 96). Importantly, analyses such as these do not deny the reality and material existence of bodies as such; however, they have resulted in a pronounced tendency to conceive of sex not as a *cause* but as an *effect*. As Lena Gunnarsson notes in a critique of Judith Butler's work, 'it is in the regulatory norms of sex that all causality and structure is located, whereas the bodily and material are understood mainly as effects' (2014, p. 27; see also Hull 2006, pp. 57–63).[14] While this not-wholeheartedly-textualist version of constructivism therefore does not – strictly-speaking – adopt a monist ontological position, its one-dimensional emphasis on socialisation/enculturation does result in a unidirectional understanding of causality. Such an understanding is, however, incompatible with interdisciplinary research as well; to the extent that interdisciplinarity involves both disciplinary differentiation/specialisation *and* the (re)integration of differentiated/specialised knowledge claims into multidirectional explanations, after all, even this toned-down version of constructivism remains at odds with it.

This is of significant importance as FSS is in clear need of integrated, interdisciplinary accounts of the events/phenomena that it studies. Its accounts of SGBV, for instance, are both incoherent and unintelligible without the ability to draw on knowledge claims from a range of disciplines, especially biology, psychology, and the sociocultural sciences. What, for instance, is rape without (1) human corporeality (as understood by biologists), (2) agency/intentionality/trauma/etc. (as understood by psychologists), *and* (3) the breaking of societal rules/norms by coercively transforming sociocultural relationships (as understood by sociocultural scientists)? All three of these disciplines – or rather, the causal powers/mechanisms that they study – must arguably be integrated if we are to provide well-rounded accounts of this phenomenon. Such accounts are ruled out, however, if FSS authors adopt a constructivist approach, as (1) references to corporeality become inadmissible when, instead of referring to women and men, we are asked to refer to 'people called women [and men]' (Sylvester

2002), and (2) references to agency must be shoehorned into accounts that are otherwise anti-humanist in orientation.

The adoption of a constructivist approach therefore has very significant – and adverse – consequences. These become especially apparent when we consider its inability to sustain an account of agency. There are few phenomena that are of concern to FSS, after all, that would remain intelligible without it having resort to the distinction between behaviour and *intentional* behaviour. The targeting of women as part of 'ethnic cleansing' (e.g. Nikolic-Ristanovic 1998), for instance, is unintelligible without this, and – troublingly – claims about both the injustice that is done to the survivors or victims and the moral responsibility of the perpetrators collapse. Moreover, the consequences of eliminating human corporeality from our analyses are clearly discernible in the work of FSS authors like Christine Sylvester and Laura J. Shepherd. The former asserts, for instance, that 'men and women are [just] the stories that have been told about "men" and "women"' (1994, 4), while the latter quotes Sharon Marcus' claim that 'rape is a question of language, interpretation and subjectivity' (2007, p. 248). Importantly, such accounts *should* play a significant role in interdisciplinary research on this topic. However, an approach that focuses solely on language and interpretation is also radically impoverished; not only does this focus provide us with a very narrow understanding of the sociocultural realm (as composed exclusively of language and its subjective interpretation) and seem to suggest that survivors could just choose to reinterpret or re-describe what happened to them, after all, it also elides human corporeality.

Overall, then, it might be concluded that constructivism tends towards a unidirectional understanding of causality. It therefore provides the FSS subfield with an 'over-socialised' analytical framework. In so doing, however, its philosophico-methodological logic is – once again – not all that different from the logic of (neo-)positivism. Specifically, the (quasi-)nomothetic understanding of causality that (neo-)positivists adopt, like the constructivist emphasis on socialisation/enculturation, tends towards unidirectionality. If we conceive of causality in terms of the universal laws that govern empirical events, after all, the act of granting something causal power suggests that it will straightforwardly determine outcomes. If genetic factors are conceived of as causal in bringing about SGBV, for instance, (neo-)positivism results in (or at least facilitates) an essentialist or biological determinist account of these factors as being its sole determinants.

Further to this, the one-dimensional understanding of being/reality that constructivist FSS authors adopt puts them at risk of further theory/praxis inconsistencies. While some of these authors have expressed scepticism about or wholly rejected the idea of biological sex at a theoretical level, for instance, they have arguably remained firmly committed to its reality in practice. Without such a commitment it seems impossible, in fact, to sustain their abovementioned claim that mainstream *Security Studies* has systematically excluded the roles/voices/experiences/interests/viewpoints/etc. of women from consideration. If this is the case, after all, even constructivists must have found some way of differentiating male from female bodies. Moreover, even the most radical FSS constructivists have commonly continued to make SGBV a key focal point in their work. It seems impossible for them to do justice to this phenomenon, however, from a perspective that denies that sex is irreducible to its sociocultural construction; for instance, it seems impossible for the proponents of such a perspective to account for the rape-based impregnations that have been perpetrated against women during periods of genocidal violence (e.g. Nikolic-Ristanovic 1998). Likewise, it seems counter-productive in the extreme to adopt a third wave feminist perspective to examine the pro-natalist policies that certain governments have adopted during times of war (e.g. Bayard de Volo 1998). Such scenarios cannot but remain unintelligible if we fail to provide philosophical space for the biological reality that (1) it is only bodies with clusters of female characteristics than can be impregnated, and (2) it is only bodies with clusters of male characteristics than can impregnate them.[15] When explicit denials of the overwhelming pervasiveness of sexual dimorphism[16] are combined with the study of issues that implicitly presuppose its reality, therefore, this results in theory/praxis inconsistencies. Indeed, this provides us with yet further illustrations of the fact that reality has a habit of biting back.

As a result, it seems clear that any satisfactory approach to grounding interdisciplinary FSS research must take this 'habit' into account; specifically, it must *reintegrate* the non-/extra-discursive features of reality that constructivism *represses* in a way that allows it to avoid theory/praxis inconsistencies. More generally, such an approach must provide a viable alternative to its one-dimensional focus on discourse/meaning and overcome (1) its inability to sustain an account of agency, (2) its anthropocentrism, and (3) its unidirectional understanding of causality. The second part of this chapter will argue that these goals can be achieved by drawing on critical realist philosophy. In particular, it will claim that this approach allows us to rethink and reclaim ontology in a way that provides interdisciplinarity – along with the broader 'studies' agenda – with a robust philosophical basis and rationale. Rather than *abandoning* or *inverting/overturning* positivism and constructivism, furthermore, it will argue that critical realism is *preservative* in nature.

On critical realism and interdisciplinarity

Situating critical realist philosophy

To provide a defence and elaboration of the abovementioned claims it is essential to begin by situating critical realist philosophy – as an internally differentiated and continuously developing approach – with reference to the foundationalism/anti-foundationalism and positivism/post-positivism debates. With regard to the second of these debates, it has adopted an explicitly post-positivist stance. It has done so, however, to rethink and reclaim the notion of science, and not – as constructivist FSS authors have done – to discard or dissolve it. With regard to the first debate, critical realist philosophy has adopted an alternative to both extremes; while it denies that there are indubitable or unassailable foundations from which absolutely secure knowledge can be developed, it also rejects the absolutist claim that this means that we cannot develop robust forms of knowledge at all. Instead, critical realism favours what this chapter will refer to as a *post-foundationalist* approach, which relies especially on the use of immanent critiques.

Indeed, with regard to (neo-)positivist philosophy of science, Roy Bhaskar – the initiator of critical realist philosophy – developed a specific type of immanent critique that he termed an Achilles' heel critique. This kind of critique seizes on 'the most important premise for a particular position' and aims to show that 'all the beautiful insights that are hoped to be sustained by it cannot in fact be sustained' (Bhaskar in Bhaskar and Hartwig 2010, p. 79). Throughout *A Realist Theory of Science* (2008 [1975]) Bhaskar applied this strategy to the archetypal activity of 'hard' science – experimentation – to show that the area in which (neo-)positivists presume they are strong, they are actually weak. While the relevance of doing so may not be immediately apparent to those readers who are primarily interested in critical realism, constructivism, and their respective ability to ground interdisciplinary FSS research, this issue will be the focus of the next section.[17] The final section of this chapter will then show that both the *power-/mechanism-based understanding of causality* and the notion of *ontological depth* which result from Bhaskar's critique of (neo-)positivism function as philosophical building-blocks for interdisciplinary (FSS) research.

Bhaskar's critique of positivism (and its implications for constructivism)

Bhaskar's work begins by posing a deceptively simple question: Why are the practical interventions into the natural world that experimentation involves required at all? The strict form of empiricism that has historically grounded positivism demands, after all, that knowledge is based exclusively on sensory experience. This foundationalist epistemological approach is therefore incompatible with situations in which experimental interventions are required. If these are the necessary feature of science that they appear to be, however, it follows that the nature of the world is not always accessible to us by means of sensory experience. Indeed, the consistent *need* for experimentation illustrates that the most emblematic practice of science is incompatible with positivist empiricism. In practice, Bhaskar argues, experimentation aims to develop forms of knowledge that (1) go beyond sensory experience (trans-phenomenal knowledge), and (2) may contradict sensory experience (counter-phenomenal knowledge). It is this, in fact, which makes science necessary, as 'without the contradiction between appearance and reality, science would be redundant, and we could [simply] go by appearances' (Collier 1994, p. 47). As this does not appear to be the case, however, positivist empiricism fails to provide us with an epistemological framework that is suitable for engaging in scientific research.

More generally, Bhaskar highlights that this one-dimensional, empiricist framework is suspect because it presupposes that what exists, or what can be legitimately spoken of/known, is exhausted by what human beings are capable of experiencing.

This is problematic because (1) it is an inherently anthropocentric presupposition, and (2) it means that positivism, despite its attempted monopolisation of the term 'science', cannot sustain the intelligibility of experimentation. To the extent that positivists value theory/praxis consistency, therefore, they are forced into a choice between the adoption of *either* a philosophical approach 'which is consistent with its epistemology but of no use to science' *or* a philosophical approach 'which is relevant to science but more or less inconsistent with its epistemology' (Bhaskar 2011 [1989], p. 57). As their lives – like the lives of constructivists – are dependent on and intertwined with scientific knowledge that has accumulated over the centuries, however, the latter option appears the more plausible. Indeed, in the (post-)modern context that contemporary proponents of positivism inhabit, choosing this option is the only way to avoid the theory/praxis inconsistencies that result from a compromise formation.

Further inconsistencies arise, however, when we expand the range of Bhaskar's analysis to include the issue of causality. As discussed, (neo-)positivists understand this phenomenon in (quasi-)nomothetic terms. Constructivists, in contrast, overturn this understanding, primarily by (1) questioning the immutability/naturalisation that it seems to suggest, and (2) adopting an idiographic/contextual approach. It is likely for such reasons that Caron E. Gentry and Laura J. Sjoberg, two prominent FSS authors, distinguish between causal, constitutive, and symbolic activities/analyses (2007, p. 218). Critical realism, instead, provides an alternative to these positions; an alternative, that is, which suggests that causality/science and context are not antithetical.

To shed light on this position we must return to Bhaskar's analysis, as this analysis suggests that an alternative, anti-anthropocentric, *depth ontology* is required for experimentation to remain an intelligible activity. The first thing to note in this regard is that the persistent need to develop and employ measuring equipment illustrates that those events which occur are not necessarily accessible to human sensory organs. It is therefore vital – in terms of the ontological stance we adopt – to distinguish between the *empirical* realm (which concerns sensory experience) and the realm of the *actual* (which concerns the broader category of events as such). Second, the nature of experimentation also suggests that scientific interventions can trigger (activate, stimulate, release, enable, etc.) causal powers/mechanisms that would have otherwise remained dormant or inactive. This is – again – of significant importance for the ontological stance we adopt, as such powers/mechanisms may therefore be described as *real*, irrespective of whether they are also triggered (actual) or experienceable/experienced (empirical). When this twofold argument is systematised, it results in Bhaskar's model of ontological depth, which is reproduced in Figure 1. This model is, of course, fundamentally at odds with the anthropocentrism and one-dimensionality of positivist empiricism, and it replaces its (implicit) ontology of *empirical events* with an (explicit) ontology of '*structurata*' (Wight 2006, p. 218). These may be conceptualised, quite simply, as the various types of 'stuff' that exist, and as possessing different sorts of *real* causal powers; powers, that is, which – when and where they are triggered – produce *actual* and *empirical* events.

	Real	Actual	Empirical
Powers/Mechanisms	✓		
Events	✓	✓	
Experiences	✓	✓	✓

Figure 1 Ontological depth (Bhaskar 2008 [1975], p. 56).[18]

It is not just at this abstract level, however, that Bhaskar's anti-anthropocentric depth ontology is of importance. Rather, it also allows us to *rethink* and *reclaim* causality/causal analysis in a way that breaks free from *both* the nomothetic/(neo-)positivist *and* the idiographic/constructivist approaches. To grasp why this is the case we must consider another seemingly simple question that Bhaskar poses: Why is experimentation required at all? He answers as follows: 'an experiment is necessary precisely to the extent that the pattern of events forthcoming under experimental conditions would not be forthcoming without it' (Bhaskar 2008, p. 33). If this is the case, however, three initial conclusions follow. First, it follows – against what (neo-)positivists claim – that scientific activities like experimentation are *not* in fact concerned with the identification of causal laws. Rather, the primary – and hence by no means sole – purpose of experimental activities is to shield or isolate the actualised causal powers of structurata from counteracting and distorting forces to produce patterns of events that would not otherwise be forthcoming. Second, it follows that *work* is commonly required to produce the regular patterns of events which (neo-) positivists aim to identify. This is the case, of course, because scientists would not need to design experiments that aim to produce such patterns if every causal relation was already spontaneously characterised by regularity. Third, if it is true that producing regular sequences of events commonly requires work on the part of scientists, it follows that that such sequences are not just *insufficient* for the purpose of identifying a causal relationship – as neo-positivists have long acknowledged, and as is clearly evidenced by the prevalence of spurious correlations – but that they are also *unnecessary*. After all, while strict *regularities* may break down outside of experimental settings where scientists are not actively engaged in producing them, *causality itself* does not. Instead, the practical work involved in setting up experiments presupposes, at a theoretical level, that causal processes *may* but *do not have to be* characterised by regularities. In fact, the persistent *need* to engage in experimentation – that is to say, the key role that this practice plays in scientific research – suggests that *strict regularities are likely to be rare in non-experimental settings.*

Building on this, both the labour-intensive nature of experimentation and the fact that regularities are an insufficient/unnecessary feature of causal processes point to the need of making two crucial distinctions. First, we must distinguish between *the existence and exercise of real causal powers*, on the one hand, and *their actual and empirical effects*, on the other. As Bhaskar notes, causal powers may 'be possessed unexercised, exercised unrealized, and realized unperceived (or undetected)' (Bhaskar 2008 [1975], p. 175). Second, we must also distinguish between *closed systems* and *open systems*. A closed system requires both intrinsic conditions (e.g. a stable structuratum with a real and actualised causal power) and extrinsic conditions (a stable external environment) for its realisation. Importantly, it is only when these two conditions are met – whether through self-conscious experimental design or mere happenstance – that empirical event (A) will *always* follow empirical event (B). In contrast, an open system describes any situation in which the intrinsic and/or extrinsic conditions for closure are *not* met. While causal processes in open systems may bring about rough-and-ready, partial 'demi-regularities' (Lawson 1997, p. 204) they are not characterised by *strict* regularities. In fact, the work involved in setting up an experiment is most commonly concerned exactly with eliminating – or any case attempting to reduce – the counteracting and distorting effects that would otherwise result from operating in an open systemic setting. If this is correct, however, we may add to the above-mentioned claim that regularities break down outside of *experimental settings* the more general claim that this is just what happens outside of *closed systems*. Nonetheless, the specific case of experimentation to which Bhaskar's work draws attention is illustrative of a wider dilemma for (neo-)positivist authors. In particular, this dilemma is that – if these authors value theory/praxis consistency – they are forced into another choice; they can *either* remain committed to nomotheticism but abandon the idea that experimentation is a scientific practice *or* remain committed to experimentation but abandon nomotheticisim. For reasons that were alluded to above, choosing the latter option appears, once again, to be the only plausible way for (neo-)positivists to avoid theory/praxis inconsistencies.

It deserves emphasis, however, Bhaskar's analysis has significant implications for idiographic/constructivist claims as well. First among these is the fact that it undermines the distinction which Gentry and Sjoberg make between causal, constitutive, and symbolic activities/analyses (2007, p. 218). What these authors have understood as existing 'outside' of causality/causal analysis can be *reclaimed* for it, after all, once we *rethink* this phenomenon from a critical realist perspective. This is the case, in short, because the powers/mechanisms that we study no longer need to produce regular sequences of empirical events for them to be included in this category. Second, because Bhaskar's analysis shows that (real) powers/mechanisms that are triggered in open systems do not produce invariant patterns of (actual/empirical) events, it also allows us to *rethink* the constructivist/idiographic claim that science is inherently and necessarily decontextualising. Even if scientists establish the operation of a universal (set of) mechanism(s) in an open system, after all, their accounts must of necessity engage with the particular spatiotemporal context in which it/they were triggered if they are to determine what are its/their effect(s).

These critical realist claims are very obviously at odds with both the scepticism or hostility towards science which characterises the constructivist consensus and the understanding of causality/causal explanation that (neo-)positivists favour.

Despite this, they sustain both the constructivist concern with contextuality and the (neo-)positivist concern with causality/causal analysis/science. As such, rather than simply *abandoning*, *overturning*, or *inverting* these approaches, a critical realist understanding of causality/causal explanation *preserves* their strengths in a distinctive (and arguably more coherent) philosophical framework. In so doing it makes an important contribution to reclaiming and rethinking ontology from an anti- or post-anthropocentric perspective.

How, though, does critical realist philosophy provide interdisciplinarity with a basis and rationale? The final section of this chapter will provide an answer to this question. In doing this it will build on the *depth ontology* and the *power-/mechanism-based understanding of causality* that were developed above by connecting them with the *emergentist/stratified account of being* that critical realism proposes. Specifically, this section will argue – first – that when these features of critical realist philosophy are brought together this provides FSS with a clear basis and rationale for (1) *disciplinary specialisation* (to understand the differentiation of reality), and (2) *interdisciplinary integration* (to make sense of its interconnection) (Holland 2013). Second, it will argue that it is only when these features are combined that is possible to avoid *both* the problems that constructivist FSS authors have identified with 'under-socialised/a-social' biological determinist or gender essentialist positions *and* the problems that were identified above with 'over-socialised' constructivist positions. Indeed, put positively, it is only in this way that it is possible to *preserve* the strengths of approaches that stress biology at the expense of socialisation/enculturation, and vice versa. Finally, this section will also contend that, when this preservative orientation is adopted, it provides feminism/FSS with a philosophical basis that (1) is able to sustain a coherent account of agency, (2) grounds both its analytical and normative aims, (3) replaces the *implicit* and *unidirectional* approach to causality/causal analysis which results from constructivism with an *explicit* and *multi-directional* approach, (4) replaces the *anthropocentric, one-dimensional ontology* of constructivist work with an *anti-* or *post-anthropocentric, multi-dimensional ontology*, and (5) avoids the theory/praxis inconsistencies which plague constructivist FSS.

Emergence, ontological stratification, and interdisciplinarity

How does critical realist philosophy ground a preservative approach? Its proponents have answered this question by drawing attention to the phenomenon of *emergence*. What, then, is emergence? This question is arguably harder to answer than it has ever been, as the term emergence has accrued various layers of (often contrasting/competing) meaning throughout its lengthy history. While disentangling these different layers and evaluating their merits is therefore a matter of some importance and urgency, regrettably this task cannot be undertaken here. Rather, this section will proceed – rather unceremoniously – by simply stating its definition, without seeking to differentiate it from other such definitions or arguing for its superiority. In short, then, emergence here refers to any situation in which:

(1) some causal/taxonomic property β is dependent for its existence on some other causal/taxonomic property α;
(2) this dependency involves forms of co-variance according to which fundamental changes in α mean fundamental changes in β (as well as vice versa), and
(3) the causal/taxonomic properties of β are irreducible to the causal/taxonomic properties of α.

A frequently used example of this phenomenon is water, as water molecules possess a number of causal/taxonomic properties that their component parts clearly do not. As opposed to the oxygen and hydrogen atoms of which it consists, for instance, water possesses the causal power to extinguish fires and the taxonomic property of liquidity. It may therefore be said to possess properties that are irreducible to those of its component parts; or, more formally, these properties may be described as emergent from the relational organisation (structuring, arranging, etc.) of hydrogen and oxygen atoms into an irreducible structuratum. The proponents of emergentism have commonly claimed, however, that the process which brings about the holistic properties of water occurs throughout the entirety of being. Reality can therefore be understood as consisting of an indeterminate[19] number of levels, all of which are characterised by irreducible causal/taxonomic properties. As these levels remain existentially dependent and build on pre-existing levels of reality for their existence, being as such may be understood – metaphorically speaking[20] – as *stratified*.

This ontology serves a wide range of purposes. The most important of these for the aims of this chapter, however, is the fact that it counters reductionist perspectives by highlighting that, even if α can *explain* the existence of β, this does not mean that β can also be *explained away*. As authors like Dave Elder-Vass have highlighted, emergentists propose a distinction between *eliminative reductions* and *explanatory* reductions (2010, p. 38). The first of these terms refers to situations in which the causal/taxonomic properties that are associated with a supposedly higher level are in fact *reducible to* – or 'nothing but' – the properties of a supposedly lower level. These properties are therefore explanatorily *redundant* and can be eliminated in favour of the properties of the supposedly lower level. This would occur, for instance, in the unlikely event that oxygen and/or hydrogen atoms were after all found to be liquids that are capable of extinguishing fires. The second term, instead, refers to situations in which higher level causal/taxonomic properties are irreducible to – or 'more than' – the properties of a lower level. The properties of this higher level are therefore explanatorily *relevant*. As oxygen is vital for the existence of fire and hydrogen is an explosive gas, for instance, the holistic properties of water molecules are clearly relevant to any account of how rainfall prevented a forest fire from burning our house to the ground.

By broadening the scope of this logic, critical realists propose an understanding of reality that is 'compositional' in nature (Elder-Vass 2005). Such an understanding conceives of being as consisting of 'real irreducible wholes which are both composed of parts that are themselves irreducible wholes, and are in turn parts of larger wholes' (Collier in Pratten 2013, p. 56). In turn, this also provides FSS (as well as feminism more generally) with the tools that it requires to avoid the weaknesses of *both* biological determinism *and* the idea that socialisation/enculturation is fully determining. While the causal/taxonomic properties to which biologists refer can be provided with philosophical space by adopting a compositional approach, after all, critical realist ontology clarifies that (1) the level of being which they study is only one among many, and (2) the powers/mechanisms that this level of being contains therefore contribute to bringing about actual/empirical events in a non-deterministic manner when they are triggered in open systems.

In addition to this, the emergentist idea that being/reality is stratified also provides an important counterpoint to Wibben's claim that feminist work which presupposes the existence of biological sex reproduces the idea that 'gender difference follows sex difference' (2010, p. 88). From a compositional, critical realist perspective this statement is problematic for two main reasons.

The first of these concerns the fact that references to biological sex need not be essentialist in the way that constructivists have generally understood this term. To make sense of this claim it is important to begin by highlighting that, while some critical realists *have* adopted the language of essences, most have chosen to refer to causal/taxonomic properties instead. This is the case because the former of these categories has – whether justifiably or not – become associated with a static, singular, and/or deterministic understanding of biology/sex and human nature, whereas the latter has remained relatively free from such associations. Making reference to properties rather than essences is therefore strategically preferable from the perspective of a philosophical approach that has actively militated against such understandings. As Andrew Sayer argues, '[i]f this is what essentialism is, it is certainly wrong, but equally certainly it is not what realism is, at least in its modern versions' (1992, p. 163; see also Sayer 1997). Second, Wibben's statement is problematic because it assumes that any approach which accepts the reality of biological sex must also understand gender relations/norms as following directly from this reality. Wibben's statement seems to imply, in other words, that – once the reality of biological sex is granted – gender relations/norms are reduced to epiphenomena. While this may well be intended as putting a final nail in the coffin of biological determinism by highlighting its unappealing analytical implications, however, Gunnarsson (2013) highlights that such claims in fact presuppose a deterministic understanding of biological properties. This is the case because arguments like Wibben's presuppose that 'if biology is admitted to be a basis of human functioning, then it must *determine* human behavior' (ibid., p. 6). This presupposition is only warranted, however, if the positivist claim that causality inheres in nomothetic processes is also warranted. Once this position is abandoned in favour of both the power-/mechanism-based approach to causality and the stratified/emergentist ontology that critical realism favours we are – instead – in a position to provide a basis for the (second wave feminist) slogan that 'biology is not destiny'.[21]

This claim is both important and true, but it has thus far remained without explicit philosophical support.

If there is no need to subscribe to the assumption that the powers/mechanisms that Fukuyama describes as 'bred in the bone' (1998, p. 27) will straightforwardly determine actual/empirical events, however, neither is there any need to succumb to (1) the broader problems that result from what Gunnarsson terms 'nature phobia' (2013, p. 4), and (2) the idea that we are guilty of adopting a dualistic or dichotomous analytical framework when we maintain the sex/gender opposition.

With regard to the first of these issues, Gunnarsson's notion refers to the idea that 'the only way to safeguard oneself against charges of biologism' within constructivist feminist circles is to subscribe to the idea 'that nature, although it might be rhetorically acknowledged, has no influence on gender and sexuality whatsoever' (ibid.). Such ideas are arguably prevalent in constructivist FSS. It seems unlikely, for instance, that a statement such as Hirschmann's – who, again, claims that 'meaning makes reality' – would be approvingly quoted by Wibben without the support of a broader nature-phobic intellectual environment (2011, p. 27). Similarly, Detraz's claim that climate change-based security threats should be understood as 'rooted in perception' (2017, p. 207) clearly resonates with the abovementioned idea that nature has no influence on gender-dynamics. The fear/anxiety in which such one-dimensional analyses are rooted is easily assuaged, however, by means of a stratified/emergentist ontology. After all, a multi-dimensional ontology of this kind – along with the power-/mechanism-based understanding of causality that informs and grounds it – provides space for any number of explanatory factors. In fact, it arguably allows us to get all the way from particles to people and politics in a philosophically coherent and non-reductionist manner.[22] From this perspective, discourse/meaning is simply one irreducible phenomenon within being as a whole; indeed, this perspective suggests that the non-/extra-discursive features of being provide the basis that is required for this phenomenon to exist or be possible. In contrast with Hirschmann's claim, then, it might be concluded – although not without a degree of embellishment and oversimplification – that it is actually reality that makes discourse/meaning.

With regard to the second issue, it is crucial that a clear contrast is drawn between terms like *binary opposition*, *dichotomy*, and *dualism* and the term *distinction*. As Gunnarsson stresses, the former terms refer 'to the kind of absolute separation which ignores any interconnection and mutual constitution between the two terms in question' (2013, p. 14). The latter, instead, suggests that two (or more) things, *whatever their similarities, forms of overlap, and interactions may be* are non-identical in some respect. When this conceptual contrast is brought to bear on the claim that any maintenance of the sex/gender opposition implicates us in dualistic forms of thought it allows us to clarify that – when such efforts are rooted in emergentism – this is not the case. After all, emergentism includes co-variance as one of its essential features, and it is therefore incompatible with ontological dualism. Rather, from an emergentist perspective, the sex/gender opposition should be understood as a distinction, thereby suggesting the existence of *both* dissimilarities *and* similarities, forms of overlap, co-variation, mutual constitution, and so on.

If critical realism does not implicate us in biological determinism, nature phobia, and ontological dualism, however, how does it ground a coherent account of agency? To provide an answer to this question we must return to the building blocks that were provided above. In particular, an effective account of agency can be easily sustained once we adopt (1) a *depth ontology* rather than a *flat (empirical or textual realist) ontology*, (2) an *emergentist/stratified ontology* rather than an *orthodox (monist or dualist) ontology*, and (3) a *power-/mechanism-based understanding of causality/causal analysis* rather than a *nomothetic* or an *idiographic understanding of causality/causal analysis*. As discussed, critical realist philosophy claims both that being has depth and that causality inheres in the *real* powers of structurata; powers, that is, which, when they are triggered, produce *actual* and/or *empirical* events. From this perspective it is therefore no longer possible to conceive of matter (or whatever can be said to be real) as the passive stuff upon which active nomothetic processes/causal laws enforce their will. Rather, this power-bearing stuff itself must now be conceived of as active, whether as already causally efficacious or – at least – as causally potent. When this perspective is brought to bear on the question of agency it suggests an understanding of this phenomenon that conceives of it – first – as the *real* power of a structuratum (typically, though not necessarily, a human being) to act in an intentional manner. Second, and building on this, the emergentist/stratified ontology that critical realism favours allows us to conceive of this distinctive power as a causally/taxonomically-irreducible feature of whole human beings, as opposed to the various parts of which they consist. As such, critical realist philosophy – in contrast with both neo-positivism and constructivism – arguably *does* provide us with the resources that are required to sustain a coherent account of agency. In so doing, importantly, it preserves both the analytical and the normative strengths of humanism for feminism/FSS.

At the same time, critical realists – like constructivists – have rejected the liberal humanist tendency to portray human beings as 'stable, bounded subject[s]' and 'autonomous, rational chooser[s]' (Marhia 2013, p. 26). This is the case, primarily, because they have argued that intentional agents must be understood as existing within an emergent sociocultural context that affects (and is internalised by) them. As above, the main argument for this position is rooted in the post-foundationalist approach that critical realism favours; specifically, it is rooted in an immanent critique of ontological individualism that adopts its claims about the centrality of intentional/agential human behaviour as its premise. As Bhaskar notes, the problem with this premise is 'how one could ever give a non-social [...] explanation of individual, at least characteristically human, behaviour' (1998 [1979], p. 30). Even the intentional/agential activities that individualists place centre-stage, after all, 'presuppose a social context for their employment' (ibid.); cashing a cheque, for instance, presupposes the existence of a banking system, while hiring and firing employees presupposes the existence of a system of property ownership and control.

Importantly, activities such as these do *depend on* the individual intentions/states of mind in which individualists root their explanations. In fact, they depend on a whole range of psychological, biological, chemical, and physical powers/mechanisms. Critical realist philosophy suggests, however, that these kinds of interactions cannot be *fully explained or accounted for* by referring exclusively to these powers/mechanisms. Whether one is a banker or an account-holder, for instance, is simply not determined by physical, chemical, or biological powers/mechanism; or, to return to the specific topic at hand, this status is not determined by one's individual intentions/state of mind. Rather, any satisfactory explanation or account of interactions such as these must also make reference to the (explanatorily relevant) positions that people occupy within them. It is only by doing so that our explanations can begin to *fully explain or account for* the fact that certain people are landlords while others are tenants, that certain people are employers while others are employees, etc. As Sayer stresses, '[y]ou cannot simply become an employed person by believing and declaring yourself to be one' (1992, pp. 32–33). Rather, one's status as an employee, tenant, account-holder, etc. depends on one's position within a sociocultural relationship. If this is the case, however, it follows that these kinds of activities are dependent on the relational organisation of parts (human beings) into a new whole (e.g. a corporation). Indeed, more generally, it follows that they are *existentially dependent on*, *causally/taxonomically-irreducible to* ('more than'), and *covariate with* the intentions/states of mind in which individualists root their explanations and accounts. In accordance with the definition of this phenomenon that was provided above, then, sociocultural structurata qualify as emergent features within being as a whole.

If this conclusion is correct, however, it means that *both* agential/intentional (human) structurata *and* sociocultural structurata are real, irreducible components of reality. In turn, this suggests that human persons are *neither* fully unitary/centred/stable/autonomous *nor* fully fragmented/decentred/unstable/dependent. FSS research that is rooted in critical realist philosophy would therefore *uphold* a basic commitment to humanism – thereby providing a basis for the analytical and normative aims of feminism – while *rejecting* its problematic (a-social/under-socialised) liberal instantiations. Furthermore, it would *uphold* the concern with socialisation/enculturation that is characteristic of anti-humanist approaches, while *rejecting* their problematic (over-socialised) reduction of human beings to the effects of texts or structures. Rather than simply *abandoning* or *inverting* the tenets of humanism and anti-humanism, therefore, critical realism again *preserves* their strengths by creating a *synthesis* of these approaches.

How, though, does this synthesis provide us with a philosophical basis and rationale for interdisciplinary FSS research? The first thing to note in this regard is that the emergentist/stratified ontology of critical realism provides FSS with such a basis and rationale for *disciplinarity*; that is to say, in contrast with the ontological monism that underpins both physicalist forms of positivism and textualist constructivism, it provides FSS with a basis and rationale for the existence of disciplines and – by extension – for disciplinary specialisation. This is the case, in short, because an emergentist/stratified ontology – as a result of its emphasis on the existence of multiple causally/taxonomically irreducible levels of being – is itself differentiated in nature. If being as such is differentiated, however, it follows that research is more likely to succeed if it is organised along differentiated lines as well. In fact, to the extent that a specific (sub-)discipline can be shown to study a range of causal/taxonomic properties that are irreducible to the range of properties of another (sub-)discipline, its existence is ontologically justified (and non-arbitrary). This range of properties is referred to by critical realists as the *domain ontology* of a (sub-)discipline and is held to consolidate it by both identifying the types of entities that are its subject and clarifying some of their more general characteristics. Crucially, the specification of such a domain ontology also helps to curtail the risk of unwarranted disciplinary reductions (Elder-Vass 2005, p. 7). If it can be established that the domain ontology of one (sub-)discipline is irreducible to the domain ontology of another by means of the kind of *a posteriori* arguments that were alluded to above, after all, it follows that a reduction is unwarranted.[23,24]

More important for the purposes of this chapter, however, is the fact that an emergentist/stratified ontology also provides a clear philosophical basis and rationale for *interdisciplinary* research. Importantly, it does this in conjunction with the distinction that critical realist philosophy makes between 'pure' and 'applied' research. The first of these terms refers to research that aims to identify/understand specific powers/mechanisms in (relative) isolation. The second, instead, refers to research that utilises ('applies') the understanding of powers/mechanisms in which such pure research results to shed light on how their interactions in open systems have brought about actual and empirical events. As these events are likely to be caused by structurata that are themselves internally stratified it is highly probable that applied researchers will have to integrate claims from different disciplines into interdisciplinary explanations. This remains, however, a contingent matter, because it is dependent on the specific event/phenomenon with which their research is concerned. When this research involves 'layered' and multiply-determined structurata like human beings in open systemic settings, however, studying and referring to varied types of powers/mechanisms that operate at different ontological levels is imperative.

Indeed, more specifically, it is essential for such research to engage with *upward*, *downward*, and *same-level* causality. This chapter has thus far focused its attention primarily on upward causality; that is to say, it has focused on 'the way in which the parts of a system [structuratum], with their properties and relationships, causally generate the emergent properties of the whole' (Mingers 2014, p. 70). However, from a critical realist perspective – in contrast with e.g. a constructivist perspective – causality should be understood as a multidirectional phenomenon. This means that it is possible for the powers of one ontological domain to both *affect* and *be affected by* the powers of other domains and the powers of the same domain to which it belongs. For instance, the broad range of powers that are currently studied by *psychology* may affect and/or be affected by other such powers (same-level causality), the powers studied by *biology* (upward causality), and the powers studied by the *sociocultural* sciences (downward causality). Importantly, it is only when we grant the reality of such multidirectional causal processes that it is possible for researchers or scientists to develop the kind of interactive, dynamic, and multi-causal models of reality which genuinely interdisciplinary research demands.

Overall, then, it might be concluded that (1) it is the differentiation of being itself that provides researchers with a justification for *disciplinary differentiation/specialisation*, and (2) it is the potential for (and likelihood of) interactions between the varied types of emergent causal powers/mechanisms that exist at different ontological strata or levels which provides researchers with a justification for *interdisciplinary research*.

This means, however, that the basis and rationale that critical realist philosophy provides for interdisciplinary research differs markedly from the one that authors like Braidotti (2013) have provided for the broader 'studies' agenda. Braidotti argues that the rise of this agenda reflects the evolution of a number of 'radical epistemologies' that offer a 'clear institutional response to the inhuman(e) structures of our times' and 'the disasters of modern and contemporary history' (ibid., p. 148). While the proponents of critical realist philosophy might agree with the idea that such institutional responses are indeed required to study the structures and disasters to which Braidotti alludes, their justification for this position would – in contrast – be rooted primarily in ontological considerations. Importantly, this is not to claim that epistemological arguments in favour of interdisciplinary research are wholly *incorrect* or that they are necessarily *incompatible* with critical realist claims about the need to ground interdisciplinarity at an ontological level. Rather, it is simply to suggest that such arguments are *insufficient* because they are unable to carry the intellectual weight that is currently placed on them. As Bhaskar et al. note, '[t]here is general agreement in the literature that contemporary approaches to interdisciplinarity are problematic' (2018, p. 9). The need for interdisciplinary research is therefore 'unlikely to be satisfied [...] as it is currently theorized' (ibid.). After all, it is only if being itself is *both* differentiated *and* interconnected that interdisciplinary research is genuinely warranted and necessary. Moreover, it is arguably only if being *does* possess this characteristic that we are in a position to explain the persistent appeal of interdisciplinarity in intellectual and institutional circumstances that are otherwise characterised by endless disciplinary fissures. From the critical realist perspective that is developed in this chapter, this continued appeal 'reflect[s] an explicit recognition – although far from [a] complete understanding – of [both] the interconnected nature of reality' and 'the need to develop forms of knowledge that express this characteristic' (Holland 2013, p. ix).

Conclusion

While FSS is by no means a completely homogenous sub-field, the proponents of constructivism – broadly defined – currently enjoy a hegemonic status within it. The rapidly *increasing* popularity of constructivism has, furthermore, correlated closely with the rapidly *decreasing* popularity of biological determinist or gender essentialist positions. Indeed, the appeal of constructivism derives to a large extent from the simple fact that it appears to provide feminist authors with a way out of these murky waters. In contrast with broader forms of contemporary feminist theorising – which are currently experiencing a *naturalistic/new materialist turn* (Gunnarsson 2013; Groff 2013, Chapter 7; van Ingen 2016b) – large numbers of prominent FSS authors have therefore remained wedded to positions that are closely aligned with the *cultural turn*. In this regard, FSS has experienced remarkably little change. As discussed, this has come at a significant price; specifically, it has resulted in the continuing dominance of a philosophico-methodological approach that is (1) anthropocentric and one-dimensional in terms of its focus on discourse/meaning, (2) unidirectional in terms of its understanding of causality, (3) incapable of sustaining an account of agency, and (4) unable to ground the interdisciplinary research that is required to account for the events/phenomena with which FSS is concerned. Remarkably, many of the same problems occur within (neo-) positivist work. Constructivist authors' efforts to distance FSS from mainstream *Security Studies* have therefore been less than successful. Indeed, their affirmation of an interdisciplinary 'studies' agenda by means of the FSS label is emphatically cancelled out by their simultaneous adoption of a constructivist philosophical framework, thereby leaving feminist researchers ill-prepared for practical, applied forms of empirical research.

In contrast, this chapter has argued that a robust basis and rationale for interdisciplinary research – along with the broader 'studies' agenda – is provided by critical realist philosophy. This philosophical approach, it has claimed, does not deny the need for and uses of disciplinary differentiation/specialisation, does not fetishise existing disciplinary boundaries, *and* allows for the (re)integration of differentiated/specialised knowledge claims into interdisciplinary outcomes. More generally, critical realism allows us to *rethink* FSS by providing it with a philosophical framework that is explicitly multi-dimensional, anti- or post-anthropocentric, and premised on a multi-directional understanding of causality. As such, it not only poses a significant challenge to the constructivist consensus but – more importantly – it provides a sophisticated alternative to it, thereby paving the way for an 'after' to the contemporary hegemony of constructivism within FSS.

In particular, this 'after' suggests that FSS authors should study the events/phenomena to which they have drawn attention by adopting a bio-psycho-sociocultural framework of analysis. As opposed to the singular emphasis on socialisation/enculturation that is characteristic of 'thick' constructivism, then, critical realist philosophy also provides space for *both* agency (by means of what we might term a critical or 'thin' humanism) *and* 'the solid kickable existence of bodies, the fleshy reality of different sorts of genitals, the pluckability of differently distributed body hair, the measurability of hormones, and so on' (New 1998, p. 362). Further to this, critical realism facilitates FSS authors tying these bio-psycho-sociocultural determinants to broader forms of (non-human/more-than-human) being, including 'physical spaces, raw materials, tools and machines, domesticated and wild animals and plants, agricultural and semi-natural ecosystems, buildings, highways and so on' (Benton and Craib 2011, p. 129). Factors such as these are, after all, 'produced, reproduced or transformed as elements in the overall metabolism of society' (ibid.).

Despite this all-encompassing orientation, the *abstract* basis and rationale that critical realist philosophy provides for interdisciplinary research is contingent; that is to say, it is dependent on the subject, question, or problem at hand. When we focus our attention on the *concrete* range of issues (e.g. SGBV) that FSS authors have investigated, however, the need to develop integrated forms of knowledge of always-already-integrated events/phenomena is unmistakable. In this particular intellectual context, it is *only* by engaging in interdisciplinary research that these authors will be able to do both analytical and normative justice to the issues they study.

As a result, the adoption of a critical realist approach to FSS makes for a significant contrast with, for instance, the adoption of Wibben's narrative approach (2011). This contrast is crystallised when Wibben quotes Michael Shapiro, who claims that we should engage in 'an interrogation of the way that form is imposed on an otherwise unruly world' (2011, p. 43). From a critical realist perspective, such statements are only partially true. Critical realist efforts to reclaim and rethink ontology suggest, after all, that being is not a *tabula rasa*; specifically, these efforts suggest that being has form *independently* of whatever form human beings may impose on it. While the kind of interrogations in which Wibben (via Shapiro) urges us to engage are certainly valuable from this philosophical perspective, critical realism therefore also urges FSS researchers to recognise that *non-human/more-than-human being* 'is not passive, [and] will not conform to whatever categories and attributions we may arbitrarily assign to it' (New 1998, p. 363). As Jane Bennett writes, we must resist the anthropocentric impulse 'to conclude the biography of an object by showing how it, like everything, is socially constituted' (2004, p. 358). Instead, it is essential that we (1) allow the non-human/more-than-human forms of being that constructivist work *represses* to *resurface*, and (2) adopt a philosophical framework which systematically *reintegrates* them.

Once again, this is not to say that 'thick' constructivist claims and insights should simply be *abandoned, discarded*, or *inverted in favour of crude (reductionist) forms of materialism.* Rather, these should be *incorporated* into a more capacious philosophical framework that also includes or encompasses what we might term a 'thin' textualist perspective. Such a framework is provided by critical realism. This approach has developed a distinctly preservative philosophical orientation that synthesises the various strengths of both constructivism and (neo-)positivism and – as a result – is very largely *both/and* rather than *either/or* in nature. Bhaskar has referred to this orientation as the 'critical realist embrace' (Bhaskar and Hartwig 2010, pp. 77–78) and – against the dogmatism that some of its critics have claimed it represents – this chapter has therefore sought to highlight the heterodox or pluralistic nature of critical realist philosophy.

It is this heterodox orientation as well that allows critical realism to reclaim and rethink science. As opposed to (neo-)positivism and constructivism – both of which fail to recognise that key scientific activities like experimentation are, in fact, incompatible with '[t]he schoolroom image of modern science' (Hollis 1994, p. 3) – it is therefore able to avoid the theory/praxis inconsistencies that result from a compromise formation. In contrast with constructivist FSS, for instance, critical realism is (1) able to incorporate scientific evidence about biological sex and climate change into its analyses without this resulting in contradictions, and (2) compatible with a commitment to the findings of medical science and the broader feminist aim of providing women (and men) with access to safe, effective, and affordable healthcare. Similarly, its depth ontology and power-/mechanism-based understanding of causality ensure that, in contrast with (neo-)positivism, it is relevant to scientific practices. Despite the fact that scarcely a dent has been made in its 'resounding unpopularity among feminist theorists' (New 1998, p. 366), critical realist philosophy therefore allows us to 'walk our talk' – or avoid 'cognitive dissonance' – in a way that constructivism and (neo-)positivism simply do not. Indeed, critical realism provides us with a much more satisfactory basis for feminist aims than do these approaches. Particularly significant in this regard is its theorisation of agency, as this provides us with an ontological basis for both the analytical and the normative aims of feminism/FSS. After all, it is only when the rational core of humanism is maintained, in however 'thin' or 'thick' a fashion, that sustaining a conception of (in)justice is possible. Moreover, it is only if agency has not gone the way of all flesh that 'we can do something to change the conditions which continue to generate profound injustices and inequalities' (Clegg 2006, p. 323). While innumerable sex-/gender-based injustices continue to lay ruin to the *actual* and *empirical* realms it is therefore of the utmost importance that critical realist philosophy provides us with an ontological basis for the idea that change is a *real* possibility.

Notes

1 The development of IR has been categorised in different ways. One popular (though by no means uncontroversial) framing is in terms of a number of 'Great Debates'. Even when this framing has been accepted, however, differences of opinion have continued to exist about their number. While some invoke three such debates, others refer to four (see e.g. Kurki and Wight 2013).
2 At the same time, feminist IR scholars have also problematised the 'common sense' assumption that, while sexual violence is certainly an unfortunate phenomenon, it is an inevitable outcome of or inextricably bound up with war (see e.g. Cohen et al. 2013).
3 For definitions of these terms please consult the section termed 'Interdisciplinary Integration: Constructivist FSS and the Fragmentation of Knowledge' below.
4 As Caroline Moser noted at the start of the third millennium:

> Despite the wealth of descriptive evidence on [sex- and gender-based] violence, theoretical analysis of its specific causes is both limited and fragmented. Analyses tend to reflect professional disciplines such as economics, biomedical sciences, criminology, epidemiology, psychology and sociology. Frequently they are compartmentalized and disarticulated with each other, and tend to perpetuate fragmented understandings of violence.
>
> (2001, pp. 30–51)

Little has changed in this regard.

5 Specifically, these earlier accounts are charged with depicting the roles of both women and men in generalising, stereotyping, de-agentialising, and dichotomising/binaristic ways. Constructivist FSS scholars regularly claim, for instance, that the writings of earlier feminists depicted men as competitive, domineering, militaristic, and/or aggressive perpetrators of (sexualised) violence who govern the public (political) realm. Women, in contrast, are argued to have been portrayed primarily as participants in anti-war movements, pacifistic 'beautiful souls' (Elshtain 1987), nurturing and life-giving mothers, and/or victims of (sexualised) violence who inhabit the private (family) realm. Contemporary research has conclusively shown that the empirical record is in fact much more complex.

6 It is widely accepted, for instance, that (1) wars are still very disproportionally fought by men, and (2) men perpetrate the vast majority of war-time sexual violence. Despite this, it is also increasingly recognised that it is generally only a small minority of men who actually participate. As Sara Ruddick writes, '[i]n all war, on any side, there are men frightened and running, fighting reluctantly and eager to get home, or even courageously resisting their orders to kill' (in Cockburn 2001, 20; see also Al-Ali and Pratt 2016; Conway 2008)

7 For example, constructivist FSS authors have increasingly criticised the fact that modern (philosophy of) science understands emotions exclusively as factors which negatively affect 'the robustness and truth' of its rational enquiries (Wibben 2011, 181). Instead, they stress the need to (re)integrate emotions into academic research and writing (see e.g. the contributions to Sylvester 2011). As Helen Basini argues, the idea that such research and writing results in claims that are 'less rigorous or important than "positivist truth" is something that [...] needs to be continually critiqued and contested' (2016, p. 181).

8 The constructivist feminist IR/FSS literature therefore mirrors a tension that is also apparent in the literature on climate change. A significant part of this literature is rooted in conceptions of the natural world that are steeped in anti-modernist and anti-scientific romanticism. At the same time, of course, this romantic rejection of modernity and science is accompanied by an embrace of scientific evidence about climate change.

9 This has resulted in some post-structuralist authors attempting to locate agency/the possibility for change *within* discourse itself. On this philosophical strategy and its limitations see e.g. Hull (2006, Chapter 4).

10 I will adopt the term multi-disciplinarity throughout this chapter. The position which this term describes has at times been referred to as cross-disciplinarity as well.

11 I will adopt the term anti-disciplinarity throughout this chapter. The position which this term describes has at times been referred to by other names – including pre- and post-disciplinarity – as well.

12 This includes, of course, its preoccupation with the prevalence and philosophical importance of intersexuality. For a critical account of post-structural claims about this phenomenon see Hull (2006, Chapter 4).

13 This equivocation is organised along a sliding scale that ranges from implicit presuppositions (see discussion in the main body) to ambivalence (e.g. Enloe 2004, p. 90) and more-or-less explicit references to the reality of biological sex and sexual dimorphism (Cockburn 2001, pp. 15, 22).

14 Furthermore, as New notes, '[f]rom a critical realist point of view, this is an instance of the epistemic fallacy' (2005, p. 66). This concept refers to the view that 'statements about being can be reduced to or analysed in terms of statements about knowledge' (Bhaskar 2008, p. 26).

15 As New (2005, ch. 3 this volume) and Gunnarsson (2011, ch. 4 this volume) suggest, categories like female/male and woman/man should, from a critical realist perspective, be understood as (good) abstractions. Importantly, this does not preclude the existence of biological diversity *within* these categories.

16 As New notes, '[s]exual difference in humans is not entirely dichotomous [...] but nearly so' (2005, p. 62). See also notes 12 and 15.

17 This section provides a summary of claims that I have defended at greater length – and with greater sophistication – elsewhere (van Ingen 2016a).

18 While Bhaskar primarily uses the terms 'mechanism' and 'generative mechanism' throughout A Realist Theory of Science (2008 [1975]) other critical realists have instead referred to 'powers'. Throughout this chapter I use both term concurrently.

19 As Danermark et al. argue, there is no 'definite, beforehand-given number of strata. Neither is there a definite answer to the question regarding how strata are organized. There is an ongoing debate regarding this' (2002, p. 65; see also New (2005)).

20 Hence, it unequivocally does *not* refer to a literal layering of β on top of α.

21 As New notes, it is clear that, in the nomothetic sense of cause,

> sexual difference does not 'cause' the institution of marriage or any particular historical form of it, nor does it 'cause' sexual regulations forbidding or permitting homosexuality. But in a critical realist sense, sexual (reproductive) difference *is* one of the mechanisms contributing to the development of such institutions and such rules. Just because it is a 'basic', lower level mechanism, its workings are compatible with many different ways of regulating reproduction and sexuality.
> (2005, 65)

22 This statement should not be interpreted to mean that emergentism necessarily relies on the existence of particles. As Tony Lawson writes:

> according to quantum field theory, or at least its seemingly more explanatory powerful interpretations, if there is anything that underpins everything else it is quantum field processes and the phenomena that appear to be particles are the resulting effects of the quantisation of field excitatory activity. The particle-like elements are in fact said to be "quanta of excitation" or "field quanta". As such they are effectively emergent forms of organisation displaying particle-like behaviour.
> (2012, 356; see also Mason 2015; Norris 2000; Pratten 2013)

23 It deserves emphasis that this remains, of course, an extremely complex and messy task. As Tuukka Kaidesoja stresses, the powers/mechanisms that are studied by different disciplines 'do not form any neat compositional or hierarchical order' (2009, 306). The powers/mechanisms that are currently studied by physics, for example, are 'greatly variable in size and organization' (ibid.). Indeed, the domain of being which this discipline studies itself contains numerous cases of emergence (Emmeche et al 1997: 91). The kind of disciplinary distinctions that are suggested throughout this chapter are therefore inevitably somewhat crude. Indeed, such divisions may well give rise to rigid accounts of disciplines which obscure that being is *both* characterised by real, emergent differences *and* 'leaky' (porous, cracked, etc.). In our attempts to organise research/science in a way that that is philosophically justified, it is therefore essential that *being itself* continues to be our point of reference. This means, first, that we should recognise that there probably do not exist clear-cut or 'hard' boundaries between different ontological strata.

As a result, it seems likely that these boundaries will continue to be subject to debate, clarification, and/or qualification. Second, it means that we should avoid conflating the labels we use when we describe some property as 'biological', 'psychological', etc. with that property itself; after all, *it is the properties of structurata which emerge and not the disciplines that study them.* Rather, disciplines should be understood as heuristic devices. Importantly, this does not mean that their existence is simply arbitrary; rather, it means that – like all the concepts we use – disciplinary distinctions should be employed reflexively. This involves committing to the idea that we may need to either abandon or refine/improve/develop them. With regard to the latter, we may wish to create both *sub-disciplines* (e.g. molecular biology, cellular biology, etc.) and *linking disciplines* (biochemistry, psychosociology, etc.). In accordance with the perspective that is advanced in the main body, however, such issues can only be decided by means of *a posteriori* evaluations that draw on the logical and empirical evidence that is available to us.

24 As such, this approach allows for the idea that some disciplinarity distinctions are indeed merely conventional or artificial/unwarranted/arbitrary/damaging impositions while avoiding an ill-advised extension of this logic to include all such distinctions. Critical realist philosophy, then, grounds a 'thin' rather than a 'thick' form of disciplinary conventionalism, and it neither fetishises nor simply eliminates/dissolves disciplinary distinctions. Rather, from this perspective, disciplinary distinctions should be understood as fallible efforts to understand and institutionalise the differentiation of being itself.

References

Al-Ali, N. and N. Pratt. 2016. "Positionalities, Intersectionalities, and Transnational Feminism in Researching Women in Post-Invasion Iraq," in A. T. R. Wibben (ed.) *Researching War: Feminist Methods, Ethics and Politics*, pp. 76–91. Abingdon, Oxon: Routledge.

Aldrich, J. H. 2014. *Interdisciplinarity: Its Role In A Discipline-Based Academy*. New York: Oxford University Press.

Alison, M. 2003. "Cogs in the Wheel? Women in the Liberation Tigers of Tamil Eelam." *Civil Wars* 6(4): 37–54.

Baldwin, J. 1998 [1966]. "A Report from Occupied Territory," in T. Morrison (ed.) *James Baldwin: Collected Essays*, pp. 728–38. Putnam: Penguin.

Basini, H. 2016. "'Doing No Harm': Methodological and Ethical Challenges of Working with Women Associated with Fighting Forces/Ex-Combatants in Liberia," in A. T. R. Wibben (ed.) *Researching War: Feminist Methods, Ethics and Politics*, pp. 163–84. Abingdon, Oxon: Routledge.

Bayard de Volo, L. 1998. "Drafting Motherhood: Maternal Imagery and Organizations in the United States and Nicaragua," in L. Lorentzen and J. Turpin (eds.) *The Women & War Reader*, pp. 240–53. New York and London: New York University Press.

Bennett, J. 2004. "The Force of Things: Steps Toward an Ecology of Matter." *Political Theory* 32(3): 347–72.

Benton, T. and I. Craib. 2011. *Philosophy of Social Science: The Philosophicl Foundations of Social Thought*, 2nd edition. Houndmills, Basingstoke and Hampshire: Palgrave Macmillan.

Bhaskar, R. 1998 [1979]. *The Possibility of Naturlism: A Philosophical Critique of the Contemporary Human Sciences*, 3rd edition. London: Routledge.

———. 2008 [1975]. *A Realist Theory of Science*. Abingdon, Oxon: Routledge.

———. 2011 [1989]. *Reclaiming Reality: A Critical Introduction to Contemporary Philosophy*. Abingdon, Oxon: Routledge.

———, B. Danermark and L. Price. 2018. *Interdisciplinarity and Wellbeing: A Critical Realist General Theory of Interdisciplinarity*. Abingdon, Oxon: Routledge.

——— and Mervyn Hartwig. 2010. *The Formation of Critical Realism: A Personal Perspective*. Abingdon, Oxon: Routledge.

Braidotti, R. 2013. *The Posthuman*. Cambridge: Polity Press.

Bueno-Hansen, P. 2016. "An Intersectional Analysis of the Peruvian Truth and Reconciliation Commission," in A. T. R. Wibben (ed.) *Researching War: Feminist Methods, Ethics and Politics*, pp. 185–202. Abingdon, Oxon: Routledge.

Butalia, U. 2001. "Women and Communal Conflict: New Challenges for the Women's Movement in India," in C. O. N. Moser and F. C. Clark (eds.) *Victims, Perpetrators or Actors? Gender, Armed Conflict and Political Violence*, pp. 99–114. London: Zed Books.

Clegg, S. 2006. "The Problem of Agency in Feminism: A Critical Realist Approach." *Gender and Education* 18(3): 309–24.

Cockburn, C. 2001. "The Gendered Dynamics of Armed Conflict and Political Violence," in C. O. N. Moser and F. C. Clark (eds.) *Victims, Perpetrators or Actors? Gender, Armed Conflict and Political Violence*, pp. 13–29. London: Zed Books.

———. 2010. "Gender Relations as Causal in Militarization and War." *International Feminist Journal of Politics* 12(2): 139–57.

Cohen, D. K., A. H. Green and E. J. Wood. 2013. "Wartime Sexual Violence: Misconceptions, Implications, and Ways Forward." 323. Washington: United States Institute of Peace.

Cohn, C. 2013. "Women and Wars: Towards a Conceptual Framework," in C. Cohn (ed.) *Women and Wars*, pp. 1–35. Cambridge: Polity Press.

Collier, A. 1994. *Critical Realism: An Introduction to Roy Bhaskar's Philosophy*. London: Verso.

Conway, D. 2008. "The Masculine State in Crisis: War Resistance in Apartheid South Africa." *Men and Masculinities* 10(4): 422–39.

Danermark, B., M. Ekstrom, L. Jakobson and J. Karlsson. 2002. *Explaining Society: An Introductin to Critical Realism in the Social Sciences*. Abingdon, Oxon: Routledge.

Detraz, N. 2017. "Gender and Environmental (In)security: From Climate Conflict to Ecosystem Instability," in S. MacGregor (ed.) *Routledge Handbook of Gender and Environment*, pp. 202–15. Abingdon, Oxon: Routledge.

Dietrich Ortega, L. M. 2012. "Looking Beyond Violent Militarized Masculinities: Guerilla Gender Regimes in Latin America." *International Feminist Journal of Politics* 14(4): 489–507.

Ehrenreich, B. 1999. "Men Hate War Too." *Foreign Affairs* 78(1): 118–22.

Elder-Vass, D. 2005. "Emergence and the Realist Account of Cause." *Journal of Critical Realism* 4(2): 315–38.

———. 2010. *The Causal Power of Social Structures: Emergence, Structure, and Agency*. Cambridge: Cambridge University Press.

Elshtain, J. B. 1987. *Women and War*. New York: Basic Books.

Emmeche, C., S. Køppe and F. Stjernfelt. 1997. "Explaining Emergence: Towards an Ontology of Levels." *Journal for General Philosophy of Science* 28: 83–119.

Enloe, C. 1988. *Does Khaki Become You? The Militarization of Women's Lives*. London: Pandora Press.

———. 2000. *Maneuvers: The International Politics of Militarizing Women's Lives*. Berkeley: University of California Press.

———. 2004. *The Curious Feminist: Searching for Women in a New Age of Empire*. London: University of California Press.

Fukuyama, F. 1998. "Women and the Evolution of World Politics." *Foreign Affairs* 77(5): 24–40.

Gentry, C. E. 2016. "Chechen Political Violence as Desperation: What Feminist Discourse Analysis Reveals," in A. T. R. Wibben (ed.) *Researching War: Feminist Methods, Ethics and Politics*, pp. 19–37. Abingdon, Oxon: Routledge.

———. and L. Sjoberg. 2007. *Mothers, Monsters, Whores: Women's Violence in Global Politics*. London and New York: Zed Books.

———. L. Sjoberg 2015. *Beyond Mothers, Monsters, Whores: Thinking about Women's Violence in Global Politics*. London: Zed Books.

Groff, R. 2013. *Ontology Revisited*. Abingdon, Oxon: Routledge.

Gunnarsson, L. 2011. "A Defence of the Category 'Women'." *Feminist Theory* 12(1): 23–37.

———. 2013. "The Naturalistic Turn in Feminist Theory: A Marxist-Realist Contribution." *Feminist Theory* 14(3): 3–19.

———. 2014. *The Contradictions of Love: Towards a Feminist Realist Ontology of Sociosexuality*. Abingdon, Oxon: Routledge.

Hansen, L. 2001. "Gender, Nation, Rape: Bosnia and the Construction of Security." *International Feminist Journal of Politics* 3(1): 55–75.

Hartwig, M. 2009. "Introduction," in R. Bhaskar *Scientific Realism and Human Emancipation*, pp. x–xxxiii. Abingdon, Oxon: Routledge.

Heartfield, J. 2002. *The Death of the Subject Explained*. Sheffield: Sheffield Hallam University Press.

Holland, D. 2013. *Integrating Knowledge Through Interdisciplinary Research: Problems of Theory and Practice*. Abingdon, Oxon: Routledge.

Hollis, M. 1994. *The Philosophy of Social Science: An Introduction*. Cambridge: Cambridge University Press.

Hull, C. 2006. *The Ontology of Sex: A Critical Inquiry into the Deconstruction and Reconstruction of Categories*. Abingdon, Oxon: Routledge.

Ibáñez, A. C. 2001. "El Salvador: War and Untold Stories – Women Guerillas," in C. O. N. Moser and F. C. Clark (eds.) *Victims, Perpetrators or Actors? Gender, Armed Conflict and Political Violence*, pp. 117–30. London: Zed Books.

Kaidesoja, T. 2009. "Bhaskar and Bunge on Social Emergence." *Journal for the Theory of Social Behaviour* 39(3): 300–22.

Khalili, L. 2012. *Time in the Shadows: Confinement in Counterinsurgencies*. Stanford: Stanford California Press.

Kirby, P. 2012. "How Is Rape a Weapon of War? Feminist International Relations, Modes of Critical Explanation and the Study of Wartime Sexual Violence." *European Journal of International Relations* 19(4): 797–821.

Kurki, M and C. Wight. 2013. "International Relations and Social Science," in T. Dunne, M. Kurki, and S. Smith (eds.) *International Relations Theory: Discipline and Diversity*, 3rd edition, pp. 14–35. Oxford: Oxford University Press.

Lawson, T. 1997. *Economics & Reality*. London: Routledge.

———. 2012. "Ontology and the Study of Social Reality: Emergence, Organisation, Community, Power, Social Relatons, Corporations, Artefacts and Money." *Cambridge Journal of Economics* 36(2): 345–85.

Leatherman, J. L. 2011. *Sexual Violence and Armed Conflict*. Cambridge: Polity Press.

Ling, L. H. M. 2000. "Hypermasculinity on the Rise, Again: A Response to Fukuyama on Women and World Politics." *International Feminist Journal of Politics* 2(2): 278–86.
Marhia, N. 2013. "Some Humans are More Human than Others: Troubling the 'Human' in Human Security from a Critical Feminist Perspective." *Security Dialogue* 44(1): 19–35.
Mason, P. S. 2015. "Does Quantum Theory Redefine Realism? The Neo-Copenhagen View." *Journal of Critical Realism* 14(2): 137–63.
Mingers, J. 2014. *Systems Thinking, Critical Realism and Philosophy: A Confluence of Ideas*. London: Routledge.
Moser, C. O. N. 2001. "The Gendered Continuum of Violence and Conflict," in C. O. N. Moser and F. C. Clark (eds.) *Victims, Perpetrators or Actors? Gender, Armed Conflict and Political Violence*, pp. 13–29. London: Zed Books.
———. and F. C. Clark. 2001. "Introduction," in C. O. N. Moser and F. C. Clark (eds.) *Victims, Perpetrators or Actors? Gender, Armed Conflict and Political Violence*, pp. 3–12. London: Zed Books.
Mulinari, D. 1998. "Broken Dreams in Nicaragua," in L. Lorentzen and J. Turpin (eds.) *The Women & War Reader*, pp. 157–63. New York and London: New York University Press.
Neugebauer, M. E. 1998. "Domestic Activism and Nationalist Struggle," in L. Lorentzen and J. Turpin (eds.) *The Women & War Reader*, pp. 177–83. New York and London: New York University Press.
New, C. 1998. "Realism, Deconstruction and the Feminist Standpoint." *Journal for the Theory of Social Behaviour* 28(4): 349–72.
———. 2005. "Sex and Gender: A Critical Realist Approach." *New Formations* 56: 54–70.
Nikolic-Ristanovic, V. 1998. "War, Nationalism, and Mothers in the Former Yugoslavia," in L. Lorentzen and J. Turpin (eds.) *The Women & War Reader*, pp. 234–9. New York and London: New York University Press.
Norrie, A. 2010. *Dialectic and Difference: Dialectical Critical Realism and the Grounds of Justice*. Abingdon, Oxon: Routledge.
Norris, C. 2000. *Quantum Theory and the Flight from Realism: Philosophical Responses to Quantum Mechanics*. London: Routledge.
Parashar, S. 2016. "Women and the Matrix of Violence: A Study of the Maoist Insurgence in India," in A. T. R. Wibben (ed.) *Researching War: feminist Methods, Ethics and Politics*, pp. 38–56. Abingdon, Oxon: Routledge.
Peterson, V. S. (ed.) 1992. *Gendered States: Feminist (Re)visions of International Relations Theory*. Boulder: Lynne Rienner Publishers.
Pratten, S. 2013. "Critical Realism and the Process Account of Emergence." *Journal for the Theory of Social Behaviour* 43(3): 251–79.
Richter-Montpetit, M. 2016. "Militarized Masculinities, Women Tortures, and the Limits of Gender Analysis at Abu Ghraib," in A. T. R. Wibben (ed.) *Researching War: feminist Methods, Ethics and Politics*, pp. 92–116. Abingdon, Oxon: Routledge.
Sayer, A. 1992. *Method in Social Science: A Realist Approach*, 2nd edition. Abingdon, Oxon: Routledge.
———. 1997. "Essentialism, Social Constructionism, and Beyond." *The Sociological Review* 45(3): 453–87.
Scheper-Hughes, N. 1998. "Maternal Thinking and the Politics of War," in L. Lorentzen and J. Turpin (eds.) *The Women & War Reader*, pp. 227–33. New York and London: New York University Press.

Sharoni, S. 2001. "Rethinking Women's Struggles in Israel-Palestine and the North of Ireland," in C. O. N. Moser and F. C. Clark (eds.) *Victims, Perpetrators or Actors? Gender, Armed Conflict and Political Violence*, pp. 85–98. London: Zed Books.

Shepherd, L. J. 2007. "'Victims, Perpetrators and Actors' Revisited: Exploring the Potential for a Feminist Reconceptualistion of (International) Security and (Gender) Violence." *The British Journal of Politics and International Relations* 9(2): 239–56.

Stern, M. and A. T. R. Wibben. 2015. "A Decade of Feminist Security Studies Revisited." *Security Dialogue Special Virtual Issue*: 1–6.

Sylvester, C. 1994. *Feminist Theory and International Relations in a Postmodern Era*. Cambridge: Cambridge University Press.

———. 2002. *Feminist International Relations: An Unfinished Journey*. Cambridge: University of Cambridge.

———. 2011. "The Forum: Emotion and the Feminist IR Researcher." *International Studies Review* 13: 687–708.

Tickner, J. A. 1992. *Gender in International Relations: Feminist Perspectives on Achieving Global Security*. New York: Columbia University Press.

———. 2005. "Gendering a Discipline: Some Feminist Methodological Contributions to International Relations." *Signs: Journal of Women in Culture and Society* 30(4): 2173–88.

———. and L. Sjoberg. 2010. "Feminism," in T. Dunne, M. Kurki, and S. Smith (eds.) *International Relations Theory: discipline and Diversity*, 2nd edition, pp. 196–212. Oxford: Oxford University Press.

van Ingen, M. 2016a. "Conflict Studies and Causality: Critical Realism and the Nomothetic/Idiographic Divide in the Study of Civil War." *Civil Wars* 18(4): 387–416.

———. 2016b. "Beyond the Nature/Culture Divide? The Contradictions of Rosi Braidotti's 'The Posthuman'." *Journal of Critical Realism* 15(5): 530–42.

Wibben, A. T. R. 2010. "Feminist Security Studies," in M. Dunn Cavelty and V. Mauer (eds.) *The Routledge Handbook of Security Studies*, pp. 84–94. Abingdon, Oxon: Routledge.

———. 2011. *Feminist Security Studies: A Narrative Approach*. Abingdon, Oxon: Routledge.

———. 2016. "Introduction: Feminists Study War," in A. T. R. Wibben (ed.) *Researching War: Feminist Methods, Ethics and Politics*, pp. 1–16. Abingdon, Oxon: Routledge.

Wight, C. 2006. *Agents, Structures and International Relations: Politics as Ontology*. Cambridge: Cambridge University Press.

Wittgenstein, L. 2009 [1953]. *Philosophical Investigations*, 4th edition. Chichester, West Sussex: Blackwell Publishing.

11 Integrating critical realist and feminist methodologies

Ethical and analytical dilemmas[1]

Sadie Parr

Introduction

Over the last decade, I have been engaged in conducting qualitative research examining policy responses to 'anti-social behaviour (ASB)', in particular, family and parenting-focussed 'solutions' such as Family Intervention Projects (Parr 2008, 2011). In working to develop knowledge regarding the governance of the 'problem' that has been labelled 'ASB', I have argued elsewhere (Parr 2009) that scholars would benefit from employing a critical realist approach in their research on the grounds that it may offer a more rigorous research framework that circumvents the shortcomings of 'social constructionist' approaches which have been dominant within the policy field. Alongside my belief in the potential benefits of critical realism, I have been committed to adopting what can broadly speaking be labelled as feminist research practices as guiding principles, given that the large majority of research participants have been single-parent women whose social experiences have made them vulnerable. However, I would argue that, in practice, feminist research principles and critical realism do not necessarily sit together comfortably. A particular concern for me has been marrying a desire to allow the 'voices' of women to be 'heard' and their knowledge valued, with a belief in the critical realist principle that some accounts of reality are better than others. This raises questions about how we do data analysis and, in turn, what constitutes knowledge. Tackling these kinds of questions has been challenging given that the critical realist literature has primarily been occupied with largely abstract philosophical discussions and epistemological debates (Satsangi 2013), and there has been less focus on how to actually carry out empirical research. This paper seeks to explore the practicalities of conducting empirical research underpinned by critical realist philosophy. It also examines the dilemmas I faced in trying to reconcile this methodological approach with the ethical and political research practices informed by feminist scholarship. In so doing, the paper draws primarily on research undertaken as part of my doctoral study where I worked through and attempted to resolve these issues.

I begin by outlining briefly my doctoral research. Section two then provides an overview of critical realism and the methodological implications of this philosophical position. In the following section, I provide a discussion of the ethical issues that were prominent in the data gathering process and the broadly feminist research principles I adopted to address these. The final section then focuses on the dilemma of how to balance feminist approaches which stress the central role of participants' knowledge, particularly those who are labelled and whose voices are not readily heard, with the critical realist position that it is possible and indeed desirable to adjudicate between different representations of reality. A central question is one that Edwards and Sheptycki (2009) have posed, that is, to what extent should researchers' 'expert' knowledge be valued over and above that of other actors?[2] I do not claim to have found an easy answer to this question about who claims to know and how (Gillies and Alldred 2002). Rather, this paper is intended as a reflective piece that documents how, in my own work, I have conceptualised and tried to resolve what I consider to be potential points of divergence between critical realist and feminist research. In so doing, I have tried to elaborate a position that seeks to provide explanatory accounts on which credible, authoritative pronouncements can be made which can seek to influence the direction of social policy.

The research

Intensive family support was the New Labour Government's (1997–2010) key strategy for changing the behaviour of the 'most challenging' families (Respect Task Force 2006) – those considered to be 'anti-social' and the 'neighbours from hell'. Since coming to power in the 2010 UK general election, the Liberal-Conservative Coalition government has remained committed to the continuation and expansion of such services as part of the 'troubled family' agenda. Families referred to intensive support projects on account of their behaviour are generally characterised as having multiple and inter-related welfare support needs, and project staff work intensively with them to help address what are considered to be the 'root causes' of the behaviour that has led to complaints. When first established, such projects were controversial as they sought to control the conduct of families, some of whom were expected to relinquish basic freedoms by moving into residential units and accept being subjected to the near constant scrutiny of project staff. Although there is now a general consensus within the policy community that intensive family support is 'fit for purpose' (White, Warrener, Reeves, and LaValle 2008, p. 146), critical commentators, from a diversity of perspectives, have questioned whether such interventions are really such an unqualified good thing (Featherstone 2004, 2006; Smith 2006). My doctoral research sought to critically explore the role of 'intensive family support' in the governance of ASB. Analytical attention was focused on the development and implementation of one case study intensive family support project aim at reducing ASB among families who are homeless or at risk of eviction on account of their conduct, named here as the Family Support Service (FSS). I was interested in looking at how power and control are exercised in intensive family support projects and with what purpose. I also wanted to establish to what extent intensive family support is a positive and beneficial or negative and repressive form of intervention. The thesis research was based on semi-structured, in depth, face-to-face interviews as the main research method.

Critical realism

My research was underpinned by the philosophical assumptions of critical realism. While the position was not used dogmatically, I drew on the ideas and principles associated with the critical realist work of Sayer (1992, 2000) and Danermark, Ekstrom, Jakobsen, and Karlsson (2002) as well as Layder (1989). Critical realists presuppose an ontology in which the world is seen to be differentiated and make a distinction between three domains of: 'the real', 'the actual' and 'the empirical'. The empirical is constituted only by that which is experienced by individuals; the actual is constituted by events which may or may not be experienced; while the real is constituted by those mechanisms or causal powers that generate the series of events that constitute the actual and experiences (Collier 1994; Danermark et al. 2002; Sayer 2000). This entails the view that the world has depth and that the real cannot be reduced simply to experience, including the experience of the subject. Social science informed by this philosophy is concerned with mechanisms, with understanding what gives rise to the messy outcomes at the level of direct experience in the everyday world of the empirical:

> Thus, early feminism inspired by the direct sharing of accounts of women's experiences began to theorise about the structures of women's oppression within society, and the nature of the mechanisms which operated so powerfully to produce inequality at all levels.
>
> (Clegg 2006, p. 316)

According to critical realists, all entities possess an intrinsic structure which endows it with dispositions and capacities to act, behave or 'work' in certain ways. It is the socially produced, lattice-work of relations between individuals and groups that constitutes the structure of the social world and which is understood to be the enabling conditions for human action (e.g. social rules and norms) (Matthews 2009). Structures are not 'things' with a material existence but are real in the sense that they possess causal powers: 'Their existence lies behind and affects manifest phenomena' (Matthews 2009, p. 352). That said, social structures are not thought to impact on individuals in a straightforward deterministic manner. Rather, concrete outcomes are understood to be conditioned by the uniqueness of geographical and historical context (Sayer 2000).

Rejecting crude realism, the crux of critical realism is that social phenomena, be it actions, texts and institutions, exist regardless of interpretations of them; the social world is both socially constructed and real. In critical realism, emphasis is therefore placed on the constitutive role of meaning and language (Sayer 1992). Realists agree with other philosophical positions (e.g. social constructionism) therefore that the naming of phenomena is of central importance but differ in their commitment to a belief in the material reality underlying discursive accounts of social phenomena.

For critical realists, although a social practice is concept dependent and socially constituted, the social world is not identical to the concepts on which it is dependent; we must assess the objectivity of different social constructions. Objectivity refers to how practically adequate different accounts are. Thus, despite the discourse-dependence of our knowledge, we can distinguish between successful and unsuccessful references and produce reliable knowledge that can be effective in informing and explaining (Sayer 2000). This approach brings to the fore normative issues and the need for social scientists to not only understand and explain the social world scientifically but to think about it normatively. Critical realists therefore accept 'epistemic relativism' in the sense that our beliefs are produced, transient and fallible but do not subscribe to 'judgmental relativism' which claims that all beliefs are equally valid and there are no rational grounds for preferring one to the other:

> We can (and do!) rationally judge between competing theories on the basis of their intrinsic merits as explanations of reality ... what critical realism does is to establish the basis of the possibility of this.
>
> (Lopez and Potter 2001, p. 9)

It has been argued that critical realism bears many similarities to research grounded in its foremost philosophical 'rival', namely, (weak) 'social constructionism' which also acknowledges the existence of a real world independent of 'constructions' (Fopp 2008a). Critical realism goes beyond social constructionism, however, by bringing to the fore that which is often tacit and underdeveloped within the latter (Fopp 2008b). Like social constructionism, critical realism acknowledges that social scientific knowledge is historically and culturally situated but it offers the possibility of being able to judge between competing theories on the basis of their merits as explanations about the social world (Lopez and Potter, 2001). Indeed, many academics, myself included, have not been able to avoid measuring dominant analyses of ASB against alternatives (Nixon and Parr 2006). Critical realism is driven by the central claim that it is unwise and erroneous to abandon the search for truth in social science which in turn enables authoritative claims to be made about how we might initiate change (Layder 1998).

Given critical realism's alternative and distinctive view of causation, in which context and individual agency is intrinsically involved in causal processes, the analytical importance of the former should be accorded analytical importance in understanding social phenomena (Sayer, 1992). Certain research designs, such as case study research, better lend themselves to analyses that are sensitive to contextual and causal circumstances. As such, in critical realist research less weight is placed on 'extensive' research (Danermark et al. 2002; Sayer 1992), typically associated with quantitative methods and concerned with the discovery of common properties and general patterns within a population as a whole, a concern with 'breadth' rather than 'depth'. Critical realists claim that other 'languages' are needed to understand the nature of social objects and the way they behave (Crinson 2001; Sayer 1992). Emphasis is therefore placed on 'intensive' research which emphasises causal explanation in a specific or a limited number of case studies, be it a person, organisation, cultural group, an event, process or a whole community (Sayer 2000). This more detailed and focused approach is necessary to understand the specific causal connections and dynamics associated with the phenomena under study (Matthews 2009). Qualitative methods are associated with this type of research strategy on the basis that they help to clarify complex relationships and processes that are unlikely to be captured by predetermined response categories or standardised quantitative measures.

Ethics in practice

The broad aim of my doctoral research was to investigate the role of 'intensive family support' in the governance of ASB. To do this, I undertook qualitative case study research in one location in order to enhance existing knowledge about the realisation of this particular policy agenda. Critical realist case study research is concerned with seeking (theoretically informed) explanations of social phenomena. The approach brings with it an assumption that there is an underlying truth that is amenable to explanation and that research should be concerned with identifying the social causes and effects of the object under study (in my research the FSS) (Danermark et al. 2002; Dobson 2001). In contrast to interpretivists, for critical realists, empirical case studies are not just a study of contingencies (that which is neither necessary nor impossible) but are also concerned with documenting structures and necessity in the world which are relatively enduring, may exist independently of the case study context and determine what it is that exists.

As part of my research, interviews with 26 research participants were conducted over four years. This included project staff, actors from a range of 'partner' agencies and interviews with five women who, with their children, had been referred to the FSS on account of allegations of ASB which had rendered them homeless or at risk of homelessness. In this chapter, I am concerned with the process of conducting research with the latter. The research was limited to a sample of five women as the intention was to 'track' families through the process over an 18-month period with each being interviewed on two or three occasions: 13 in-depth interviews in total were carried out with the women.

There were certain ethical considerations to consider given the sensitive nature of the research topic and the social positions that the women occupied. There is no precise definition of the 'vulnerable' but often the term is underpinned by notions of diminished autonomy and increased risk to adverse social outcomes. As such, people who are identified as being 'vulnerable' will include those who are 'impoverished, disenfranchised and/or subject to discrimination, intolerance, subordination and stigma' (Nyamathi 1998, p. 65 in Liamputtong 2006, p. 2). The women who agreed to take part in the research could be considered as facing social vulnerability. Indeed, the women suffered stigma associated with the label 'anti-social', and as a result were often alienated from the wider communities in which they lived. A number of them suffered long-term health problems, they survived on low incomes and lived in areas of deprivation and high crime. Extreme care was therefore demanded during the research in order to ensure they were not left worse off after taking part. The approach I adopted in undertaking the study drew on feminist-inspired research practices in an attempt to ensure that my research was ethically responsible.

Feminism can be conceived of as part of a broader political project concerned with power and social change for the benefit of women, yet there is no universal definition of feminism as theory or practice. I use the notion broadly here and draw on the 'moments of agreement' (Franks 2002) between feminisms to refer to research which aims to 'capture women's lived experiences in a respectful manner that legitimates women's voices as sources of knowledge' (Campbell and Wasco 2000, p. 783 in Liamputtong 2006, p. 10). This is about validating women's experiences and using their experiences as a basis for building knowledge in order to challenge oppression and effect social change in order to improve women's lives. In terms of qualitative empirical work, and while recognising that there are tensions and debates amongst feminists, feminist work generally has in common an approach that emphasises care and responsibility over outcomes (Edwards and Mathner, 2002). Feminists who have conducted qualitative research have documented the numerous ethical dilemmas that arise during the data collection process which revolve around issues of power and the quality of the relationship between the researcher and the researched. This has led to an accumulated knowledge on what constitutes 'good' research relationships based on: empathy and mutual respect; the need for a less rigid conception of 'method' that allows the researcher flexibility; and for the researcher to not be constrained by an imperative for impersonal, neutral detachment (Birch and Miller 2002). Furthermore, it is acknowledged how our subjectivity, our different personal histories and our lived experiences influence our research. As such, feminists have argued for a self-critical reflexivity in order to make transparent the process of knowledge production (Broom, Hand, and Tovey 2009; Rose 1997).

Reflecting on my own research, during interviews with the women receiving intensive family support, I was conscious of the particularly pronounced unequal power relations that framed the interview context. This was not only the power imbalance that is often inherent in the research interview as a consequence of the researcher's role in deciding what questions to ask and more or less directing the flow of the conversation, but the disconnection that was a consequence of class differences. I recognised a significant contrast between my own social location and that of the interviewees. My education and salary, and the access to social, cultural and material resources that the latter affords stood in contrast to the women I interviewed who were unemployed, living on low incomes, in deprived neighbourhoods and in poor-quality housing. Some were homeless at the time interviews were conducted and living in temporary accommodation. Despite this, I made connections with the women, tried to develop trust and minimise the effects of these signs of difference (while acknowledging the impossibility of creating a non-hierarchical situation).

I chose not to, as it would have been somewhat disingenuous (Duncombe and Jessop 2002), to feign naivety of the FSS but did acknowledge the women's expertise in an attempt to foster a more egalitarian relationship. I explained that I was there to learn from them as they had knowledge and experience that I lacked. Although power was not shared equally, this began each interview by signalling to the interviewee that she was in a position that carried some power. The interviews followed a semi-structured format to allow discussion on questions, topics and issues that were of pertinence to the research. This reflects the critical realist view that prior theoretical ideas are important in guiding the research, including the questions posed (Layder 1998). The interviews did not, however, follow a rigid format but were dynamic and adaptive and the women were offered the opportunity to expand on questions, raise new topics and, in part, determined where the interview went. Thus, if the women did not want to address a certain topic, it was not discussed and by the same token if they were particularly interested in another topic, it was discussed more than intended or even desired (Hoffmann 2007). The latter was important given that the women were allowing me access to private, sensitive and intimate knowledge about themselves and their family, and it seemed ethically just to give them the space to talk at length on matters of particular significance to them, sometimes if it was not directly pertinent to the research.

I tried to positively influence the research relationships by fostering a two-way relationship through an element of self-disclosure (Oakley 1981), where I tried to give something back to the women in return for the information they gave me. I was not concerned this would 'taint' the research. Rather, being open and engaging in a dialogue felt the only and most ethically just approach to take. This included sharing information about myself, my personal life and my opinions with participants; giving the participants the opportunity to ask questions; and engaging in small talk and humour. Despite the differences that clearly existed between myself and these women, through these strategies we sometimes managed to forge common ground. In one interview this was through our similar experiences of working as a cleaner and we exchanged stories as well as tips on cleaning. Through this we laughed together and developed a good rapport. This is not to assert that commonalities led to sameness or shared identities, indeed there were obvious differences between myself and the women. The condition of some of the women's homes in particular brought into sharp relief the privilege of my own class position. I had not before come into direct contact with such extreme poverty and was disturbed by the circumstances within which some families were surviving.

Notwithstanding this, the women and I built good research relationships. No doubt my gender and ethnicity (all the women were white British) was also an important factor which helped facilitate the research process. Although one of the women in particular was somewhat shy, less self-assured and perhaps did not possess the 'linguistic capital' that enabled her to feel at ease in the interview situation, on the whole the woman were forthcoming and I did not encounter any difficulties in arranging subsequent meetings. Some claimed to have found the interview a positive experience.

There were times during interviews when the women became agitated, upset and angry, and expressed acute feelings of sorrow, frustration, guilt, fear and hope. This brought to the fore my ethical responsibility to find ways to not only respond in an appropriate manner but manage the women's emotions and ensure their emotional well-being was not harmed in any way by the experience or that they did not feel that the interview was a painful or distressing experience. Rather than be indifferent, detached and not responsive to emotional moments for fear of getting 'too close' to the participant or endangering the validity of the response, whenever sensitive and difficult topics were raised by the women I offered comfort and responded as humanly and kindly as possible. Notwithstanding this, when very emotional and traumatic events were talked about I was careful not to probe on these sensitive subjects, offer any opinion or advice, nor try to solve the participants' problems conscious of the fact that I am not trained to engage in 'therapeutic' conversations which could potentially inflict damage upon an individual (Parr 1998). This said, I was also careful not to move on too quickly and avoid difficult stories that had great significance for the women and which they wanted to tell, even if the interview subject was moving forward in a direction that was not particularly productive for my own research purposes.

Although I tried to manage the interviewees' emotional well-being, there were times where I felt uncomfortable when I left the women once the interview had drawn to a close, particularly where the interview had elicited emotional responses. It was on these occasions when I felt that the process was akin to what Yoland Wadsworth (1984) refers to as a 'data raid', where researchers 'smash and grab': get in, get the data and get out. As such, I felt I wanted to assure the women that their participation might prove worthwhile (in the longer term) and that what they were doing could lead to greater understanding and go some way to effecting positive change with regard to legislation, policy or the behaviour of agencies, yet I was not convinced of this myself. Rather, I was acutely aware that the research may have little benefit (other than to myself through enhancing my own educational capital in terms of gaining academic publications and a PhD) and I was also pretty certain that the interviewees on the whole were not 'empowered' by the experience nor would personally benefit from the research. For all of these reasons, the research work was often emotionally draining. This raises further ethical dilemmas that there is not that space here to discuss about the notion and politics of 'participation' and even the process of doing 'rapport' building and 'fake' friendship (Duncomb and Jessop 2002; Holland 2007).

Knowledge production

When it came to analysing the data and constructing knowledge about the FSS, like other feminist researchers, it was important to me that the 'voices' of the women taking part in my research were 'heard'. This was particularly pertinent given that the policy field of ASB impacts disproportionately on already disadvantaged women. A key feature of the discourse is a demonising rhetoric about those who fail to regulate their behaviour in line with normalised standards whereby the 'problem family' are distinguished as an uncivilised minority distinct from the 'hard-working, law-abiding majority'. Consequently, although the official ASB discourse remains largely un-gendered, it is as a direct result of the way in which the 'problem' is framed that women have become legitimate targets of state intervention:

> … In the wider context of ASB policy discourses which vilify particular segments of the population it is striking that a majority of families defined as anti-social are headed by single mothers. The empirical evidence clearly illustrates how women-headed households have become the target group for disciplining technologies such as FIPs.
>
> (Nixon and Hunter 2009, p. 120)

I and my colleagues have consequently published work that has tried to give a platform for the demonised 'other', the 'neighbours from hell', to have their voices heard (Hunter, Nixon, and Parr 2010; Nixon and Parr 2006; Parr 2011). Indeed, women who have told us their stories have often resisted and contested the dominant demonising analysis apparent within official discourses. Listening to women's 'voices' and stories, and understanding their lives, 'in and on their own terms' was important therefore and has indeed been a long-standing concern amongst feminist researchers (Finch 1984; Mauthner and Doucet 1998; Oakley 1981).

Although prioritising the 'voices' of women was a key moral and political concern, operationalising this methodological principle within the actual research process and, in particular, in terms of data analysis and knowledge construction is complex, and within feminism there are tensions and debates about how best we represent women in order to make their voices heard (Gillies and Alldred 2002; Letherby 2002; Mauthner and Doucet 1998). The influence of critical realism with its emphasis on the possibility of objective knowledge made the question of whose claims to the truth count, even more pertinent.

Many feminist methodologies recognise how any effort to give research participants a 'voice' reflects not only the participant's interpretation of the phenomena under study but the researcher's interpretation as well; the contingent and situated nature of knowledge. Research is not only infused with our own identities but wider theoretical and academic debates (Mauthner and Doucet 1998). As such, it is acknowledged that research only ever tells a partial and fallible story about the lives of the people under study and that it is impossible to capture 'raw', 'pure' or 'authentic' experiences:

> We pay attention to what we think this person is trying to tell us within the context of this relationship, this research setting, and a particular location in the social world.
>
> (Mauthner and Doucet 1998, p. 21)

This endeavour encompasses a willingness to recognise and document our involvement in the process of research in order to legitimate particular representations. This is an argument for objectivity in that our work, if not value-free, is 'value-explicit' (Letherby 2003b). Yet notwithstanding this, for many feminists the goal is to give respondents the authority to define themselves and their position (Letherby 2002). They attempt to hear more of respondents' voices and understand more of their perspectives to ensure they are appropriately represented (Mauthner and Doucet, 1998).

Bringing together the desire to give women a voice, with the acknowledgement of the impossibility of full representation, together with the assertion that our work can produce a valid account on which to effect change is a challenge (Layder 1989). Satsangi (2013) suggests that since the mid-1980s and despite their differences, feminist approaches have tended to have either an explicit or implicit endorsement of methodological assumptions characteristic of the broadly interpretivist realm. These approaches share a number of general ontological assumptions including the belief that there is no one objective reality, nor fundamental truth, but multiple realities that are locally and culturally specific (contingent and non-generalisable) and can be altered by the knower (Denzin and Lincoln 2000). Some, such as those inspired by recent developments in grounded theory seek to reduce the voice of the researcher as much as possible and their role in representing women in order to maximise the authority of the participants. This means 'representing as faithfully as possible the words and experiences of the study participants' (Allen 2011, p. 36). In doing so, however, it could be argued that researchers fall foul of the shortcomings of empiricism; they continue to prioritise experience as the foundation for knowledge and appear to aspire to value neutrality. In post-modern or post-structuralist feminism, epistemic privilege is rejected and, with it, objective truth as well, emphasising instead the contingency and instability of the social identity of respondents, and consequently of their representations. This latter position has been criticised, however, as paralysing practical efforts at effecting social and political change (Gilles and Allderd 2002). Put simply, if one version of events is no more adequate than another, this, by implication, means that there can be no advances in knowledge, a particular problem for normative and policy-orientated research. These philosophical debates were pertinent to me as I sought both to represent my respondents and tell their stories, yet I also placed an emphasis on providing explanations and the possibility of adjudicating between accounts. The remainder of this section reflects on how I tried to reconcile these priorities through the lens of critical realism.

Like feminist researchers, critical realists accept that the study of social phenomena requires a 'double hermeneutics' which involves interpreting others' interpretations (Danermark et al. 2002).[3] However, critical realism goes a step further. For critical realists, although concepts and meanings are necessary for an actors' explanation of their situation, they are likely to not only be flawed but may misrepresent certain aspects of what happens (Sayer 2000). Indeed, social actors may be unable to explain objectively and to account fully for their actions, for instance, when social actors are constrained and bound by social structures, and the conceptual tools and discursive resources available to them in their culture which provide them with ways of interpreting their circumstances (Sayer 1992; Skeggs 1997). Moreover, while people are always knowledgeable about their conduct, and, in turn, respondents' knowledge enables the researchers' knowledge claims, they can never carry total awareness of the entire set of potential consequences of their action (Pawson and Tilley 1997). As such, research participants' experience, or the things they say may not provide reliable grounds for knowledge claims about relationships and structures. Furthermore, it is argued that social reality is not just composed of individuals' meanings; individual reasoning or intention is only one mechanism within a wider process of causes, for example, social positions, norms and rules (Danermark et al. 2002; Layder 1998). However, information regarding these is not always obtainable directly from individual experience or indeed research interviews. Thus, it is not enough to collect and repeat the interpretations and explanations that people themselves have of various phenomena – there would arguably be no need for social science if explanations were self-explanatory. For critical realists, it is necessary for the researcher to look beyond the data to gain a broader understanding. Moreover, it is researchers' access to information (theoretical and experiential or data) that respondents are unlikely to have, which allows them to adjudicate between accounts and provide fuller and more adequate explanations:

> I have access to more narratives of experience and more interpretative tools than my respondents and I have also been 'given' more time to think and particularly to theorise about these issues than many of the people I spoke and wrote to. My presentation is filtered through my understandings, but at the same time I have made a self-conscious attempt to understand my respondents' understandings in their own terms.
>
> (Letherby 2002, p. 53)

In trying to resolve a tension between critical realism and the commitment to valuing women's stories and wanting their voices to be heard, in my analysis, I began with the experiences of women. I tried to represent the voices of my respondents and I valued their analysis: I listened to their self-conceptions and the meanings they attached to the FSS intervention in their lives. However, I selected extracts from the interview transcripts that, for me, were most salient for the purposes of answering my research questions. In so doing, some respondents had more to 'say' than others and so they appeared more often in my subsequent findings. Moreover, I did not always necessarily accept their accounts as straightforward 'evidence' but sought to reconstitute the women's experiences through sociological conceptualisation and theorising (Parr 2011). This means that I have taken the accounts of my interviewees and analysed them according to my political, personal and intellectual perspective (Letherby 2002, 2003a; Skeggs 1997). In turn, I had the final say in deciding what participants' experiences revealed and my research findings represented my, not my respondents, interpretations.[4] 'My' interpretation is one that has emerged out of an engagement with the collective knowledge of a community of experts (Edwards and Sheptycki 2009). This approach combines an emphasis on prior theoretical ideas and models that feed into and guide research while at the same time attending to the generation of theory from the ongoing analysis of data (Layder 1998).

I chose not to involve respondents in interpreting, verifying or (re)writing the findings of my research. This decision stands in contrast to feminists who have discussed ways of including participants throughout the research process and many feminist researchers argue for the active participation of women in research in order to remove the notion of ownership of knowledge. This is not because I considered the respondents to be a subordinated mass who require 'de-programming' and 'bringing to truth' (Clarke 2004), nor do I believe that I have produced something that respondents would not recognise at all. My research, I hope will ensure a version of their experiences, views and concerns are heard. Rather, my position was driven in part by an anti-relativism which suggests that as researchers, with access to more narratives of experience, theoretical explanations and interpretive tools, while not being intellectual superior, we may be intellectually privileged and this enables a critique of accounts (Letherby 2002, 2003a). Furthermore, I was concerned that their participation would be undertaken on 'stigmatising terms': that is, the acceptance by participants of a disempowered identity or social location. The women may have been reluctant, for instance, to see their social location as vulnerable (in the way I have described them) or subject to punitive sanction (as some commentators have defined intensive family support). Their participation could potentially have further disempowered them and could have had a detrimental impact on the relationship between the families and the FSS (Taylor 2005). That said, despite the difficulties associated with explaining theoretical interpretations, providing explanations which linked the women to structures not of their making may have helped counter feelings of inadequacy as Skeggs (1997) found in her study of how women experience class. Furthermore, discussion of findings does enable participants to contradict, confirm or challenge leading to reassessment, abandonment and reassertion. In *Formations of Class and Gender*, Skeggs (1997) listened to what working class women said about their own lives, but ultimately rejected how they interpreted their activities and their rejection of class. Instead, she retained and reasserted her own interpretation insisting on 'the centrality of class', even though this is something which they consciously tried to disclaim (ibid., p. 94). My conclusions do therefore represent a fragmented representation of my respondents' lives and may indeed stand in opposition to their accounts or may be viewed as inaccurate. I retained power and control in the research process; in the end, I am the one that spoke for my participants (Mauthner and Doucet 1998).

The process I have presented here with regard to the way in which my empirical research was conducted, written about and presented, will be familiar to many qualitative researchers working from a variety of perspectives. This methodology is not therefore distinctly critical realist: the majority of qualitative researchers use similar techniques of data collection and take as their starting point experiences. Yet, they conceive of the information obtained in different ways. What critical realism does is bring to the fore that which is often tacit and underdeveloped within other approaches (Fopp 2008b). There is, for instance, a clear overlap between critical realism and other philosophical positions that draw on (weak or 'soft' versions of) post-structuralism as the latter often contains an implicit realist ontology (Matthews 2009; Sayer 1997; Wai-Chung Yeung 1997). Likewise, there are some implicit if not overt realist themes of argument made by some standpoint feminists (Satsangi 2013). What critical realism does is put issues of validity, reliability and truthfulness in the foreground and provides a firm and coherent philosophical foundation on which to make methodological choices and establish truth claims. I would agree with Edwards and Hughes (2009) and argue that social science is better cultivated through a direct engagement with, rather than circumvention of, the 'burdens of sociological realism' (Rose and Miller 1992).

Conclusion

This chapter has examined the practicalities of conducting empirical research that is both underpinned by a critical realist philosophical position and the ethical research practices and political concerns associated with feminist scholarship. There are many complex philosophical and methodological dilemmas that the marrying of these two approaches raises and I do not suggest to have addressed all of these within this chapter. However, this chapter is an attempt to reflect on how, as a feminist researcher, I conceptualised and resolved the methodological issues raised by adopting a critical realist position in my own research. Particular emphasis was placed on how to balance approaches which stress the central role of participants' knowledge particularly those 'labelled' and whose voices are not readily heard with the 'expert' knowledge of the researcher.

With regard to the production of knowledge, I acknowledged that judgements about reality are always situated in and relative to the context within which they are produced, and maintained that research should be respectful of respondents' experiences and understandings. However, in line with the underpinning tenets of critical realism, I also maintained a position that does not dispute the existence of a material reality but assumes the existence of the real and, with that, truth (Letherby 2003a). As such I did not automatically accept women's accounts as straightforward 'evidence' but 'reconstituted' their experiences through sociological conceptualisation and theorising. I believe this approach is necessary if research is to make authoritative claims, have normative and social policy implications, and not be concerned solely with issues of accurate representation rather than reality itself. My research is therefore a social scientific truth-claim but one that is fallible and, like the viewpoints of my respondents, open to public scrutiny, criticism and corroboration.

Notes

1 This chapter was originally published as: Sadie Parr (2015) "Integrating critical realist and feminist methodologies: ethical and analytical dilemmas." *International Journal of Social Research Methodology*, 18(2): 193–207, DOI: 10.1080/13645579.2013.868572. © Taylor & Francis Ltd, http://www.tandfonline.com. Reprinted by permission of the publisher.
2 In the field of disability studies, Danieli and Woodhams (2007) raise a similar concern when they ask whether the aim of emancipatory research should be to provide 'accurate accounts' that honour the views of disabled people as valid or to produce research which supports the social model of disability but which may reflect the researchers views rather than those of the researched.
3 This is also recognised in work associated with post-modernism, post-structuralism within hermeneutic and interpretive traditions.
4 A discussion of my findings is published elsewhere (Parr, 2011).

References

Allen, M. 2011. "Violence and voice: Using a feminist constructivist grounded theory to explore women's resistance to abuse." *Qualitative Research*, 11, 23–45.

Birch, M. and T. Miller. 2002. "Encouraging participation: Ethics and responsibilities," in N. Mauthner, M. Birch, J. Jessop, and T. Miller (eds.) *Ethics in qualitative research*, pp. 123–145. London: Sage.

Broom, A., K. Hand and P. Tovey. 2009. "The role of gender, environment and individual biography in shaping qualitative interview data." *International Journal of Social Research Methodology*, 12, 51–65.

Clarke, J. 2004. "Subjects of doubt: In search of the unsettled and unfinished." Paper prepared for CASCA Conference, London, Ontario, May 5–9.

Clegg, S. 2006. "The problem of agency in feminism: A critical realist approach." *Gender and Education*, 18, 309–324.

Collier, A. 1994. *Critical realism: An introduction to Roy Bhaskar's philosophy*. London: Verso.

Crinson, I. 2001. "A realist approach to the analysis of focus group data." Paper presented at the 5th Annual IACR Conference, Roskilde University, Denmark, August 17–19.

Danermark, B., M. Ekstrom, L. Jakobsen and J. Karlsson. 2002. *Explaining society: Critical realism in the social sciences*. London: Routledge.

Danieli, A. and C. Woddhams. 2007. "Emancipatory research methodology and disability: A critique." *International Journal of Social Research Methodology*, 8, 281–296.

Denzin, N. and Y. Lincoln. 2000. *Handbook of qualitative research*. Thousand Oaks, CA: Sage.

Dobson, P. J. 2001. "Longitudinal case research: A critical realist perspective". *Systemic Practice and Action Research*, 14, 283–296.

Duncombe, J. and J. Jessop. 2002. "'Doing rapport' and the ethics of 'faking friendship'," in M. Mauthner, M. Birch, J. Jessop, and T. Miller (eds.), *Ethics in qualitative research*, pp. 107–122. London: Sage.

Edwards, A. and G. Hughes. 2009. "Inventing community safety," in P. Carlen (ed.) *Imaginary penalties*, pp. 64–83. Cullompton: Willan.

———. and M. Mathner. 2002. "Ethics and feminist research: Theory and practice," in N. Mauthner, M. Birch, J. Jessop, and T. Miller (eds.) *Ethics in qualitative research*, pp. 123–145. London: Sage.

———. and J. Sheptycki. 2009. "Third wave criminology: Guns, crime and social order." *Criminology and Criminal Justice*, 9, 1–19.

Featherstone, B. 2004. *Family life and family support: A feminist analysis*. London: Palgrave Macmillan.

———. 2006. "Re-thinking family support in the current policy context." *British Journal of Social Work*, 36, 5–19.

Finch, J. 1984. "'It's great to have someone to talk to': The ethics and politics of interviewing women," in C. Bell and H. Roberts (eds.) *Social researching: Politics, problems, practice*, pp. 70–87. London: Routledge and Kegan Paul.

Fopp, R. 2008a. "From weak social constructionism to critical realism in housing theory: Exploring issues." Paper presented to the Australian Housing Researchers Conference, RMIT, Melbourne.

———. 2008b. "Social constructionism and housing studies: A critical reflection." *Urban Policy and Research*, 26, 159–175.

Franks, M. 2002. "Feminisms and cross-ideological feminist social research: Standpoint, situatedness and positionality – Developing cross-ideological feminist research." *Journal of International Women's Studies*, 3, 38–50.

Gillies, V. and P. Alldred. 2002. "The ethics of intention: Research as a political tool," in M. Mauthner, M. Birch, J. Jessop and T. Miller (eds.) *Ethics in qualitative research*, pp. 32–52. London: Sage.

Hoffmann, E. 2007. "Open-ended interviews, power, and emotional labor." *Journal of Contemporary Ethnography*, 36, 318–346.

Holland, J. 2007. "Emotions and research." *International Journal of Social Research Methodology*, 10, 195–209.

Hunter, C., J. Nixon and S. Parr. 2010. "Mother abuse: A matter of youth justice, child welfare or domestic violence?" *Journal of Law and Society*, 37, 264–284.

Layder, D. 1989. *Sociological practice: Linking theory and social research*. London: Sage.

———. 1998. *Sociological practice: Linking theory and social research*. London: Sage.

Letherby, G. 2002. "Claims and disclaimers: Knowledge, reflexivity and representation in feminist research." *Sociological Research Online*, 6, 4.

———. 2003a. *Feminist research in theory and practice*. Buckingham: Open University Press.

———. 2003b. "Reflections on where we are and where we want to be: Response to 'Looking back and looking forward: Some recent feminist sociology reviewed'." *Sociological Research Online*, 8, 4.

Liamputtong, P. 2006. *Researching the vulnerable: A guide to sensitive research methods*. (New edition). London: Sage.

Lopez, J. and G. Potter. 2001. *After postmodernism: An introduction to critical realism*. London: The Athlone Press.

Matthews, R. 2009. "Beyond 'so what?' criminology: Rediscovering realism." *Theoretical Criminology*, 13, 341–362.

Mauthner, N. S. and A. Doucet. 1998. "Reflections on a voice-centred relational method of data analysis: Analysing maternal and domestic voices," in J. Ribbens and R. Edwards (eds.) *Feminist dilemmas in qualitative research: Private lives and public texts*, pp. 119–144. London: Sage.

Nixon, J. and Hunter, C. 2009. "Disciplining women and the governance of conduct," in A. Millie (ed.), *Securing respect: Behavioural expectations and anti-social behaviour in the UK*, pp. 119–138. Bristol: Policy Press.

———. and Parr, S. 2006. "ASB: Voices from the front line," in J. Flint (ed.) *Housing, urban governance and ASB: Perspectives, policy and practice*, pp. 79–98. Bristol: Policy Press.

Oakley, A. 1981. "Interviewing women: A contradiction in terms," in H. Roberts (ed.) *Doing feminist research*. pp. 30–61. London: Routledge and Kegan Paul.

Parr, H. 1998. "The politics of methodology in 'post-medical geography': Mental health research and the interview." *Health & Place*, 4, 341–353.

Parr, S. 2008. "Family intervention projects: A site of social work practice." *British Journal of Social Work*, 39, 111–122.

———. 2009. "Confronting the reality of anti-social behaviour." *Theoretical Criminology*, 13, 363–381.

———. 2011. "Family policy and the governance of anti-social behaviour in the UK: Women's experiences of intensive family support." *Journal of Social Policy*, 40, 717–737.

Pawson, R. and N. Tilley. 1997. *Realistic evaluation*. London: Sage.

Respect Taskforce. 2006. *Respect action plan*. London: Home Office.

Rose, G. 1997. "Situating knowledges: Positionality, reflexivities and other tactics." *Progress in Human Geography*, 21, 305–320.

Rose, N. and P. Miller. 1992. "Political power beyond the state: Problematics of government." *British Journal of Sociology*, 43, 173–205.

Satsangi, M. 2013. "Synthesizing feminist and critical realist approaches to housing studies." *Housing Studies*, 30, 193–207.

Sayer, A. 1992. *Method in social science: A realist approach*. London: Routledge.

———. 1997. "Essentialism, social constructionism, and beyond." *The Sociological Review*, 45, 453–487.

———. 2000. *Realism and social science*. London: Sage.

Skeggs, B. 1997. *Formations of class and gender: Becoming respectable*. London: Sage.

Smith, R. 2006. "Parent education: Empowerment or control?" *Children and Society*, 11, 108–116.

Taylor, D. 2005. "Governing through evidence: Participation and power in policy evaluation." *Journal of Social Policy*, 34, 601–618.

Wadsworth, Y. 1984. "Do-it-yourself social research." Melbourne: Victorian Council of Social Services.

Wai-Chung Yeung, H. 1997. "Critical realism and realist research in human geography: A method or a philosophy in search of a method." *Progress in Human Geography*, 21, 51–74.

White, C., M. Warrener, A. Reeves and I. LaValle. 2008. *Family intervention projects: An evaluation of their design, set-up and early outcomes*. London: Department for Children, Schools and Families.

12 Critical Realist Discourse Analysis, motherhood, and gender

A systematic methodological approach to analysis

Wendy Sims-Schouten

Introduction

In this chapter I will propose a methodological approach for undertaking applied Critical Realist Discourse Analysis (CRDA) with a specific focus on talk around motherhood, female employment and day-care. This approach was generated on the basis of interviews with Dutch and English mothers (N = 40) and is rooted in the critical realist approach to philosophy that was initiated by Roy Bhaskar (1989, 1997, 2014). The chapter will argue that this methodological approach allows us to make sense of the participants' narratives about (or accounts of) their lives by means of three distinctive phases. These are (1) a scaffolding phase, (2) a data collection phase, and (3) a synthesised discourse analysis phase.

By focusing on the role of abduction and retroduction, as well as incorporating Bhaskar and Danermark's (2006) notion of 'laminated systems' (a multiplicity of mechanisms that operate at a multiplicity of irreducible ontological levels) this chapter will provide insight into the causal variables and structures that 'scaffold' (or contribute to) the participants' narratives. 'Laminated systems', then, functions as a metaphor that allows us to acknowledge insights from various disciplines, account for different scales and temporalities, and highlight the irreducibility of specific 'layers' of reality to one another. This enables us to take into account a wide range of factors that influence the phenomenon under investigation. In the present case, for instance, there exists significant evidence to suggest that women's perceptions of motherhood and female employment are subject to a range of influences; maternal well-being being one of these. Maternal well-being, in turn, is influenced by fatigue (e.g. see Cooklin et al. 2011; Dunning and Giallo 2012) as well as being affected by expectations that derive from the broader society in which mothers are situated (e.g. concerning their ability to multi-task, how to be a 'good' parent, etc. see Brady et al. 2015; Sims-Schouten and Riley 2014). Research has shown, furthermore, that emotional support plays a significant role in how women engage with issues around motherhood and female employment (Luthar and Ciciolla 2015). Aspects relating to hegemonic masculinity (control, power, dominance), socioeconomic position, roles, social status, and access to resources are also of critical importance here (e.g. see Bergin et al. 2008; Cromby and Harper 2009; Pilgrim and Bentall 1999). By using the metaphor of 'laminated systems' the methodological approach that is proposed in this chapter therefore aims to develop an integrated, holistic understanding of such factors.

Before doing this, however, the next section will provide a brief overview of some of the key differences between CRDA and conventional discourse analysis. While this chapter is mainly intended as providing its readers with a *methodological* rather than a *philosophical* argument – and it is therefore primarily designed as a starting point for researchers who are (or might become) interested in contextualising talk around motherhood and gender – providing such an overview is, nonetheless, of significant importance; specifically, this serves the purpose of situating my methodological claims within much broader philosophical discussions.

Critical Realist Discourse Analysis vs discourse analysis

The CRDA methodological approach draws on the tradition of 'multi-level synthesised' discourse analysis (e.g. see Edley and Wetherell 1999; Riley et al. 2010; Sims-Schouten and Hayden 2017). More specifically, it combines discourse analysis with principles and practices that derive from discursive psychology and applied critical realism. Discourse analysis is an umbrella term for a group of methodological approaches that are generally grounded in some form of social constructionism. These approaches share (1) a focus on analysing language, and (2) an understanding of knowledge as socio-historically specific, as produced through social processes, and as linked to social action (Burr 2003). The term 'discourse' itself is most commonly associated with the work of Michel Foucault (2002 [1969]). However, a variety of approaches that seek to analyse the semiotic content of social interactions have been developed across the social sciences and humanities. Discourse analytic approaches generally assume that (social) reality is not an unproblematic given but, rather, that (social) phenomena are constructed in assemblages of language and practice which together constitute a particular 'discourse'. For example, the pain of childbirth might seem to an undisputed, unmediated, and wholly natural fact, but social constructionists might point to a popular book that rejects the term 'contraction' in favour of 'rushes' in order to reconceptualise it (Gaskin 2002). Discursive psychology is a particular strand of discourse analysis that was developed by Potter and Wetherell (1987). Whilst discourse analysis focuses on how people construct the world and make sense of themselves by drawing on common sense discourses and ideologies (Billig 1989, 2001), discursive psychology, in line with conversation analysis, is concerned with the interactional accomplishments of talk (Hepburn and Wiggins 2007). For example, in their study on racist discourse in New Zealand, Potter and Wetherell (1992) identified different interpretative repertoires by means of which culture was flexibly and locally constructed to perform various types of activities.

Finally, Bhaskar's critical realist approach draws both on constructionist claims about the role of social processes in constituting the social world and the realist position that people's actions will be influenced by personal, societal and institutional mechanisms that are independent of (or at least irreducible to) their understanding (Bhaskar 1989; Sims-Schouten and Riley 2014). Thus, unlike 'hard' social constructionists, critical realists assert that the social world is also made up of non-discursive structures that have an impact on people's lives irrespective of whether they are (fully) aware of this. Bhaskar's dialecticised version of critical realism ('dialectical critical realism') suggests, furthermore, that causal mechanisms (whether discursive or non-/extra-discursive) must be situated within a dialectically interconnected totality which includes within itself historical processes and concrete events (Roberts 2014; Scambler and Scambler 2015). Some of these claims have been developed further by other critical realists. For example, Banta (2012) has placed discourse in a dialectical relation to the wider realm of social relations, thereby analysing it as a causal mechanism that is involved in the generation of social phenomena alongside other (non-/extra-discursive) mechanisms (also see e.g. Fairclough 2010; Flatschart 2016; Joseph and Roberts 2004). In this way, it becomes possible to argue that social phenomena are created through the interplay of discursive and non-discursive factors.

In accordance with this approach, the CRDA approach that this chapter proposes views non-discursive factors (embodied, material and institutional) as causal mechanisms that operate alongside discursive factors. The starting point for this position is the idea that, while people draw on a set of (culturally specific and potentially contradictory) common sense discourses to make sense of reality (in line with Potter and Edwards 1999; see also Billig 1991), both this talk and the wider forms of discourse in which it is embedded occur within the generative boundaries of embodied, material and institutional factors. This claim is informed by the anti-anthropocentric view that discourse does not constitute or create our world independently but, rather, that it *co*-constitutes the realities that we experience (see also Nightingale and Cromby 2002). Non-discursive aspects linked to embodiment (e.g. post-natal depression), materiality (e.g. family income) and institutions (e.g. educational systems, employer's maternity leave policies) are therefore understood as shaping the constructions that people adopt and live through and as having an impact on their discursive utterances. In this way, CRDA is able to incorporate both the discursive and the non-discursive aspects of being by engaging in a systematic, phased method of analysis. This phased approach incorporates (1) the rhetorical strategies that participants employ (by drawing on discursive psychology), (2) the wider discourses on which participants draw to make sense of themselves, and (3) participants' embodied, material and institutional contexts, including how these provide the conditions of possibility for sense making (Sims-Schouten and Riley 2014).

In order to study the beliefs, constructions, and ideologies around motherhood, then, these need to be analysed in light of the complex, diverse and multi-layered realities of women's lives (Laney et al. 2015). With regard to the development of motherhood, gender, and female employment over the past 150 years, this chapter will argue that this has been influenced by three main factors. These are (1) the role of governments and their various policies and forms of legislation, (2) the role of psychology, especially psychological models of motherhood and attachment (e.g. Spock and Needlman 2012; Van Oudenhoven and Wazir 2006), and (3) the role of the feminist movement and its various 'waves' (starting with the first feminist wave in approximately 1860). All three could be understood – in CRDA terms – as a kind of scaffolding milieu, providing insight into the conditions that give rise to how mothers account for themselves and their choices regarding female employment, day-care, and motherhood. The next few sections will provide an overview of these three factors.

Governments and governmental institutions

Until the start of the 1900s, England and the Netherlands showed similar tendencies in terms of developments around female employment. For example, in both countries day-care was a privilege for the rich who – despite commonly not having to work – hired paid personnel to look after their offspring. In poorer families children would, instead, be taken to women in the neighbourhood (e.g. widows). These too were paid for the care they provided, while the children's parents worked (e.g. see Clerkx and van IJzendoorn 1992). Thus, whilst paid care was a convenience for the rich, it was – as a result of the near-absence of workers' protections – a necessity for the poor. From the 1900s onwards, however, some differences started to appear between the two countries. These resulted primarily from the fact that the Netherlands was, at the time, a vertically organised society (a so-called 'pillarised' society which was dominated by various ideological groups, ranging from, for example, Roman Catholicism to Protestantism and liberalism), whereas England was a horizontally layered society, as manifested especially in the British class system (Martens 1997). These structures influenced perceptions around motherhood and female employment: for example, pillarisation in the Dutch context meant that parenting practices and female employment were very much informed by the ideological groups to which parents belonged, including especially the social institutions and organisations (e.g. labour unions, political parties, churches, newspapers, and radio stations) that were linked to these groups. In contrast, the status of female employment in England more strongly corresponded to class, with especially working-class women having little effective choice but to pursue employment to provide for their families.

In both countries, female employment and the demand for day-care increased from the 1980s onwards (although the Netherlands was somewhat lagging behind England on this front). While day-care is in part subsidised by employers and the government in the Netherlands, the rise of neoliberal economics in England since the 1980s ensured that it has mostly been contained within the private (market) sphere. Starting in the 1990s, the English government introduced a number of schemes that aimed to facilitate access to this market, especially by means of 'childcare vouchers' (a tax saving scheme). As a result, all three and four-year-olds in England are currently eligible for 15 hours of free nursery education per week. Providing this service is, however, the responsibility of local authorities, meaning that the actual availability of this type of support has – especially since the 2008 crisis – been negatively impacted by a succession of cuts to public funding. As it stands, many smaller nurseries cannot afford to offer free time, while others restrict the number of places they provide (e.g. see Torjesen 2016). While it is common for mothers to work part time both in the Netherlands and England, Dutch employers are legally obligated to offer part-time contracts on the employee's request (Wielers and Raven 2013). In contrast, part-time work is often perceived as a constraint in England. As opposed to the Netherlands (Miani and Hoorens 2014), it therefore tends to be available only for women on low and middle incomes.

Psychology and psychological models

Institutionalised forms of psychology, like governmental bodies, have created a scaffolding milieu, generating conditions in which it makes sense to account for motherhood and female employment in one way rather than another. In fact, a number of key psychological models of child development and motherhood have strongly influenced policies and popular conceptions around female employment and day-care in both the Netherlands and England.

Consider, for example, the popularity of Benjamin Spock's ideas around motherhood – ideas that were influenced by Freud's theory regarding the crucial importance of infant-mother relationships – in the *Baby and Child Care* (Spock and Needlman 2012). Further to this, consider attachment theory, resulting from the pioneering research of Bowlby and his colleagues at the Tavistock Clinic in London between 1948 and 1956 (e.g. see Bowlby 2005), which continues to be a frequently cited approach within contemporary forms of developmental psychology. This theoretical approach is commonly understood – whether justifiably or not – as presupposing the existence of a naturally-given maternal bond that is deemed necessary for healthy psychological growth. It was widely embraced in post-WWII Britain and served to reinforce gendered parenting roles by emphasising the crucial role of attachment to a main caregiver, usually understood to be the mother, for the developing child (Polat 2016). Bowlby's work around attachment and maternal deprivation continues to play an important role in decisions around day-care; for instance, his focus on the crucial early years (the 'sensitive period') is often used to explain why, especially in England, mothers choose to reduce their working hours substantially in the year of childbirth (Miani and Hoorens 2014). Despite this, the influence of attachment theory is ambivalent: while it can, on the one hand, serve to bolster legal protections (such as parental leave) for working mothers, it can also be instrumentalised to argue that mothers who choose to return to work shortly after birth are jeopardising the future well-being of their offspring.

Whatever the truth of the matter, a number of prominent psychological models have been deeply implicated in creating and maintaining dominant constructions of child development, particularly by constructing gender templates and role definitions of motherhood that position women as the 'natural' carers for their child.

The feminist movement

The role of feminism in shaping discourse around child-care needs to be understood in light of the four successive waves of feminism that constitute its history. The first wave is commonly held to have begun in the late nineteenth century and was primarily concerned with women's civil rights (Pankhurst 2013). The second wave (also known as the Women's Liberation Movement or 'Women's Lib') started in the 1960s, and expanded feminist discussions to include equality in marriage and the workplace, as well as to sex, sexuality and violence against women (Setch 2001). Growing out of critiques of the perceived inadequacies of the second wave, third-wave feminism (from the 1970s until about 2000) focused less on laws and the political process and more on individual identity, inspired by the notion that women are of many colours, ethnicities, nationalities, religions and cultural backgrounds (Mann and Huffman 2005). This wave was not just concerned with cultural and sexual politics, however, but also engaged with various political and social issues, ranging from on-going wage discrimination to education, domestic violence, eating disorders, globalisation and the effects of racism and classism on the movement (Gillis et al. 2004, pp. 5–6).

Finally, social media and the internet are commonly seen as the catalyst for fourth wave feminism. This wave is sometimes understood as a continuation of the third wave, especially its emphases on micropolitics and challenging sexism/misogyny insofar as these appear in everyday rhetoric, advertising, film, television, literature, and social media. One of the achievements of feminism has been to undermine the association between women's social position and the supposed biological aspects of mothering. Feminists have commonly rejected this biological connection and, instead, have argued that gender roles are governed by distinctly social/cultural rules and meanings. As such, feminists have played an important role in the study of labour markets, work, and employment by drawing attention to the inequality and exploitation that is inherent to both traditional mothering roles and androcentric social structures more generally (Benjamin 2002; Hattery 2001).

Method: 'doing applied CRDA'

This section will develop a multi-level, 'synthesised' form of discourse analysis which draws on Bhaskar's critical realist approach, especially his model of ontological depth. This model employs a distinction between the realms of the 'real' (structures and their causal powers), the 'actual' (the events or processes that result when causal powers are triggered), and the 'empirical' (the sub-category of actual events that are accessible by means of human senses) (Bhaskar 1989; Leca and Naccache 2006). This model suggests a mode of inquiry that asks – by using retroductive and abductive forms of logic – which 'real' powers have been triggered that cause the observable phenomena under study to exist as they do; or, in simple terms, 'what has to be the case for this outcome to be possible?' Further to this, CRDA also draws on the aforementioned notion of 'laminated systems' to engage with the multiplicity of mechanisms that operate at a multiplicity of irreducible ontological levels. Hence, it is dependent on an emergentist/stratified understanding of being which suggests that – in open systems – causal powers interact in complex ways that make the existence of specific phenomena or events more or less likely. The notions of 'ontological depth' and 'laminated systems' therefore function as philosophical vehicles that enable us to account for causation without succumbing to either determinism or voluntarism.

In the current context, this means that motherhood and female employment should be understood *neither* as wholly determined by causal structures such as biological necessity, *nor* as mere 'social constructs' without any connection to non-discursive reality. Rather, these are here conceptualised in terms of the World Health Organization's biopsychosocial model. As Bhaskar (2014) has suggested, this model is in line with the critical realist idea that there exist various irreducible strata within being, all of which contain causal powers. When these *real* powers a triggered they interact to produce *actual* and *empirical* events. As such, the CRDA approach allows us to conceive of discourse, embodiment, materiality and social structures as interacting in complex, iterative ways, with none of these factors taking absolute precedence over the others in understanding motherhood and female employment.

My research is based on a total of 40 interviews – 20 with Dutch mothers and 20 with English mothers. In each sample, half of the mothers were employed, and all participants either used formal or informal (e.g. through relatives) forms of day-care at the time of the interview. In addition to this, both of the national samples included a number of full-time mothers who used day-care facilities either so the children could socialise or to give themselves a break from child-minding duties (N = 2 for the Dutch and N = 4 for the English participants). Participants had between 1 and 3 children and came from a variety of social and economic backgrounds; the sample was predominantly white, a total of four participants (three in England and one from the Netherlands) were from an ethnic minority background. The interviews were semi-structured and lasted for up to one hour. Ethical guidelines were adhered to and informed consent was obtained at the start of each interview.

Data collection consisted of three phases:

Phase one – this phase focused on 'discovery', or what critical realists term abduction, and aimed to develop a broad understanding of what factors might be relevant for my investigation. It then proceeded by testing these factors, in an iterative manner, against new information. This phase involved conducting a thorough literature review from as wide a perspective as possible, thereby allowing me to identify the most commonly recurring elements of embodiment, institutions and materiality that – according to the wider literature on these issues – had a significant impact on motherhood, female employment and day-care (see also Sims-Schouten and Riley 2014).

Phase two – once key factors in the discursive and non-discursive context of motherhood, female employment and day-care were identified, I developed a research design which allowed me to explore these issues in greater depth by using a range of data collection tools, including questionnaires and semi-structured interviews. The questionnaires asked for information about the participants' age, income, local day-care facilities and other factors that were relevant to the research topic. The data that resulted was cross-referenced with selected quantitative information, especially data on the quality of day-care facilities in the area and/or regional and national government policies. Semi-structured interviews, which sought to deepen my understanding of the participants' lives, took place in their homes.

Phase three – semi-structured interviews were then analysed by using a multi-level, synthesised form of discourse analysis (Sims-Schouten and Riley 2014; Wetherell 1998). Because CRDA draws on discursive psychology the initial focus was on the interactive accomplishments of talk, such as managing facts, blame, and accountability (Potter 1997).[1] The second level of discourse analysis focused on the wider discourses on which participants drew in order to make sense of themselves, including common sense discourses and ideologies (Billig 1989, 2001). The data were then transcribed in detail, drawing on Jefferson (1985); attention was paid, for instance, to aspects of talk in relation to intonation (↑↓ in the extracts for rising and lowering intonation), pauses, speeded up talk (> <), quiet speech (° °), etc.[2] The third level of the synthesised discourse analysis introduced the critical realist aspect of my work by examining talk with regard to how participants' embodied, material and institutional contexts provide their conditions for sense-making.

Applied CRDA – examples of analysis

The Netherlands and England have the highest rates of female part-time employment in Europe. This was often referred to by the participants of my study in order to identify a situation that amounted to 'the best of both worlds' (i.e. the optimal possible combination of employment and motherhood) and which helped them to establish a balance between the moral demands of being a 'good mother' and somebody who has 'their own life' and 'identity'. Non-discursive aspects – relating to how Dutch and English society are organised when it comes to their facilities for parents, income/economic class, and the quality of day-care – also appeared to play a 'scaffolding' or generative role in their reasoning.

The quality of English day-care has traditionally been low. Between 1997 and 2010, however, the then Labour government sought to improve this situation by making funding available to improve the qualifications of the workforce. The quality of 'early years' settings has, however, continued to vary

(Nutbrown 2012). Dutch day-care is similarly of variable quality, with some research suggesting that its quality has deteriorated over the years (Helmerhorst et al. 2015). Below is an excerpt from an interview with an English participant who is currently a full-time mother and cites quality issues in the day-care provided as a factor in her considerations. The specific institution to which she refers was rated as 'unsatisfactory' by the Office for Standards in Education, Children's Services and Skills (Ofsted) and had mistakenly placed her two-year-old son in the three to four year-old group, resulting in an experience of disempowerment and a lack of trust in the day-care provided:

1. W: What are you doing at the moment?
2. P: .h I am at h↑ome (1.0) I gave up work eventua↓lly,
3. P: and decided to stay at home with them (1.0) >I think< after I tried nursery
4. P: and it fai:led, that I j↓ust thought I'd rather be at home with them and
5. P: know exa↑ctly °sort of, you know°
6. W: hm[m
7. P: [I can gui↓de them, or decide what I want them to be do↓ing,
8. P: What activities I want them to be do↓ing

The participant clearly indicates that there is a connection between her decision to stay at home and the fact that day-care did not work out for her and her children (lines 3, 4). The broader literature on this issue shows that, aside from general supply issues, the difficulty of finding *suitable* day-care commonly features as a material constraint upon women's opportunities to return to work (see Nightingale and Cromby 1999); this was evident in both of the national samples. The fact that the participant's decision to stay at home was not taken lightly is made clear by the emphasis on 'eventua↓lly' in line 2. By referring to her experience of day-care and linking it directly to her decision to stay at home this participant is aligning herself with the traditional caring role of mothers (see also Phoenix and Woollett 1991) – this is also made clear in the 'three-way-list' completer (using three arguments to strengthen a point, see Antaki and Wetherell 1999) in lines 7 and 8: 'I can gui↓de them', 'decide what I want them to be do↓ing', and '[w]hat activities I want them to be do↓ing'. The fact that, as a mother, she considers herself to be fully responsible for the development of her children is made apparent by the focus on 'exa↑ctly' which precedes the three-way-list completer in line 5. Here the participant makes an appeal to common knowledge, evident from the softly uttered '°sort of, you know°' in line 5 (see also Billig 2001). Importantly, this appeal also ties in with attachment theory/psychology, especially its aforementioned emphasis on the crucial importance of early child–mother relationships.[3]

The choice of whether to return to work or not is further informed by the financial situation of the family. In England, compared to the Netherlands, mothers take more time off from work after childbirth (Miani and Hoorens 2014). Moreover, while part-time work is popular among women in both countries, in England this is often associated with lower-skilled jobs, whereas in the Netherlands there is a greater likelihood that both parents (regardless of job level and skill) will work part-time (Miani and Hoorens 2014). The participant in the extract below is Dutch and has a five months old daughter; she returned to work two months after the child was born. She is married and the family are on a low to average income.

1. W: *Vertel me over je werk*
   W: Tell me about your job
2. P: *Nou, ik werk dus ook voor de financiele onafhankelijkheid, he*
   P: Well, I also work to be financially independent, you know
3. P: *.hh dat je jezelf kunt onderhouden, dat vind ik be↑langrijk*
   P: .hh being able to support oneself, I find that important
4. P: *ook omdat het dan financieel wat makkelijker is*
   P: also because it means that it is a bit easier, financially
5. P: *en ik mijn eigen geld heb, ik hoef geen verklaring*
   P: and I have my own money, which means I don't have to explain
6. P: *-inaudible- also ik iets koop*
   P: -inaudible- when I buy something

Despite several waves of feminism, women are still perceived as being more responsible for their offspring than men. This means that women are often left to justify why they are making certain decisions, such as carrying on with work. The participant in the extract above, for instance, draws on a financial discourse, referring to financial independence (emphasised through the word '*onafhankelijkheid*' in line 2) in order to justify her decision to return to work. While this could be intended to show that she does not want to be a financial burden on her husband (line 3) or that she believes such financial dependence to be potentially harmful to her own well-being, it can also be understood in terms of an effort to portray herself as an independent, modern woman who can look after herself. Similarly, the link between female employment and monetary income can be evaluated both in light of feminist discourses about independence and equality and as a non-discursive scaffolding factor. As a discourse, 'financial independence' is used (in the case of this participant) to portray herself as a modern woman who does not lean on or need others (see Himmelweit and Sigala 2003). More generally, this discourse allows women to justify their return to work without being frowned upon, at least to an extent. Yet, from a non-discursive viewpoint, women who refer to financial needs in order to justify their return to working life may simply be experiencing a situation in which their husband's salary is insufficient to provide for the family.

Not only do women have to justify returning to work, however, once they do so they are also paid less on average and they are less likely to be promoted (see also Lebowith 2015). The participant in the extract below is self-employed and her husband is a computer technician; the couple have three children, two teenagers from the mother's previous relationship and an 18-month-old. It follows a section of the interview in which the mother explained that, before she was self-employed, she commonly felt that she had to prove herself in front of her colleagues by showing that she could be both a good mother and a career woman.

1. P: ; >you won't get the pro↑mo↓tion<, and you won't get
2. P: the respect that other p↑eople get. So a m↑a:[n
3. W: [right
4. P: >a man might get in at seven in the mor↑ning<, and go
5. P: home at seven at n↓ight, but his work (1.0) may not be,
6. P: (1.0) as high a standard as yours
7. W: hmm
8. P: but be↑cause he is always seen to be sitting in the o↓ffi:ce,
9. P: (1.0) because he c↑a:n
10. W: Yes
11. P: >because he hasn't got that< home life to worry a↑bout (2.0)
12. P: So, I think it's a bit, of both, it's from the work pla:ce, you
13. P: get the pres↓sure .hh and its from me:, b'cause (1.0) >I want
14. P: to be able to do both<, and I want to be able to do them both as
15. P: well as each other
16. W: right
17. P: >which is why I went< (1.0) that's why I now work for myself
18. P: because I (1.0) if I want to not do anything to↓da:y, I can, >and (if?) I want
19. P: to be with G {child}<, then I make the decision for myself

As with the previous extract, this participant takes her position as an independent woman who knows her own mind as a starting point. This is apparent especially in her emphasis on 'I' and 'myself' in lines 18, 19: 'then I make the decision for myself'). Yet, within these lines, she also constructs herself as responsible for her children. Here she argues from the point of view that gender inequalities (lines 1–9 – see the emphasis on 'man' in line 4 and the rising intonation in 'because he c↑a:n' in line 9), together with her caring duties ('home life' in line 11), are responsible for her decision to become self-employed (see line 17: 'that's why I now work for myself'). Interestingly, while this mother talks in negative terms about gender inequality at work – for example by arguing that '>you won't get the pro↑mo↓tion<' (line 1) – she appears to take her caring role for granted ('>because he hasn't got that< home life to worry a↑bout', line 11); both are said quickly (indicated by the ><), as if they are simply a given. As such, she indicates that there are two issues that play a fundamental role in women's oppression. First, the unequal division of household and childcare tasks within the family (see also Fahlen 2016), which means that mothers have to be 'superwomen' if they want to combine employment with family-life. Second, the notion that 'you won't get the respect that other p↑eople get' (lines 1,2). This suggests that gender inequalities are also caused by a lack of respect for (and patience with) women who have to fulfil both their roles as employees and mothers (lines 12–15). The above should furthermore be seen in light of the fact that, in England, part-time work is often associated with lower skilled jobs and fewer opportunities for promotion (Miani and Hoorens 2014).

Some participants referred to the lack of government support for women who want to stay at home – being a full-time mother is a privilege that is still reserved only for the few families whose male breadwinner earns an income that is sufficient to provide for all of its members. The next extract comes from an interview with an English mother; she is a full-time mother who has one child, an 18 months old girl. Her husband is a salesman.

1. P: you, you're definitely a non-person if you
2. P: just started to (1.0) .hh to stay at h↓ome, I means °it's it's
3. P: like° you have absolutely no .hh {clear throat} no help or,
4. P: or recognition from the government as it w↓ere
5. P: .hh >you know<, you get (1.0) >I mean< you get your
6. P: ch↓ild bene↓fit, which is next to no↓thing (1.0)
7. W: right
8. P: and you do have to: (1.0) you know, tell yourself that actually
9. P: you are, you know, you, it's just as valuable a job you
10. P: you're doing, staying at home and looking after your b↑aby

In England, more so than in the Netherlands, day-care is considered a private responsibility, and the quality of day-care provision has improved only minimally to date (see also Osgood and Robinson 2017; Sims-Schouten and Riley 2014). In fact, family support and benefits have been cut in recent years to contribute to the Conservative government's manifesto promise to reduce welfare spending by £12bn by the end of parliament. This factor functions as scaffolding, a generative mechanism, in this mother's argument that you are 'definitely a non-person' (line 1) when you stay at home; from line 4 ('recognition from the government as it w↓ere') it is clear that she holds the government responsible for this. Note, furthermore, that she strengthens this argument through the use of extreme case formulations (see Pomerantz 1986), 'definitely' (line 1) and 'absolutely' (line 3). She turns this external pressure from the government into internal pressure, linked to self-worth, in the latter part of the extract ('tell yourself' and 'you're doing, staying at home', see lines 8–10). In fact, she is making sense of her 'stay-at-home status' by constructing this in terms of doing a 'valuable' 'job' (line 9), suggesting that motherhood can only be on a par with employment if it is understood as 'doing a job'.

Phase one of the three-part analysis showed that there exist significantly fewer mother and toddler and infant groups/places (which provide opportunities for both to socialise) in the Netherlands than in England. This was also evident from the interviews with Dutch mothers, who referred to social interaction as a benefit of being employed to a far greater extent than the English participants. The extract below provides an example of this. This section comes from an interview with a Dutch participant who has one child, a 15-month-old boy; this mother works part-time as a pharmacy assistant and her husband is a project manager.

1. W: kun je je belangrijkste reden om kinderopvang te gebruiken samenvatten?
   W: *could you summarise your most important reason for using day-care?*
2. P: eh:m (1.0) .h j↓a, mijn allerbelangrijkste reden is graag,
   P: *erm (1.0) well, my most important reason is really*
3. P: dat ik wil w↑erken, °gewoon toch° (1.0) °die tijden die ik net z↓ei°
   P: *that I still want to work (1.0) those hours that I mentioned earlier on*
4. W: Ja
   W: *Yes.*
5. P: °j↓a dat vind ik g↓ewoon° (1.0) °ja, voor mezelf heel be↑langrijk°
   P: *yes I just find that (1.0) yes, very important for myself*
6. P: Ik zie het gewoon niet zitten om eh,h J↑a dat zit gewoon
   P: *I just can't face to er Yeah that is just*
7. P: in m'n kar↑akter, denk it
   P: *part of my character I think*
8. W: ja.
   W: *yes*
9. P: ik vind het gewoon heel erg leuk om eh
   P: *I just really like it very much to er*
10. P: JA >om toch nog met< ↓andere men↓se:n, in contact te ko↓men
    P: *YES, to still be in contact with other people.*

This participant refers to her own stake and interests when asked what the most important reason is for her choice to use day-care (line 1). As opposed to some of the other participants in the sample, who focused mostly on benefits for the child (i.e. that day-care is good for a child's development), she refers to the benefits for herself (see line 5, with emphasis on 'heel belangrijk' = very important). By referring to her character ('part of my character I think', line 7) she emphasises authenticity and accuracy, because nobody knows her better than she does (see also Speer and Potter 2000). Moreover, this statement works to show that the decision is, to an extent, beyond her control, not something that she can help; it is part of her 'character' rather than a specific choice that she has made. Himmelweit and Sigala (2003, p. 7) call this the 'constraint of identity', referring to the fact that mothers' identities inform how they construct the decisions they face so that they do not consider options that are not in accordance with their identities. By constructing employment as a category-bound activity (see Silverman 2001) of being in 'contact with other people' (line 9, 10 – the significance of this is highlighted by the loudly uttered 'YES, to still be in contact with other people') and socialising she suggests that being a full-time mother reduces her options in this regard.

Discussion and conclusion

The above examples illustrate how discursive and non-discursive causal mechanisms at different levels of reality interact to produce specific experiences of motherhood. The women cited refer to these mechanisms in an integrated and interconnected way; for example, by accepting women's 'natural' role as the main carer while, at the same time, decrying specific discursive framings of it (e.g. denial of respect by work colleagues). Crucially, the interview excerpts show that non-discursive and discursive constraints are not understood as clearly separable – the women want to think of themselves as independent, rational actors, but they are aware of the fact that their ability to realise this understanding is contingent on material conditions such as the availability of day-care and/or part-time work. It is here, in particular, that the adoption of a CRDA approach is useful, as this approach allows us to side-step the age-old structure/agency and materialism/idealism (or constructivism) dualisms in favour of an approach that conceives of these as dialectically co-constituted. The wish for independence, expressed by a number of participants, thus becomes legible as neither simply financial necessity nor a purely discursive construction of an idealised self, but, rather, a specific way of constructing a self *within* the constraints of material circumstance. Similarly, a desire to be employed may be composed of both the material necessity to earn an income and an individual's striving for independence, with neither factor (necessarily) being reducible to the other. Finally, the idea that women are best suited to taking care of small children draws both on non-discursive elements (such as the fact that women are biologically predisposed to be able to give birth and breastfeed) while also containing discursive elements such as the social construction of women as particularly caring and/or nurturing.

Untangling these 'blended' factors and assigning them to their respective levels of reality is the domain of philosophy and is, therefore, a matter of data analysis only to a limited extent. However, the three-phased methodological approach that was developed in this chapter demonstrates how such philosophical distinctions can inform empirical research. This approach therefore provides a starting point for researchers who wish to avoid *both* the anthropocentric social constructionist tendency to reduce all dimensions of our existence to discourse *and* biological reductionism or materialist determinism. In this way, CRDA (1) allows us to develop a dynamic and integrated/holistic understanding of women's talk about employment, motherhood, and day-care, and (2) provides us with a practical blueprint for applying the dialectic understanding of reality that critical realist philosophy adopts.

Transcription notions

° °	*Encloses speech that is quieter that the surrounding talk.*
(1.0)	*Pause length in seconds.*
Hyphen	*Word broken off.*
↑	*Rising intonation.*
↓	*Lowering intonation.*
CAPITAL LETTERS	*Talk that is louder than the surrounding talk.*
Underline	*Stress/emphasis.*
> <	*Encloses speeded up talk.*
()	*Encloses words the transcriber is unsure about. Empty brackets enclose talk that is inaudible.*
.hhh	*In-breath.*
[]	*Overlapping speech.*
[	*Onset of overlapping speech.*
{}	*Clarification, referring to tone or gesture, e.g. {laughs}*
:::	*Extended sound.*
=	*Marks the immediate 'latching' of successive talk, whether of one or more speakers, with no interval.*

(Edwards 1997; Jefferson 1985)

Notes

1 Discursive psychologists are affiliated with the conversation analytic traditions (Sacks 2001), and are primarily concerned with documenting and analysing what people do with their talk, e.g. disclaiming and making extreme statements (Pomerantz 1986)
2 Please see the transcription notes at the end of this chapter for further information.
3 See, for example, the work by Bowlby and Spock and, more recently, the work done by researchers linked to the Anna Freud centre in London (e.g. Granqvist et al. 2017) and Dutch scholars such as Van IIzendoorn (e.g. Van IJzendoorn and Sagi-Schwartz 2008).

References

Antaki, C. and M. Wetherell. 1999. "Show Concessions." *Discourse Studies* 1(1): 7–27.
Banta, B. 2012. "Analysing Discourse as a Causal Mechanism." *European Journal of International Relations* 19(2): 379–402.
Benjamin, J. 2002. "The Question of Sexual Difference." *Feminism & Psychology* 12(1): 39–44.
Bergin, M., J. S. G. Wells and S. Owen. 2008. "Critical Realism: A Philosophical Framework for the Study of Gender and Mental Health." *Nursing Philosophy* 9: 169–179.
Bhaskar, R. 1989. *Reclaiming Reality*. London: Verso.
Bhaskar, R. 1997. *A Realist Theory of Science*. London: Verso.
Bhaskar, R. 2014. "Foreword," in P. Edwards, J. O'Mahoney and S. Vincent (eds.) *Studying Organisations Using Critical Realism. A Practical Guide*, pp. V–XV. Oxford: Oxford University Press.

Bhaskar, R. and B. Danermark. 2006. "Metatheory, Interdisciplinarity and Disability Research: A Critical Realist Perspective." *Scandinavian Journal of Disability Research* 8(4): 278–297.

Billig, M. 1989. "The Argumentative Nature of Holding Strong Views: A Case Study." *European Journal of Social Psychology* 19: 203–223.

Billig, M. 1991. *Ideology and Opinions. Studies in Rethorical Psychology*. London: Sage Publications.

Billig, M. 2001. "Discursive, Rhetorical and Ideological Messages," in M. Wetherell, S. Taylor and S. J. Yates (eds.) *Discourse Theory and Practice. A Reader*, pp. 210–222. London: Sage.

Bowlby, J. 2005. *The Making and Breaking of Affectional Bonds*. London and New York: Routledge.

Brady, G., P. Lowe and S.O. Lauritzen. 2015. *Children, Health and Well-being: Policy Debates and Lived Experience*. Malden, Oxford and Chichester: Wiley Blackwell.

Burr, V. 2003. *Social Constructionism*. London and New York: Routledge.

Clerkx, L. E. and M. H. van IJzendoorn. 1992. "Child Care in a Dutch Context: On the History, Current Status and Evaluation of Nonmaternal Child Care in the Netherlands," in M. E. Lamb, K. J. Sternberg, C.-P. Hwang, and A. G. Broberg (eds.) *Child Care in Context: Cross Cultural Perspectives*, pp. 55–77. New Jersy: Lawrence Erlbaum Associates.

Cooklin, A. R., R. Giallo and N. Rose. 2011. "Parental Fatigue and Parenting Practices during Early Childhood: An Australian Community Survey." *Child: Care, Health and Development* 38(5): 654–664.

Cromby, J. and D. J. Harper. 2009. "Paranoia: A Social Account." *Theory & Psychology* 19(3): 335–361.

Dunning, M. J. and R. Giallo. 2012. "Fatigue, Parenting Stress, Self-efficacy and Satisfaction in Mothers of Infants and Young Children". *Journal of Reproductive and Infant Psychology* 30(2): 145–159.

Edley, N. and M. Wetherell. 1999. "Imagined Futures: Young Men's Talk about Fatherhood and Domestic Life." *British Journal of Social Psychology* 38(2): 181–194.

Edwards, D. 1997. *Discourse and Cognition*. London: Sage.

Fahlen, S. 2016. "Equality at Home –A Question of Career? Housework, Norms, and Policies in a European Comparative Perspective." *Demographic Research* 35(48): 1411–1440.

Fairclough, N. 2010. *Critical Discourse Analysis: The Critical Study of Language*. London: Routledge.

Flatschart, E. 2016. "Critical Realist Critical Discourse Analysis: A Necessary Alternative to Post-Marxist Discourse Theory." *Journal of Critical Realism* 15(1): 21–52.

Foucault, M. 2002 (1969). *The Archaeology of Knowledge*. London and New York: Routledge.

Gaskin, I. M. 2002. *Spiritual Midwifery*. Summertown, TN: Book Publishing Company.

Gillis, S., G. Howie and R. Munford (eds.). 2004. *Third Wave Feminism*. New York: Palgrave Macmillan.

Granqvist, P., L. A. Sroufe, M. Dozier, E. Hesse, M. Steele, M. van IJzendoorn and R. Duschinsky. 2017. "Disorganized Attachment in Infancy: A Review of the Phenomenon and Its Implications for Clinicians and Policymakers." *Attachment and Human Development* 19(6): 534–558.

Harré, R. 1990. "Exploring the Human Umwelt," in R. Bhaskar (ed.) *Harré and His Critics: Essays in Honour of Rom Harré, with His Commentary on Them*, pp. 297–364. Oxford: Blackwell.

Hattery, A. 2001. *Women, Work and Family. Balancing and Weaving*. London: Sage.

Helmerhorst, K. O. W., J. M. A. Riksen-Walraven, M. J. J. M. Gever Deynoot-Schaub, L. W. C. Tavecchio and R. G. Fukkink. 2015. "Child Care Quality in the Netherlands over the Years: A Closer Look." *Early Education and Development* 26(1): 89–105.

Hepburn, A. and S. Wiggins 2007. "Discursive Research: Themes and Debates," in A. Hepburn and S. Wiggins (eds.) *Discursive Research in Practice: New Approaches to Psychology and Interaction*, pp. 1–28. Cambridge: Cambridge University Press.

Himmelweit, S. and M. Sigala. 2003. "Internal and External Constraints on Mothers' Employment: Some Implications for Policy." *ESRC Future of Work Programme*. Working Paper no 27.

Jefferson, G. 1985. "An Exercise in the Transcription and Analysis of Laughter," in T. A. van Dijk (ed.) *Handbook of Discourse Analysis. Discourse and Dialogue. Volume 3*, pp. 25–34. London: Academic Press.

Joseph, J. and J. M. Roberts 2004. *Realism, Discourse and Deconstruction*. London: Routledge.

Laney, E. K., M. E. Lewis Hall, T. L. Anderson and M. M. Willingham. 2015. "Becoming a Mother: The Influence of Motherhood on Women's Identity Development". *Identity: An International Journal of Theory and Research* 15(2): 126–145.

Lebowith, S. 2015 "A New Study from Lean-in and McKinsey Finds Exactly How Much More Likely Men are to Get Promoted than Women." *Business Insider UK*, 1st of Oct. Available from: http://uk.businessinsider.com/women-are-less-likely-to-get-promoted-2015-10.

Leca, B. and P. Naccache. 2006. "A Critical Realist Approach to Institutional Entrepreneurship." *Organization* 13(5): 627–651.

Luthar, S. S. and L. Ciciolla. 2015. "Who Mothers Mommy? Factors that Contribute to Mothers' Well-being." *Developmental Psychology* 51(12): 1812–1823.

Mann, S. A. and D. J. Huffman. 2005. "The Decentering of Second Wave Feminism and the Rise of the Third Wave." *Science & Society* 69(1, Special issue): 56–91.

Martens, L. 1997. *Exclusion and Inclusion: The Gender Composition of British and Dutch Worksforces*. Avebury: Aldershot.

Miani, C. and S. Hoorens. 2014. "Parents at Work: Men and Women Participating in the Labour Force." *Short Statistical Report No. 2, Prepared for the European Commission, Directorate-General of Justice and Fundamental Rights*, Santa Monica: RAND Offices.

Nightingale, D. J. and J. Cromby (eds.) 1999. *Social Constructionist Psychology: A Critical Analysis of Theory and Practice*. Milton Keynes: Open University Press.

Nightingale, D. J. and J. Cromby. 2002. "Social Constructionism as Ontology. Exposition and Example." *Theory & Psychology* 12(5): 701–713.

Nutbrown, C. 2012. *Foundations for Quality. The Independent Review of Early Education and Childcare Qualifications. Final Report*. Runcan: Department of Education. Available from: www.education.gov.uk/nutbrownreview.

Osgood, J. and K. H. Robinson 2017. *Feminists Researching Gendered Childhoods*. Feminist Thought in Childhood Research Series. Bloomsbury: London.

Pankhurst, E. S. 2013. *The Suffragette Movement: An Intimate Account of Persons and Ideals*. Redditch: Read Books Ltd.

Phoenix, A. and A. Woollett. 1991. "Motherhood, Social Construction, Politics and Psychology," in A. Phoenix, A. Woollett and E. Loyd (eds.) *Motherhood, Meanings, Practices and Ideologies*, pp. 13–28. London: Sage.

Pilgrim, D. and R. Bentall. 1999. "The Medicalisation of Misery: A Critical Realist Analysis of the Concept of Depression." *Journal of Mental Health* 8(3): 261–274.

Polat, B. 2016. "Before Attachment Theory: Separation Research at the Tavistock Clinic, 1948–1956." *Journal of the History of the Behavioral Sciences* 53(1): 48–70.

Pomerantz, A. 1986. "Extreme Case Formulations: A New Way of Legitimating Claims". *Human Studies* 9: 219–230.

Potter, J. 1997. "Discourse Analysis as a Way of Analysing Naturally Occurring Talk," in D. Silverman (ed.) *Qualitative Research: Theory, Method and Practice*, pp. 144–160. London: Sage.

Potter, J. and M. Wetherell. 1987. *Discourse and Social Psychology. Beyond Attitudes and Behaviour.* London: Sage Publications.

Riley, S., Y. Morey and C. Griffin. 2010. "The 'Pleasure Citizen' Analyzing Partying as a Form of Social and Political Participation." *Young* 18(1): 33–54.

Roberts, J. M. 2014. "Critical Realism, Dialectics, and Qualitative Research Methods." *Journal for the Theory of Social Behaviour* 44(1): 1–23.

Sacks, H. 2001. "Lecture 1: Rules of Conversational Sequence," in M. Wetherell, S. Taylor and S. J. Yates (eds.) *Discourse, Theory and Practice. A Reader*, pp. 111–119. London: Sage.

Scambler, G. and S. Scambler. 2015. "Theorizing Health Inequalities: The Untapped Potential of Dialectical Critical Realism." *Social Theory & Health* 13(3–4): 340–354.

Setch, E. G. 2001. *The Women's Liberation Movement in Britain, 1969–79: Organisation, Creativity and Debate* (Doctoral dissertation, Royal Holloway, University of London).

Silverman, D. 2001. *Interpreting Qualitative Data. Methods for Analysing Talk, Text Interaction*. London: Sage.

Sims-Schouten, W. and C. Hayden. 2017. "Mental Health and Wellbeing of Care Leavers: Making Sense of Their Perspectives." *Child & Family Social Work* 22(4): 1480–1487.

Sims-Schouten, W. and S. Riley. 2014. "Employing a Form of Critical Realist Discourse Analysis for Identity Research: An Example from Women's Talk of Motherhood, Childcare and Employment," in P. Edwards, J. O'Mahoney and S. Vincent (eds.) *Studying Organizations Using Critical Realism*, pp. 46–66. Oxford: Oxford University Press.

Speer, S. A. and J. Potter. 2000. "The Management of Heterosxist Talk: Conversational Resources and Prejudiced Claims". *Discourse & Society* 11(4): 543–572.

Spock, B. and R. Needlman. 2012. *Dr Spock's Baby & Childcare 9th Edition.* London: Simon & Schuster UK.

Torjesen, I. 2016. "Austerity Cuts are Eroding Benefit of Sure Start Children's Centres." *BMJ* 2016(352): i335.

Van IJzendoorn, M. and A. Sagi-Schwartz. 2008. *Cross-Cultural Patterns of Attachment: Universal and Contextual Dimensions*. New York: Guildford Press.

Van Oudenhoven, N. J. A. and R. Wazir. 2006. *Newly Emerging Needs of Children: An Exploration*. Antwerp and Apeldoorn: Garant publishers.

Wetherell, M. 1998. "Positioning and Interpretative Repertoires: Conversation Analysis and Post-structuralism in Dialogue." *Discourse & Society* 9(3): 387–412.

Wetherell, M. and J. Potter. 1992. *Mapping the Language of Racism: Discourse and the Legitimation of Exploitation*. London and New York: Harvester Wheatsheaf and Columbia University Press.

Wielers, R. and D. Raven. 2013. "Part-Time Work and Work Norms in the Netherlands." *European Sociological Review* 29(1): 105–113.

Further reading

The debate between Tony Lawson and others on ontology, critical realism, and feminism (chronological order)

Lawson, T. 1997. "Feminism, Realism, and Universalism." *Feminist Economics* 5(2): 25–59.

Harding, S., 1999. "The Case for Strategic Realism: A Response to Lawson." *Feminist Economics* 5(3): 127–133.

Peter, F., 2003. "Critical Realism, Feminist Epistemology, and the Emancipatory Potential of Science: A Comment on Lawson and Harding." *Feminist Economics* 9(1): 93–101.

Barker, D., 2003. "Emancipatory for Whom? A Comment on Critical Realism." *Feminist Economics* 9(1): 103–108.

Nelson, J., 2003. "Once More, With Feeling: Feminist Economics and the Ontological Question." *Feminist Economics* 9(1): 109–118.

Lawson, T., 2003. "Ontology and Feminist Theorizing." *Feminist Economics* 9(1): 119–150.

Harding, S., 2003. "Representing Reality: The Critical Realism Project." *Feminist Economics* 9(1): 151–159.

Lawson, T. 2003. "Theorizing Ontology" *Feminist Economics* 9(1): 161–169.

Poutanen, S., 2007. "Critical Realism and Post-Structuralist Feminism: The Difficult Path to Mutual Understanding." *Journal of Critical Realism* 6(1): 28–52.

The debate between David Pilgrim and Jason Summersell on critical realism and trans women/'transgenderism' (chronological order)

Pilgrim, D., 2018a. "Reclaiming Reality and Redefining Realism: The Challenging Case of Transgenderism." *Journal of Critical Realism* 17(3): 308–324.

Summersell, J., 2018a. "Trans Women are Real Women: A Critical Realist Intersectional Response to Pilgrim." *Journal of Critical Realism* 17(3): 329–336.

Pilgrim, D., 2018b. "The Transgender Controversy: A Reply to Summersell." *Journal of Critical Realism* 17(5): 523–528.

Summersell, J., 2018b. "The Transgender Controversy: Second Response to Pilgrim." *Journal of Critical Realism* 17(5): 529–545.

The debate between Andrew Sayer and John Holmwood on critical realism, gender, and associational vs counter-factual thinking (chronological order)

Sayer, A., 2000. "System, Lifeworld and Gender: Associational Versus Counterfactual Thinking." *Sociology* 34(4): 707–725.

Holmwood, J., 2001. "Gender and Critical Realism: A Critique of Sayer." *Sociology* 35(4): 947–965.

Sayer, A., 2001. "Reply to Holmwood." *Sociology* 35(4): 967–984.

The broader literature on critical realism, feminism, and gender (alphabetical order)

Albritton, R. and D. Badeen. 2017. "Political Economy and Childcare: A Levels-of-Analysis Approach." *Rethinking Marxism: A Journal of Economics Culture & Society* 29(3): 384–404.

Assiter, A. 1996. *Enlightened Women: Modernist Feminism in a Postmodern Age*. Routledge, Abingdon, Oxon.

Bergin, M., J. S. G. Wells, and S. Owen. 2008. "Critical Realism: A Philosophical Framework for the Study of Gender and Mental Health." *Nursing Philosophy* 9(3): 169–179.

Clegg, S. 2016. "Agency and Ontology within Intersectional Analysis: A Critical Realist Contribution." *Journal of Critical Realism* 15(5): 494–510.

———. 2006. "The Problem of Agency in Feminism: A Critical Realist Approach." *Gender and Education* 18 (3): 309–324.

Elder-Vass, D. 2012. "Categories, Essences, and Sexes," in D. Elder-Vass (eds.), *The Reality of Social Construction*, pp. 121–142. Cambridge University Press, Cambridge.

Falconer Al-Hindi, K. 1997. "Feminist Critical Realism: A Method for Gender and Work Studies in Geography," in J. P. Jones III, H. J. Nast, and S. M. Roberts (eds.), *Thresholds in Feminist Geography: Difference, Methodology, Representation*, pp. 145–164. Rowman & Littlefield, Lanham.

Flatschart, E., 2017. "Feminist Standpoints and Critical Realism. The Contested Materiality of Difference in Intersectionality and New Materialism." *Journal of Critical Realism* 16(3): 284–302.

Fletcher, A. J. 2017. "Applying Critical Realism in Qualitative Research: Methodology meets Method." *International Journal of Social Research Methodology* 20(2): 181–194.

Gillman, L., 2016. "Critical Realist and Postpositivist Realist Feminisms: Towards a Feminist Dialectical Realism." *Journal of Critical Realism* 15(5): 458–475.

Gunnarsson, L. 2018. "'Excuse Me, But Are You Raping Me Now?' Discourse and Experience in (the Grey Areas of) Sexual Violence." *Nora-Nordic Journal of Feminist and Gender Research* 26(1): 4–18.

———. 2018. "Love, Feminism and Dialectics: Repairing Splits in Theory and Practice," in A. Garcia-Andrade, L. Gunnarsson, A. G. Jonasdottir (eds.), *Feminism and the Power of Love: Interdisciplinary Interventions*, pp. 169–187. Routledge, London and New York.

———. 2016. "The Dominant and its Constitutive Other: Feminist Theorizations of Love, Power and Gendered Selves." *Journal of Critical Realism* 15(1): 1–20.

———. 2015a. "Nature, Love and the Limits of Male Power." *Journal of Critical Realism* 14(3): 325–332.

———. 2013. *The Contradictions of Love: Towards a Feminist-Realist Ontology of Sociosexuality*. Routledge, London.

———. 2013. "The Naturalistic Turn in Feminist Theory: A Marxist-Realist Contribution." *Feminist Theory* 14(1): 3–19.

———. 2011. "Love – Exploitable Resource or 'No-Lose Situation'? Reconciling Jónasdóttir's Feminist View with Bhaskar's Philosophy of MetaReality." *Journal of Critical Realism* 10(4): 419–441.

———, A. Martinez Dy and M. van Ingen. 2016. "Critical Realism, Gender and Feminism: Exchanges, Challenges, Synergies." *Journal of Critical Realism* 15(5): 433–439.

———., A. Martinez Dy, and M. van Ingen (eds.) 2018. *Gender, Feminism and Critical Realism: Exchanges, Challenges, Synergies*. Routledge, London and New York.

Hordyk, S.R., S. Ben Soltane, and J. Hanley. 2014. "Sometimes you have to go Under Water to Come Up: A Poetic, Critical Realist Approach to Documenting the Voices of Homeless Immigrant Women." *Qualitative Social Work* 13(2): 203–220.

Hull, C. 2006. *The Ontology of Sex: A Critical Inquiry into the Deconstruction and Reconstruction of Categories*. Routledge, Abingdon, Oxon.

———. 1997. "The Need in Thinking: Materiality in Theodor W. Adorno and Judith Butler." *Radical Philosophy* 84(July/August): 22–35.

———. 2003. "Poststructuralism, Behaviorism and the Problem of Hate Speech." *Philosophy & Social Criticism* 29(5): 517–535.

———. 2003. "How Sexually Dimorphic Are We? Review and Synthesis." *American Journal of Human Biology* 15(1): 112–115.

Jessop, B. 2004. "The Gender Selectivities of the State: A Critical Realist Analysis." *Journal of Critical Realism* 3(2): 207–237.

Jonasdottir, A.G. and K. B. Jones. 2009. "Out of Epistemology: Feminist Theory in the 1980s and Beyond," in A. G. Jonasdottir, K. B. Jones (eds.) *The Political Interests of Gender Revisited: Redoing Theory and Research with a Feminist Face*, pp. 17–57. Manchester University Press, Manchester.

Kvarnhall, V. 2017. "Utilizing Critical Realism in Empirical Gender Research: The Case of Boys and the Reproduction of Male Dominance within Popular Music Life." *Journal of Critical Realism* 16(6): 26–42.

Lawson, T. 2009. "Feminism, Realism and Essentialism: Reply to van Staveren," in E. Fullbrook (ed.), *Ontology and Economics: Tony Lawson & His Critics*, pp. 311–323. Routledge, Abingdon, Oxon.

Mader, D. 2016. "Theorizing Agency and Domination through a Critical Realist Perspective on Gender Positionality." *Journal of Critical Realism* 15(5): 440–457.

Martinez Dy, A., L. Martin., and S. Marlow. 2018. "Emancipation through Digital Entrepreneurship? A Critical Realist Analysis." *Organization* 25(5): 585–608.

Mussell, H. 2016. "The Truth of the Matter." *Hypatia: A Journal of Feminist Philosophy* 31(3): 537–553.

New, C. 2003. "Feminism, Critical Realism and the Linguistic Turn," in J. Cruickshank (ed.), *Critical Realism: The Difference It Makes*, pp. 57–74. Routledge, London and New York.

———. 2001. "Oppressed and Oppressors? The Systematic Mistreatment of Men." *Sociology* 35(3): 729–748.

———. 1998a. "Feminism and Critical Realism." *Alethia* 1(1): 2–4.

———. 1998b. "Realism, Deconstruction and the Feminist Standpoint." *Journal for the Theory of Social Behaviour* 28(4): 349–372.

———. 1995. "Sociology and the Case for Realism." *The Sociological Review* 43(4): 808–827.

Rouse, J., H. Woolnough. 2018. "Engaged or Activist Scholarship? Feminist Reflections on Philosophy, Accountability and Transformational Potential." *International Small Business Journal: Researching Entrepreneurship* 36(4): 429–448.

Satsangi, M., 2013. "Synthesizing Feminist and Critical Realist Approaches to Housing Studies." *Housing Theory & Society* 30(2): 193–207.

Smirthwaite, G., Swahnberg, K., 2016. "Comparing Critical Realism and the Situated Knowledges Approach in Research on (In)equity in Health Care: An Exploration of their Implications." *Journal of Critical Realism* 15(5): 476–493.

Sweet, P.L., 2018. "The Feminist Question in Realism." *Sociological Theory* 36(3): 221–243.

van Ingen, M., 2016. "Beyond the Nature/Culture Divide? The Contradictions of Rosi Braidotti's 'The Posthuman'." *Journal of Critical Realism* 15(5): 530–542.

Wimalasena, L., 2017. "Reflexivity and Women's Agency: A Critical Realist Morphogenetic Exploration of the Life Experience of Sri Lankan Women." *Journal of Critical Realism* 16(4): 383–401.

Index